ESSENTIAL MEDICINE

A guide to important principles

Essential
Medicine

R. G. Brackenridge
M.B., Ch.B., M.R.C.P., M.R.C.P. Ed.

MTP
MEDICAL AND TECHNICAL PUBLISHING CO LTD
1971

Published by

MTP

Medical and Technical Publishing Co Ltd
Chiltern House, Oxford Road, Aylesbury, Bucks

Copyright © 1971 R. G. BRACKENRIDGE

ISBN 978-0-85200-023-6   ISBN 978-94-011-7939-3 (eBook)
DOI 10.1007/978-94-011-7939-3

FIRST PUBLISHED 1971

Books in the "Essential knowledge" series:

Essential Anatomy

Essential Medicine

Essential Physics, Chemistry and Biology

**Essential Biochemistry, Endocrinology and
  Nutrition**

Essential Diagnostic Tests

Essential Physiology

Essential Cardiology

LETCHWORTH, HERTFORDSHIRE SG6 1JS

Contents

Contents

THIS SERIES REPRESENTS A NEW APPROACH TO medical education. Each book has been written by a leading expert who is closely concerned with education.

These books do not cover any particular examination syllabus but each one contains more than enough information to enable the student to pass his or her examinations in that subject. The aim is rather to provide the understanding which will enable each person to get the most out of and put the most into his or her profession. Throughout we have tried to present medical science in a clear, concise and logical way. All the authors have endeavoured to ensure that students will truly understand the various concepts instead of having to memorize a mass of ill-digested facts. The message of this new series is that medicine is now moving away from the poorly understood dogmatism of not so very long ago. Many aspects of bodily function in health and disease can now be clearly and logically appreciated: what is required is a thoughtful understanding and not a parrot-like memory.

Each volume is designed to be read in its own right. However, four titles—*Physics, Chemistry and Biology*; *Anatomy*; *Biochemistry, Endocrinology and Nutrition*; and *Physiology*—provide the foundations on which all the other books are based. The student who has read these four will get much more out of the other books which relate to clinical matters.

We hope that a feature of this series will be regular revision. Critical comments from readers will be much appreciated as these will help us to improve later editions.

1

Health and the hospital

Definition of health

Health is a state of physical, mental and social well-being.

The object of a medical service is the promotion of good health, not simply the treatment of disease. Adequate nutrition, satisfaction at work, proper hours of sleep, and physical recreation help to promote good health.

The changing emphasis of medicine

THE PAST

Plague, cholera and smallpox were the scourges of the Middle Ages. Three hundred years later, in the nineteenth century, infections remained rampant in hospitals, and patients stood a better chance of survival if they could afford to be treated at home.

The understanding of the causes and transmission of infection, the provision of sanitation, and a fresh water supply lowered the incidence of disease dramatically in Western countries. In some developing countries, where sanitation may be non-existent and the water contaminated, cholera, typhoid and dysentery are still common.

THE PRESENT

Public health measures, then immunization, made their contribution to progress. Now we are in the era of chemotherapy and antibiotics, and tuberculosis has been conquered in the developed countries. The disease remains a scourge in the tropics, not because of climate but because of poor social conditions, inadequate education and lack of medical care. Diseases of deprivation such as malnutrition occur in many parts of the world.

The important diseases in developed countries include degenerative arterial disease, causing coronary thrombosis and strokes, malignant disease, chronic arthritis, and depressive illness—much research is devoted to their understanding, but their cause remains uncertain.

THE FUTURE—PREVENTIVE MEDICINE

Preventive medicine is concerned with the early recognition of disorder, before it has become 'disease'. Thus cytology (cell examination) helps to detect early cancer of the womb, blood examination detects anaemia, and urine testing may reveal diabetes. At the earliest stages of life, examination of the blood of the mother may indicate that her baby is at risk from a preventable disorder such as haemolytic anaemia (destruction of red cells) from Rhesus-group incompatibility. Enzyme-deficiency disorders, correctable by a suitable diet, can be diagnosed in infancy. In some inherited conditions, genetic counsellors may advise on family planning in the prevention of disease.

Preventive medicine has an important application in the care of the elderly, who form an increasing proportion of our population. Early detection of disease such as cataract (causing blindness) or anaemia allows old people to continue to live a full life.

We have a duty to remember three preventable causes of suffering —obesity (over-weight), road-traffic accidents and cigarette smoking (causing chronic bronchitis, and lung cancer)—and to do what we can to eliminate them.

We have a wider duty to prevent spoilage of the land and pollution of the atmosphere and to preserve natural resources for future generations.

The part played by the hospital

OUTPATIENTS

The hospital is part of the community health service. It is a diagnostic and treatment centre rather than a collection of beds. The patient may be referred by his family doctor, and he must be met by kindness and efficiency.

The physician takes a careful history, and previous case-notes should be available. Occupation, visits abroad, smoking and drinking habits and family history are noted. Today it is also essential to ascertain if the patient is already receiving drugs—such as aspirin sleeping tablets or the contraceptive 'pill', for the patient may not realize the importance of a drug habit.

Physical examination is carried out, and height, weight, blood pressure and urine tests recorded. Additional investigations include blood count and biochemistry, chest x-ray, peak flow rate (a test of respiratory function using the Wright meter), electrocardiogram (E.C.G.) and special tests such as barium meal x-ray of the stomach. These are within the scope of most hospitals. Special diagnostic facilities are available in cardiac and neurological units, and central reference laboratories deal with the more complicated blood tests for virus diseases and endocrine disorders.

ADMISSIONS

It may be necessary to admit the patients for observation and further investigation to reach an accurate diagnosis, essential for proper management.

Seriously ill patients will be admitted directly to hospital, and special care facilities may be required in the ambulance and in the medical unit for a condition such as coronary thrombosis (heart attack), or severe blood loss.

Admission may also be required for elderly people who have no one to look after them at home—an adequate social service often avoids such an emergency.

MANAGEMENT

Few conditions require prolonged bed rest. Its hazards include venous thrombosis (clotting), wasting of the muscles, and a depressing effect on morale. It is usually possible to let patients up to the toilet or to a bedside commode.

Many dietary regimes have been relaxed, and understanding of metabolic requirements has guided fluid balance. Urine examination has been simplified with paper strip tests. Disposable catheters and presterilized packs have made treatment safer for the patient and easier for the staff.

MODERN THERAPY

Techniques such as controlled artificial respiration, and electrical defibrillation in heart disease, demand new skills.

Drugs may cure where no treatment was possible a few years ago.

SCIENTIFIC AND HUMAN UNDERSTANDING

The nurse must accept the challenge to keep her knowledge abreast of modern medicine. She must question that which she does not understand. With her medical colleagues, she must help in the application of current therapy, and learn for the benefit of future patients.

Scientific understanding has to be balanced against human understanding. The nurse has a unique opportunity for personal contact with the patient, and a kind word may do more to help than another bottle of tablets. Time should be made available for senior staff to discuss the patient's management with his relatives.

TEAMWORK

Doctors and nurses play the principal part in patient care. Proper management now requires the assistance of many hospital departments—x-ray, biochemistry, bacteriology, physiotherapy, dietetic, social work and administration—working as a team.

THE OBJECTIVE OF HOSPITAL CARE

The objective is to have the patient up and about and restored to health as soon as possible. Following his discharge, he may be reviewed at the out-patient department or returned to the care of his family doctor before resuming work.

2

Mechanisms of ill-health

Injury (Trauma)

Road traffic accidents, and accidents at work and in the home are common causes of hospital admission. They are the province of the surgeon. However in many cases it may be difficult to know whether a medical condition such as stroke or coronary thrombosis has caused a collapse precipitating the accident.

The division between surgical and medical specialities is further blurred by the necessity for combined management in certain cases; thus patients with crushed-chest injury may require assisted ventilation and cardiac care. Pulmonary embolus (clot passing to the lungs) may follow severe injuries, and requires 'medical' advice.

It may be helpful to remember that the healing process in a medical condition such as myocardial infarction (damaged heart muscle after coronary thrombosis) is rather similar to that which occurs after an injury, the wound requiring several weeks to heal.

Heredity and environment

HEREDITY (INHERITANCE)

Each body cell contains forty-six chromosomes. There are twenty-two pairs of chromosomes (the autosomes) plus the sex-chromosomes —X plus Y in a male, or two X's in a female. One of each pair of autosomes plus one sex chromosome has been acquired from each parent at conception. The process may go wrong at this stage— mongolism is due to an extra autosome, and certain rare disturbances of stature and fertility are due to extra or deleted sex chromosomes.

Genetic disorders are due to faults in the 'genes' carried by the chromosomes. They may be 'dominant' or 'recessive'. Dominant disorders are those requiring only one of each pair of chromosomes to be affected before disease is produced, usually a rare disease such as Huntington's chorea (disturbance of movements and mental deterioration), in adult life. Recessive disorders need both members of the pair of chromosomes to be affected before disease is manifest, though some abnormality, e.g. enzyme deficiencies, may be detectable. Recessive disorders therefore occur in the offspring of near relatives who may be carrying similar traits—such intermarriage is undesirable. Some inborn errors of metabolism (e.g. phenylketonuria in infants) are inherited in this manner. 'Sex-linked' disorders such as haemophilia (failure of blood clotting) are transmitted by the X chromosome, and usually only the male manifests the disease, for his other Y sex chromosome does not constitute a pair. The female with her two X's, may carry the trait on one X, but does not suffer from the disease.

Congenital disorders are disorders present at birth, and may arise from the above genetic factors, from intra-uterine infection, or from birth injury.

Multifactorial inheritance is a term applied to diseases which seem to run in families, but their mode of inheritance is unknown. This applies to many common diseases, including arteriosclerosis, hypertension and possibly diabetes and duodenal ulcer. The fact that the latter is commoner in those of blood group O implies a genetic basis.

ENVIRONMENT

Environmental disorders are caused by external factors and include undernutrition from lack of food and over-population. Hazards at work, and atmospheric pollution are considered later as causes of disease.

Infections are obvious environmental disorders and their spread is easiest where there is overcrowding and lack of sanitation.

MIXED HEREDITARY AND ENVIRONMENTAL DISORDERS

It is often difficult to know how far a disease is inherited, and how far it is due to environmental factors. Thus there may be a pre disposition to lung cancer, but the disease will occur only if an external stimulus such as heavy cigarette-smoking is added.

Obesity tends to run in families and may have a genetic basis. Alternatively the cause may be environmental, the children being brought up to over-eat, as do their parents.

Infections and immunity

Infections are due mainly to bacteria and viruses. They are transmitted by nasal and throat secretions or the dust from handkerchiefs (e.g. influenza and pneumonia), by faecal contamination (e.g. typhoid) or by contact (e.g. smallpox).

The body mounts an immunity response to repel bacterial or virus invasion. While the immunity response has been considered mainly in connection with infection, it has an important part to play in the integrity of body tissues. Where the mechanism goes wrong, external factors may provoke a harmful 'allergic' reaction. In some cases the allergic reaction occurs without obvious external stimulus, resulting in tissue destruction—the body reacts against its own tissues, as though failing to recognize 'self'. This results in a group of disorders called the 'auto-allergic' or 'auto-immune' disorders.

When infection gains a hold, the 'inflammatory response' occurs—there is pain, redness, swelling and fever. White blood cells arrive to scavenge the infecting organism followed by the process of healing, which may be complete or result in the formation of fibrous, scar tissue.

Tumours

These may be benign, or malignant—cancer. Benign tumours remain localized but may cause pressure symptoms. Malignant tumours are composed of abnormal cells which invade surrounding tissues and spread by the bloodstream or lymphatics to distant organs as secondary tumours—metastases. Malignant tumours cause destruction, haemorrhage, wasting (cachexia) and death. Cancer may have several causes, including disturbance of immunity, the foreign cells failing to be rejected, the action of chemical carcinogens (e.g. coal tar) and genetic and hormonal factors.

Carcinoma is a cancer of epithelial cells, such as those lining the bronchi and the stomach. *Sarcoma* is a malignant tumour of bone or muscle. The *leukaemias* may be regarded as malignancy involving white blood cells, and cytotoxic drugs may help in treatment. Drugs and x-ray therapy are of some value in other growths, but surgical removal, where possible, is the main treatment. By the time a 'lump' is palpable, a cancer is very advanced. Early detection may be assisted by cytology, special x-rays, and new techniques such as thermography (recording of heat emitted) and the use of ultrasound.

Degenerative vascular disease

Arteriosclerosis (literally 'hardening of the arteries') affects middle-aged men and the elderly of both sexes. The term atheroma is applied to plaques of fatty material deposited in the arterial lining, minute clots form on the plaques and are incorporated into the vessel, narrowing it. There may be ulceration and calcification of the plaques. The process is called atherosclerosis, which, for clinical purposes, can be accepted as synonymous with arteriosclerosis. It is uncertain whether the disease is due to disturbance of fat metabolism or the coagulation mechanism, or both. The arteries may be diffusely or patchily involved, and the process is worsened by hypertension (high blood pressure). Arteriosclerosis is a most important cause of illness, for the coronary, cerebral and leg arteries are principally involved. The effects include ischaemia (lack of blood), thrombosis with infarction (death of tissue), embolus (clot-detachment), and haemorrhage from rupture of the diseased vessel. Arteriosclerosis is the subject of much research: its prevention would eliminate many cardiac and cerebral diseases discussed in later chapters.

Nutrition

Half the world's population may suffer from lack of food, but the main trouble in Britain is obesity (overweight) from too much food. A normal diet provides adequate quantities of proteins, carbohydrates, fats and minerals, with the possible exception of iron in a pregnant woman. Isolated vitamin deficiencies are rare, except in the elderly who may have scurvy from vitamin C deficiency. Gastric operations may be followed by malabsorption of iron and vitamin B_{12}, causing anaemia.

Metabolic and endocrine diseases

The most important metabolic disease is diabetes mellitus. The sign of diabetes is glycosuria (sugar in the urine) from failure to utilize sugar, but protein and fat metabolism are also affected. The disease may present as 'complications' ranging from vaginal irritation to gangrene of the feet. Thus the urine must be routinely tested for sugar in all patients attending hospital.

Classical endocrine diseases include overactivity or underactivity of glands such as the thyroid and adrenals. Other organs have been discovered to have endocrine function, however. Thus some forms of hypertension may be due to excessive production of the hormone renin by the kidney, which in turn affects the adrenal production of aldosterone, causing salt and water retention.

Mental disorder

The term 'mentally disordered persons' covers both the mentally ill (i.e. those with psychiatric disturbances) and the mentally subnormal or handicapped. Inherited enzyme defects are being increasingly recognized as causes of mental subnormality, giving the hope of prevention. Many mentally handicapped persons can be managed in their own homes, with help from social and educational services— this is preferable to confining such persons to institutions.

The commonest psychiatric disturbance is depressive illness. Patients may present with a variety of physical complaints, plus tiredness and sleep disturbance. The anti-depressive drugs (such as amitriptyline) are a major contribution to therapy.

Infection, arteriosclerosis and anaemia cause impaired mental function in the elderly, and some of these factors are treatable.

Hazards of therapy—jatrogenic disease

Rest in bed, drugs, transfusions and even oxygen have their dangers if wrongly applied. We must balance the potential benefits against any possible harm. Antibiotics, tranquillizers and steroids are such two-edged weapons. The term jatrogenic disease is applied to disease caused by 'treatment', or engendered by the attitude of doctor or nurse so that the patient feels ill yet no physical trouble exists. About 10 per cent of patients are in hospital from jatrogenic disease ranging from aspirin-induced haematemesis (vomiting of blood) to cardiac neurosis. Clearly we have a duty to do our patients no harm!

3

Infections and immunity

Causes of infection

BACTERIA

Bacteria are tiny living organisms visible under the ordinary light microscope and able to grow on 'culture media' when incubated at a suitable temperature.

They are classified by their shape—cocci are round, bacilli are rectangular, by their staining properties—Gram's stain positive or negative, and by their effect on the culture medium—thus certain streptococci destroy red cells in the medium and are called haemolytic streptococci.

Bacterial infections were formerly very common in hospitals. Thus epidemics of 'childbed fever', erysipelas and scarlet fever, occurring in the early part of the century, were due to streptococcal infection. Good hygiene, and drugs such as the sulphonamides and penicillin largely eliminated the streptococcus. Its place was taken by the staphylococcus, strains of which were penicillin-resistant. Staphylococci cause wound infection and post-influenzal pneumonia. Fortunately newer antibiotics such as cloxacillin are effective in the treatment of penicillin-resistant staphylococcal infections.

'Gram-negative' bacteria such as Bacillus proteus and Pseudomonas pyocyanea are now important causes of hospital infections, and severe illness may follow bloodstream invasion in debilitated patients, as may occur at surgical operations. Again, fortunately, new antibiotics such as carbenicillin (Pyopen) are available for treatment.

VIRUSES

Viruses are much smaller than bacteria, visible only under the high magnification possible with the electron microscope. They grow only in living cells, a technique for the specialist laboratory.

Viruses may be classified by shape, by their protein make-up, or by the parts of the body in which they multiply—thus enteroviruses (which include the poliomyelitis and Coxsackie viruses) colonize in the gut—in poliomyelitis, the nervous system is involved by secondary spread. Enteroviruses may be cultured from the faeces.

Viruses take over the metabolic processes of the cells they invade, and there is a long incubation period, during which the viruses are multiplying, before the production of symptoms. Thus chemotherapy against virus diseases is not nearly so successful as in the case of bacterial disease. Vaccination to prevent virus infection is a much more satisfactory approach.

Virus infection often opens the door for bacterial invasion—thus influenza, caused by a virus, may be followed by staphylococcal pneumonia.

There has been recent evidence showing that some virus infections (e.g. measles) may in fact persist long after clinical cure—the process has been called 'slow-virus' affection and may be associated with disturbance of immunity and neurological disease.

FUNGI

Fungi are larger than bacteria. They may cause skin infections such as ringworm. The fungus monilia causes 'thrush' of the mouth especially in patients receiving antibiotics such as tetracycline which kills bacteria, but allows fungi to grow. In debilitated patients, fungal infection may involve the lungs and spread to the bloodstream.

PROTOZOA

Protozoa are tiny living parasites. Many tropical infections are protozoal, for example amoebic dysentery, an infection of the large bowel, and malaria, where the parasite is transmitted by the bite of an infected mosquito.

Prevention of infection

A. Prevention of spread of the organism
B. Immunity

PREVENTION OF SPREAD OF THE ORGANISM

The viruses and bacteria which invade the respiratory tract are spread by droplets from sneezes and coughs, by handkerchiefs, and by dust in which bacteria may survive for days or weeks. Quiet conversation does not disseminate organisms to any important extent. Facemasks may help to prevent spread, but if they are fingered or rubbed, they do more harm than good.

Intestinal infections such as typhoid, dysentery and many virus illnesses spread by faecal contamination of hands, food and water, and by flies.

Hand-washing is by far the most important rule in preventing infection. Infective patients should ideally be nursed in isolation. Attempts to 'barrier nurse' patients in an open ward are usually unsuccessful, for infected dust contaminates clothes, bedding and the surroundings. Elaborate facilities, available only in specialized units, are necessary to achieve a germ-free environment, and to nurse patients suffering from smallpox.

IMMUNITY

Immunity means resistance to disease. The immune response occurs when an 'antigen' gains access to the body. The antigen may be an infecting organism, or a foreign substance or protein. The immune response involves the production of antibodies, or 'immune-globulins' by plasma cells and lymphocytes, and there is an additional 'cellular immunity' mediated by lymphocytes dependent on the thymus gland.

Immunity is partly inherited, and partly acquired from exposure to a small dose of organisms insufficient to produce severe infection. Immunity may also result from infection.

IMMUNIZATION (VACCINATION)

The principle of active immunization is to produce an immune response without actually causing infection. This can be achieved by modifying the organisms.

It was observed that exposure to cows suffering from cowpox produced immunity to smallpox. The virus causing cowpox is sufficiently like that of smallpox to produce such immunity.

Viruses and bacteria can be modified by culture or chemicals, and even the toxins from some bacteria can be used to produce immunity. Such active immunity is more effective and of longer duration than the immunity produced passively by injection of antibody from another person or animal.

Vaccination is carried out in infancy against diphtheria, tetanus and pertussis (whooping cough), and poliomyelitis (oral vaccine), smallpox and measles in the second year, with booster doses in the school years. German measles vaccination in girls prevents infection in pregnancy with risk of foetal damage.

B.C.G. is given to those at risk from tuberculosis.

Typhoid, cholera and yellow fever vaccines are given to those visiting the tropics. The possibility of vaccination against malaria is being investigated.

Disorders of immunity

ALLERGY (HYPERSENSITIVITY)

Allergy means altered reactivity, and the term is used to describe undesirable effects of the immune response.

Allergic reactions occur as the result of exposure to foreign proteins or substances to which the individual has previously been sensitized. However allergic reactions may occur without evidence of previous exposure. Certain individuals are especially prone to allergic reactions; this predisposition has a hereditary basis, and is often accompanied by eczema (an irritant skin condition) in infancy. Such individuals are called 'atopic' persons.

Allergic reactions occur after contact, inhalation, ingestion or injection of the offending antigen.

Types of reaction

A. IMMEDIATE REACTION. *Cause:* Antigen reacts with preformed antibodies, and powerful chemicals such as histamine are released.

Symptoms and signs: 1. Anaphylactic shock—a violent systemic reaction with pallor, vomiting, chest tightness, fall in blood pressure, and collapse.

Anaphylactic shock was seen in the days when injections of animal serum, containing much foreign protein, were used in treatment, but such therapy is now seldom given. The reaction may however occur after the injection of any foreign substance, e.g. penicillin.

2. Lesser allergic reactions—these include skin wheals (urticaria), swelling of eyelids, face and tongue (angioneurotic oedema), hay fever, and a running nose (allergic rhinitis).

3. Asthma—bronchospasm with wheezy breathing, other causes of which are discussed later, page 94.

Skin reactions such as urticaria may follow contact with plants, e.g. primula, and pollens may precipitate hay fever and asthma.

Dusts containing a house-mite, found in bedding, are especially prone to provoke asthma in allergic subjects.

Treatment: Adrenaline 0·5 ml of 1/1,000 solution by intramuscular injection, and hydrocortisone 100 mg intravenously are given immediately in anaphylactic shock, and resuscitative measures such as artificial ventilation and cardiac massage may be necessary.

Antihistamine drugs such as mepyramine (Anthisan), chlorpheniramine (Piriton) and triprolidine (Actidil) are effective by mouth, or by injection, in the lesser reactions such as urticaria and hay fever, but not in asthma.

Disodium cromoglycate (Intal) by inhalation blocks the allergic response and relieves this type of asthma. Its value in the other allergies is not yet known.

Desensitizing injections, prepared from pollens or dusts to which the patient is known to be sensitive, may be helpful if given before the pollen season.

B. SERUM SICKNESS REACTION (DELAYED SERUM REACTION). *Cause:* antigen-antibody complexes are formed in the circulation, and cause an inflammatory and sometimes destructive reaction in various organs.

Symptoms and signs: these occur 10–14 days after an injection of serum, though the reaction may occur without known precipitating factor.

There is fever, joint pain and lymph gland swelling.

Treatment: severe cases require hydrocortisone 100 mg intravenously followed by steroids such as prednisone 10 mg 6-hourly by mouth.

C. DELAYED HYPERSENSITIVITY. *Cause:* a disturbance of cellular immunity mediated by lymphocytes dependent on the thymus gland.

Symptoms and signs: drug reactions, often presenting as skin rashes and with a previous history of reaction, and *eczema* caused by nickel and chemicals, may represent delayed hypersensitivity reactions.

Treatment: withdrawal of the offending substance; steroids may be of value in severe cases.

AUTO-IMMUNE OR AUTO-ALLERGIC DISEASES

The term auto-immune diseases has come into use to describe diseases associated with abnormal antibodies in the blood. There need not be a definable external antigen, and it is uncertain how the antibodies arise. These antibodies belong to a group of proteins known as the immunoglobulins. They are associated with destruction of certain body tissues hence the name *auto*-immune diseases.

The mechanism of such diseases may be similar to the Serum Sickness reaction described.

Types

A. CONNECTIVE-TISSUE (COLLAGEN) DISEASES. Rheumatoid arthritis, systemic lupus erythematosus and scleroderma are diseases of connective tissue with certain factors in common—abnormal immunoglobulins, raised E.S.R. and tissue destruction, and suppressibility by steroid drugs.

Rheumatic fever, and acute nephritis. These diseases are an allergic reaction to streptococci, but the mechanism is similar to the above, and they may be classed in this context.

B. FARMER'S LUNG and certain types of HAEMOLYTIC ANAEMIA are auto-immune diseases.

C. ORGAN-SPECIFIC AUTO-IMMUNE DISEASES. *Myxoedema* from underactivity of the thyroid gland is associated with specific antibodies causing destruction of thyroid tissue.

Pernicious anaemia—antibodies destroy the lining cells of the stomach, resulting in lack of 'intrinsic factor' necessary for the absorption of vitamin B_{12} lower in the intestine. Lack of vitamin B_{12} affects the marrow causing pernicious anaemia.

Tissue and organ transplantation

When a tissue such as skin, or an organ such as the kidney is transplanted from a healthy donor to a patient, the host's tissues mount an immune reaction just as they do to any antigen as described above. This is mainly a cell-mediated reaction carried out by the lymphocytes, and results in rejection of the donor organ unless the immune reaction is suppressed.

TUMOUR IMMUNITY

It is possible that certain malignant tumours grow because the body fails to recognize that their cells are 'not-self' and therefore does not reject them. If immunity could be stimulated, the growth would be destroyed.

Suppression of the immune reaction

Suppression may be required in severe allergic reactions and in auto-immune diseases such as rheumatoid arthritis and haemolytic anaemia.

The following agents cause suppression:

1. Hydrocortisone and steroids such as prednisone—act by hindering antibody formation and the development of the immune response.

2. Cytotoxic drugs such as azathioprine (Imuran)—destroy rapidly dividing cells such as lymphocytes.

3. Anti-lymphocytic serum (prepared by injecting a horse with human lymphocytes)—destroys lymphocytes.

4. Removal of lymph (containing antibodies and lymphocytes) from the thoracic duct.

All these methods may be employed in suppressing the rejection reaction in kidney and other organ transplants.

Anti-inflammatory drugs such as aspirin, phenylbutazone (Buta-zolidin) and indomethacin (Indocid) have a certain immunosuppressive effect.

Patients on immunosuppressive drugs have a lowered resistance to infection. They may also become more susceptible to certain tumours.

Infectious diseases

MEASLES

Measles is a virus infection of toddlers. The child is fevered and miserable with stuffy head and running nose, the secretions spreading the infection. There is a rash involving the face and neck, spreading over the body and fading within a week. White spots in the mouth near the molar teeth, Koplik's spots, may appear earlier, and are diagnostic. Secondary bacterial invasion causes middle-ear infections and pneumonia, and while such complications are rare in previously healthy children, they are a common cause of death in measles outbreaks in under-developed countries.

Antibiotics combat these complications but the best approach, to measles is to prevent it by vaccination at the age of $1\frac{1}{2}$–2 years.

Measles virus may linger in the brain, causing a form of encephalitis some years later, though this is rare.

GERMAN MEASLES (RUBELLA)

Rubella is a virus infection of children and young adults, causing mild malaise, a rash of pink spots about the neck, and lymph gland swellings, especially the glands at the back of the neck. It is not serious in itself, its importance is when it occurs in early pregnancy. The virus infects the developing embryo, resulting in congenital defects in the heart, brain, eye and ear.

Thus girls who have not had rubella in childhood (rendering them immune) should be vaccinated against the infection whilst still at school.

SCARLET FEVER

This is a scarlet rash, mainly affecting the trunk, occurring at the height of a haemolytic streptococcal sore throat—the organism produces a toxin which affects the skin. Its incidence was maximum in children 3–6 years, but it is now rarely seen with prompt antibiotic treatment of the throat infection.

WHOOPING COUGH (PERTUSSIS)

Vaccination prevents or modifies this bacterial infection of small children. The upper respiratory passages are affected, with appearances of a cough and cold, but the cough is followed by an inspiratory 'whoop' from laryngeal narrowing, and there may be vomiting. Antibiotics are indicated in severe cases with complicating pneumonia, and though tetracycline has been used, a side-effect is discoloration of the teeth.

'Croup' is a different condition, a virus infection of the larynx causing 'grunting' breathing and a wheezy cough.

DIPHTHERIA

This is rare in Britain, due to the success of vaccination, which prevents it. It is however, a serious disease, a bacterial infection of the throat causing pain, a dirty grey membrane at the tonsillar region, gland swellings, and the production of a toxin affecting the heart and nervous system. Any suspicion of this infection indicates the need for a throat swab to confirm diagnosis, immediate administration of antitoxin and penicillin by injection, and search for the carrier who has been the source of the infection. Diphtheria may occur as an infection of the larynx alone and should be borne in mind in cases of hoarseness with systemic upset.

CHICKEN-POX (VARICELLA)

Chicken-pox is commonest in children under 10 years. Though immunity is long-lasting, infection can occur at any age. The virus is the same as that causing herpes zoster (shingles) in adults. Susceptible children may develop chicken-pox following contact with cases of shingles, but the reverse is unusual. The chicken-pox lesions are mainly in the skin, but it is possible that the virus lurks on in the nervous system in some cases, for adult shingles is an infection of the cells of the posterior nerve roots, occurs in the debilitated, or where there is root irritation or disturbance of immunity (as in Hodgkin's disease).

Chicken-pox is a mild febrile disease with a rash that comes in crops, going through stages of red spots, then fluid-containing vesicles, pustules—with much itching—and scabs which fall off without leaving a scar. The neck, shoulders and trunk are especially affected. Calamine lotion relieves the itch. Secondary infection is rare.

While the condition may be mistaken for skin infections such as impetigo, or infestation with the mite causing scabies, the important differentiation is from smallpox.

SMALLPOX (VARIOLA)

This is an important and highly infectious disease, preventable by vaccination. It is always liable to be re-introduced into a country free from the disease (such as Britain) by travellers and immigrants from Asia and South America, where smallpox is still common. Thus epidemics in Britain have arisen following the arrival in this country of infected persons, who were still in the 'incubation period' (12 days), and of contacts. One must therefore always be on the alert for an odd-looking chicken-pox-like rash in someone who has just flown in from abroad. There are of course, international vaccination regulations demanding a certificate with proof of smallpox vaccination within the previous 3 years.

Symptoms and signs: The onset is abrupt with fever (like influenza'), headache and vomiting followed by the characteristic rash going through stages of red spots and plaques, vesicles and pustules, quite deeply set in the skin and affecting the face more than the trunk, and all at the same stage, unlike the crops of chicken-pox. These lesions may coalesce or become haemorrhagic, and are extremely infectious being laden with the virus. There is severe toxaemia, the respiratory tract is also involved, and complications include pneumonia and cardiac failure.

Management: The first essential is to isolate the patient and notify the Medical Officer of Health. Scrapings from skin lesions, and a throat swab will be sent to the nearest special laboratory with electron microscopy facilities. This will distinguish chicken-pox from smallpox right away, and the diagnosis of smallpox from other virus infections that may cause similar lesions can be made by special tests in the next 48 hours.

The patient will be nursed in a special Smallpox hospital. Until recently, there was no specific therapy against the virus of smallpox, but the new drug methisazone may be of value in the very early stages. Skilled nursing is vital, with especial attention to the care of the mouth, eyes and skin, fluid requirements and sedation for delirium (toxic confusional state). Antibiotics such as penicillin may be of value in secondary bacterial skin infections and pneumonia.

All previous contacts with the patient must be sought and vaccinated—methisazone may be of value in preventing smallpox in previously unvaccinated contacts, but the slight risk of encephalitis (which may follow primary vaccination in adults) is outweighed, in smallpox epidemics, by the proven value of vaccination.

MUMPS (PAROTITIS)

Mumps is a virus infection of the parotid glands at the angle of the jaw and infection is transmitted in the saliva. It is a relatively trivial infection in children, and epidemics tend to occur in schools—incubation period is up to 3 weeks. There is fever, difficulty in opening the mouth and chewing with parotid gland swelling, and the virus may invade the nervous system causing a form of meningitis, but the condition usually settles without trouble and there is no specific treatment. Vaccination is being evaluated.

Adults may be more seriously affected by mumps and complications include orchitis (inflammation of the testis, usually unilateral) and pancreatitis, for the pancreas has cells similar to those in the parotid gland. Steroids may afford symptomatic relief.

INFLUENZA

Influenza is a virus infection, mainly affecting the upper respiratory tract, with cough, sneezing and sore throat. There is fever, headache and limb pains, and often prostration out of proportion to the respiratory signs. It is a short, sharp illness, but in those with lung disease there is risk of secondary, often staphylococcal pneumonia.

Epidemics have spread from the Far East recently due to influenza virus A2, Hong Kong strain. The virus frequently changes its character, so that vaccination is not entirely successful against a new strain. Moreover, protection may depend more on antibody in the respiratory tract than in the bloodstream, and vaccination by the nasal route may yet be more effective.

HAEMOLYTIC STREPTOCOCCAL INFECTION

Sore throat and tonsillitis

Symptoms and signs: Fever, rapid pulse, malaise, red painful throat with pus spots on the tonsils and tender swollen tonsillar lymph glands.

Virus infection and glandular fever may give the same picture.

The diagnosis is confirmed by throat swab.

Complications: Scarlet fever—from effect of toxin on skin—now rare

Rheumatic fever and Chorea ⎱see below
Acute nephritis   ⎰

Treatment: Penicillin 1 mega unit by intramuscular injection, repeated in 12 hours and followed by oral penicillin rapidly clears the throat infection—but see below.

Erysipelas

This is now a rare streptococcal infection of the skin around the nose or lips, seen in elderly or debilitated patients and responding to penicillin.

Puerperal fever

This was a serious infection of the post-partum uterus with bloodstream invasion, and is an important reason for keeping carriers of streptococci out of maternity wards.

POST-INFECTIVE COMPLICATIONS

RHEUMATIC FEVER AND CHOREA; ACUTE NEPHRITIS

These should be regarded as allergic reactions in distant organs, to certain strains of haemolytic streptococcal throat infection. They occur 1–3 weeks after the sore throat, which may be quite mild, and the antibodies formed cause an inflammation (not an 'infection') of these distant tissues.

Rheumatic fever (acute rheumatism)

Symptoms and signs: Commonest in children but can occur at any age, especially if previous attacks; fever, general malaise, painful swellings of large joints such as knees, ankles and elbows in succession. The heart rate is rapid and severe cases have carditis, an inflammation of all the heart tissues, pericardium (outer covering), myocardium (muscle) and endocardium (inner lining). The heart may dilate and fail, or involvement of the valves may result in subsequent scarring, the mitral and aortic valves being especially affected, so that heart failure may follow in later years.

The joints settle without residual disability.

Rheumatic nodules may be palpable in the skin near the elbows; erythema marginatum—a fleeting ringed eruption on the wrists is characteristic, and erythema nodosum—tender red raised patches—may occur over the shins.

Diagnosis: Rheumatoid arthritis may give a similar joint picture in adults, but usually affects smaller joints. Acute joint infection (e.g. after injury or bone infection) should be distinguished.

In rheumatic fever there is a raised anti-streptolysin (A.S.O.) titre in the blood, and a high Erythrocyte Sedimentation Rate (E.S.R.).

Treatment: Bed rest until the temperature settles.

Padded splints to the affected joints.

Aspirin 600 mg 4- or 6-hourly eases pain and has an anti-inflammatory effect.

Steroids, e.g. prednisone, 10 mg 6-hourly are used in severe cases.

Penicillin 1 mega unit by intramuscular injection 12-hourly for a few days, followed by oral penicillin, continued in modified dosage for at least a year to prevent reinfection with the streptococcus.

Such measures produce benefit within a few days. Subsequent management depends on whether heart damage has occurred, detectable as murmurs heard with the stethoscope, or increased heart size on chest x-ray. Cautious resumption of activity is indicated here.

Second attacks increase the risk of heart damage.

Subacute bacterial endocarditis may occur on a damaged heart valve.

Chorea (*St. Vitus dance*)

This is a variant of rheumatic fever, affecting children—there are jerky purposeless movements of the limbs, face and tongue from affection of the basal ganglia of the brain, and carditis may occur. Sedation may be required, and penicillin as recommended above.

Acute (glomerulo-) nephritis

This is an inflammation causing increased permeability of small blood vessels, especially in the glomeruli of the kidneys. There is fever, haematuria (blood in the urine) oedema (fluid in the subcutaneous tissues) and raised blood pressure—again occurring 1–3 weeks after streptococcal throat infection, for which penicillin is indicated. The condition is considered further under Disorders of the Kidney.

It should be noted that the haemolytic streptococcus remains sensitive to penicillin, which is therefore the antibiotic of choice in streptococcal infection.

GLANDULAR FEVER (INFECTIOUS MONONULEOSIS)

Cause: Probably a virus, related to that of 'Burkitt's lymphoma'— a glandular swelling recently described in East African children. Outbreaks of glandular fever tend to occur in young people living communally, and infection may spread by kissing.

Symptoms and signs: Sore red throat, often with tonsillar exudate is common, and distinguishable from streptococcal throat only by the negative throat swab in glandular fever. There is lymph gland swelling, especially in the neck, and the spleen may be palpable. Liver involvement may cause jaundice. Most cases are mild and settle in a week or two but may be followed by a period of depression.

Diagnosis is confirmed by blood film, which shows 'mononuclear' cells—really altered lymphocytes; the 'Paul Bunnell' test in the serum is diagnostic if positive.

Treatment: Antibiotics do not help—indeed ampicillin causes increased risk of a skin rash which sometimes occurs in glandular fever. Severe cases with grossly swollen glands and difficulty in swallowing respond quickly to steroids such as prednisone over a few days.

TUBERCULOSIS

Tuberculosis is due to infection with the tubercle bacillus, Mycobacterium tuberculosis, termed an 'acid-fast' bacillus as it resists the decolorizing effect of acid used to stain the organism for identification under the microscope. It can be cultured on special media, or if the organisms are scanty, guinea-pig inoculation (the animal manifesting the infection after 6 weeks) may establish their presence. There are two main groups of tubercle bacilli, the bovine, and the human. The bovine strain was found in the milk of affected cows, and caused intestinal, glandular and sometimes joint tuberculosis. Bovine T.B. has been eradicated from British herds, and pasteurization (heat sterilization) of milk also prevents infection. Thus only the human strain is of importance, but chemotherapy has been so successful that the disease is now uncommon in the British population and is found in the elderly rather than the young. Risk of infection arises therefore from a hidden reservoir in old people (who may neglect symptoms, regarding cough and weight-loss as the accompaniments of ageing), and from immigrants from under-developed countries where infection is rampant.

Mode of infection: This is by inhalation of droplets of infected sputum into the lungs. A *primary focus* occurs in the lung tissue, with involvement of lymph glands near the root of the lung. When tuberculosis was common, this occurred in most young people; usually the infection would heal and the subject became immune to further infection.

If resistance were low, dissemination throughout the body—miliary tuberculosis—could occur. This might result in tuberculous meningitis, previously fatal, or chronic infection in bones and kidneys.

Alternatively the primary infection might become reactivated, following a lowered resistance or reinfection, in adult life, leading to tuberculous pneumonia or to chronic fibro-caseous tuberculosis of the lungs, with much destruction cavity formation, and the expectoration of purulent sputum containing the tubercle bacilli.

Undiagnosed tuberculosis of this type is the present source of infection.

Symptoms and signs: Cough sputum and weight-loss are late signs, and early recognition depends on chest x-ray. X-ray is mandatory in all undiagnosed fevers, even if chest symptoms are minimal. T.B. meningitis may present as headache and mild neck stiffness, lumbar puncture showing increased cells, decreased sugar and the T.B. bacillus in the spinal fluid.

Frequency of micturition and dysuria may be the presenting symptoms of bladder T.B., as part of genito-urinary tuberculosis following inadequate treatment in the pre-chemotherapy era.

Diagnosis is confirmed by finding the organism on direct staining, culture, or guinea pig inoculation of sputum, cerebro-spinal fluid, or urine. Treatment should start pending these results.

Treatment: Streptomycin 1 G by intramuscular injection, and isoniazid 300 mg with para-aminosalicylic acid (P.A.S.) 12 G (sachets are available combining these oral drugs) daily. These three drugs are given for 8–12 weeks, then isoniazid and P.A.S. are continued for at least one, and probably two years. A few patients develop side-effects or the organism may be resistant, in which case second-line drugs such as ethambutol and rifampicin are used.

Prevention: Most young people in Western countries today have not been exposed to 'natural' infection with tuberculosis. They are susceptible if exposed. Their tuberculin (Mantoux) skin-test is negative. B.C.G. (Bacille Calmette-Guerin) vaccine protects against infection and is given to school leavers and to young people at risk, such as nurses. Successful vaccination converts the Mantoux test to positive (raised red plaque).

Infants and young people who spontaneously change from Mantoux negative to Mantoux positive must be suspected of having been exposed to infection, and chest x-ray and chemotherapy are indicated—such precautions may be necessary if there has been a case of tuberculosis in a family, or contact at work.

Immigrants should have a chest x-ray. Mass x-ray screening campaigns have been helpful, but now that the infection is rarer, such campaigns should probably be replaced by ones directed at sources of infection such as vagrants, alcoholics and drug-addicts, and the neglected elderly.

SARCOIDOSIS

Sarcoidosis is a condition which occurs in the 20–40 age group, and it is slightly commoner in females. The cause is uncertain, and though the lesions in the involved organs are similar to the 'tubercles' that occur in tuberculosis, the tubercle bacillus is not found in the sarcoid lesions, and the tuberculin skin test is negative.

Skin involvement includes rashes, and erythema nodosum (tender red coin-sized lesions over the shins). There may be diffuse lymph gland swelling.

Chest x-ray shows bilateral gland swellings at the hilum (root of the lung). There may be diffuse involvement of the lung fields, but only in severe cases is there complaint of breathlessness. Iritis (inflammation of the iris diaphragm of the eye) may occur.

A skin test called the Kveim test (using sarcoid tissue) may aid diagnosis.

Usually the condition is self-limiting and clears over a few months, but the patient should be kept under observation, and chest x-ray repeated, especially to make sure that one is not dealing with a tuberculous process.

Steroids are used (anti-tuberculous chemotherapy often being added as a precaution) in severe cases of sarcoidosis involving the lungs or the eye.

BRUCELLOSIS (UNDULANT FEVER)

Cause: Brucella Abortus—a small bacterium named after Bruce (who discovered a similar organism causing Malta fever), and the tendency of infected cattle to abort their young. Veterinary surgeons, farmers, and those who drink the milk of infected animals may contract the disease, which has been eradicated in some progressive farming countries, but still occurs in many British herds. Pasteurization is a stop-gap measure to render existing milk supplies safe.

Symptoms and signs: Vague ill-health, aches and pains, fever and night-sweats. Severe cases may have inflammation of spinal and other joints. The infection may be acute, or may grumble on for months, and should be considered in any vague pyrexia.

Diagnosis may be confirmed by positive tests for antibodies in the blood (e.g. agglutination test) and Brucellin skin test.

Treatment: Trimethoprim—sulphamethoxazole (Septrin, Bactrim) tablets may prove effective. Current treatment is Streptomycin 1 G daily intramuscularly plus tetracycline 500 mg 6-hourly for 2 weeks, then tetracycline alone 240 mg 6-hourly for a further 2 weeks. Cure is not invariable and relapse may occur with vague ill-health over a period of years.

Gastro-intestinal infections

These include TYPHOID and PARATYPHOID (Enteric Fever), FOOD POISONING, DYSENTERY and CHOLERA.

TYPHOID AND PARATYPHOID

Cause: Bacillus typhoid, and B. paratyphoid A, B, and C (milder infection). These organisms belong to the Salmonella group, but in the case of typhoid and paratyphoid they are human pathogens only.

Mode of infection: Faecal contamination from a patient or carrier, who may be symptomless. Water and foods such as meat products and milk transmit the infection where hygiene is poor as in some tropical and Mediterranean countries.

Symptoms and signs: Typhoid is initially a bloodstream infection and during the first week the symptoms are *not* gastro-intestinal, but systemic ones—fever, with pulse slow in relation to the temperature, headache, weakness, fatigue and a rose-spot rash of the abdomen. There is constipation rather than diarrhoea at this stage and diagnosis may be difficult unless the condition is borne in mind. Cough and bronchitis may occur.

Blood culture is positive during the first ten days, and white cell count shows decreased polymorphs, instead of the increase in most infections.

If the condition is allowed to proceed, the patient becomes extremely ill with diarrhoea, pea-soup stools, abdominal distension and risk of bowel haemorrhage and perforation. Stool culture is positive now.

Diagnosis may be confirmed by the Widal agglutination test, which demonstrates the presence of the antibodies that develop after 2–3 weeks.

Treatment: Chloramphenicol 500 mg orally 6-hourly for two weeks. Ampicillin is less effective but does not carry the risk of agranulocytosis with repeated courses of chloramphenicol.

The patient should preferably be nursed in isolation, but as the infection spreads in faeces the most important precautions are hygienic ones, and handwashing.

Prevention: Care in where and what one eats abroad!

T.A.B. vaccination should be given to those at risk.

FOOD POISONING

Causes: (a) Salmonella organisms other than those of the Enteric group above.

(b) Bacillus (Clostridium) welchii.

(c) Staphylococcal—from preformed toxin.

The food poisoning Salmonella are pathogens of men and animals, and poultry, so that infection is acquired from human and animal cases, and meat and poultry products such as improperly cooked broiler chickens. These organisms are not invasive like the typhoid ones and cases present with gastric or intestinal symptoms rather than generalized disease, about 24 hours after infection: abdominal pain, vomiting and diarrhoea, with fever and malaise.

Cl. welchii grows in improperly cooked or reheated meat and symptoms start usually with diarrhoea 8–24 hours after ingestion.

The staphylococcal toxin is formed when the organisms multiply in food contaminated with pus from a food handler with a boil or abscess, or staphylococcal nasal discharge, and vomiting occurs 2–5 hours after the infected meal.

Treatment: No drugs are of proven value. Antibiotics may upset the intestine's natural defences and make matters worse. Generally all that is required is rest and a light fluid diet for a day or two.

Prevention: Seek the carrier. Good hygiene in food preparation.

DYSENTERY

BACILLARY DYSENTERY: *Cause:* Bacilli of the Shigella group, of which Sh. sonnei is much the commonest in Britain, though other organisms cause more severe dysentery, especially in the tropics. They are purely human pathogens, causing inflammation of the large bowel (colon).

Mode of infection: From the faeces of cases, and carriers, usually by the hands, from objects such as lavatory seats. This is how Sonnei dysentery spreads in nursery schools, where infection is common, and in hospital wards. Contamination of food and water may cause epidemics.

Symptoms and signs: Lower abdominal discomfort, fever and diarrhoea often with blood mucus in the stools, with malaise from toxaemia in severe cases.

Treatment: Usually none is required. Simple remedies such as kaolin mixture may alleviate the diarrhoea. There is some evidence that chemotherapy and antibiotics upset the natural resistance of the bowel, and prolong the carrier state. The organisms are now usually resistant to sulphonamides—tetracycline, oral streptomycin or nalidixic acid (Negram) may be used, depending on stool-sensitivity reports, in severe cases.

Prevention: is by hygienic measures, and exclusion of faecal carriers from food processing.

AMOEBIC DYSENTERY: This is due to bowel infection with the small parasite Entamoeba histolytica, which occurs in the tropics and spreads in cystic form from the stools. There is diarrhoea with bleeding and bowel ulceration, but the symptoms may be mild. There may be spread to the liver, causing amoebic abscess, which may discharge through the diaphragm and be coughed up as pus likened to anchovy sauce.

Metronidazole (Flagyl) 800 mg orally three times daily for 5 days is probably now the treatment of choice, replacing emetine and chloroquine.

CHOLERA

This disease of the Far East is caused by a bacillus (Vibrio) spreading by contamination of water supplies. It is a fulminating bowel infection, with copious fluid 'rice-water' stools. Treatment demands large quantities of intravenous fluids. Tetracycline is of limited value. Vaccination is advised for those visiting an endemic area such as India.

Venereal disease

The venereal diseases are acquired from infected persons at sexual intercourse, and their increase in recent years is attributed to promiscuity, decline in moral principles with a freer attitude towards sex, separation from family ties when abroad, and ignorance. The legally defined venereal diseases are gonorrhoea, syphilis, and soft chancre, but other sexually-transmitted diseases include non-specific urethritis and some cases of vaginitis from the trichomonas parasite.

GONORRHOEA

Cause: The gonococcus, a Gram-negative bacterium seen on microscopy, or by culture.

Symptoms and signs: Purulent urethral discharge in males, with dysuria. Females may have vaginal and urethral discharge, and infection may involve the ovarian tubes causing sterility, but many female carriers are symptom free and the organism may not be found until several smears are taken. Occasionally there is an acute gonococcal arthritis. The eyes of newborn babies may be infected from contact with vaginal secretions at birth.

Treatment: One injection of procaine penicillin 2·4 mega units intramuscularly. Some strains are resistant, and higher doses of penicillin, with probenecid to block renal excretion, kanamycin and trimethoprim/sulphamethoxazole (Bactrim, Septrin) may be used.

SYPHILIS

Cause: A bacterium of spirochaete (corkscrew-like) group called Treponema pallidum. Like the gonococcus, the organism fails to survive outside the body and is acquired only by contact with an infected lesion, usually at intercourse. There is a delay of up to a month, during which the treponemes have spread throughout the body, before signs appear.

Symptoms and signs:

Primary stage —a syphilitic sore or chancre on the penis, or the vulva.

Secondary stage—skin rashes and generalized lymph gland enlargement with involvement of blood vessels and nervous system—meningo-vascular syphilis.

—occurs up to two years later, during which may have been 'quiescence'.

Tertiary stage —follows after a latent period of up to fifteen years.

—heart involvement—syphilitic inflammation of the root of the aorta causing aortic valve incompetence, and dilatation (aneurysm) of aorta.

—central nervous system—tabes dorsalis (ataxia, shooting pains)

—general paralysis of the insane (dementia).

—gumma—abscess-like swelling affecting any organ.

Congenital syphilis occurs from infection in the uterus, the baby being stillborn or with deformities of brain, teeth and bones.

Diagnosis: The spirochaete may be seen under the microscope (dark-ground illumination) in smears from early lesions. Later diagnosis depends on blood antibody tests, such as the V.D.R.L. (Reference Laboratory), W.R. (Wassermann reaction) and treponemal fluorescent antibody and immobilization tests. Cerebrospinal fluid tests are also helpful.

Treatment: Procaine penicillin 600,000 units intramuscularly daily for 10 days in primary infection. More prolonged and repeated courses are used in later stages, though there may be severe reactions (Herxheimer reaction) in cardio-vascular cases.

NON-SPECIFIC URETHRITIS

This presents as a urethral discharge, from which gonococci are absent, up to two months after sexual intercourse—the cause is infective, but the organism uncertain. There may be associated conjunctivitis (inflammation of the outer covering of the eye) and arthritis (lumbar spine and joints of the feet being involved), the condition called Reiter's syndrome.

Treatment is tetracycline 500 mg 6-hourly for a week but the response is not always satisfactory.

SOFT SORE (CHANCROID) and LYMPHOGRANULOMA INGUINALE are rare venereal infections in Britain.

INCIDENCE AND PREVENTION OF VENEREAL DISEASE

Gonorrhoea is one of the commonest transmissible diseases in the world and its incidence has risen in Britain after a period of decline. Syphilis has increased in many countries, but not in Britain where treatment facilities are good. The disease may involve any system, however, and it is still important to carry out blood tests in patients with vascular or neurological symptoms especially if they are 'tattoo'ed and travelled the world'.

Control of V.D. may be achieved by better diagnostic and treatment facilities, the tracing of contacts, health education and respect for moral standards.

Tropical diseases

MALARIA

Incidence and cause: Malaria is a most important tropical disease, and should be remembered as a cause of fever in travellers from such parts. The name comes from 'bad air', but the condition is due to infection with a parasite, of which there are several types, which undergoes part of its life cycle in certain mosquitoes which bite man. There mosquitoes do not survive in temperate climates. They breed in stagnant water, and preventive measures include draining of such breeding grounds, and the use of insecticides such as D.D.T. The parasite passes from the salivary glands of the mosquito to the bloodstream of man, invading the liver and the red blood cells, destruction of the latter coinciding with the bouts of fever characteristic of the infection. Native populations develop a natural immunity, and those carrying the 'sickle-cell' trait (from an abnormal haemoglobin) are protected against severe malaria.

Symptoms and signs: There is a 'cold stage' with shivers and rigors, followed by high fever with headache and malaise, then the temperature subsides with marked sweating. The spleen may be palpable. Diagnosis is confirmed by finding the parasites in blood films. In severe cases there may be drowsiness, fits and coma—cerebral malaria, and sometimes hypotension and collapse, with severe haemolysis (breakdown of red cells) and darkly pigmented urine (blackwater fever).

Treatment: Chloroquine (as base) 600 mg, 300 mg 6 hours later, then 300 mg daily for the next 3 days. Cerebral malaria is treated with quinine, and severe illness may require intravenous fluids, steroids and dialysis (peritoneal, or with artificial kidney).

Follow-up: In some varieties of malaria, the parasites persist in the body—thus in 'benign tertian' malaria, relapses may occur up to three years later. Primaquine added to the treatment regime prevents such relapse.

Prevention (Prophylaxis): Visitors to a malarial zone should take proguanil (Paludrine) 100 mg daily or pyrimethamine (Daraprim) 25 mg weekly, before and during their stay, and continue for a month after returning to the temperate zone.

OTHER INSECT-BORNE (VECTOR-BORNE) DISEASES

Leishmaniasis (Kala-azar) occurs in the Middle East and parts of Africa, is transmitted by sandflies and is characterized by fever and swelling of spleen and liver, with anaemia. In the South American form, transmitted by bugs, there is involvement of oesophagus and heart.

Trypanosomiasis (Sleeping-sickness) occurs in East Africa from bites of the tsetse fly, and animals such as the cow may be reservoirs of the protozoa causing the disease.

Yellow Fever occurs in Central America and parts of Africa, and is due to a virus transmitted by certain types of mosquitoes. Vaccination prevents Yellow Fever and an International Certificate may be required of those who have passed through Yellow Fever zones.

Filariasis presents as massive swellings of the legs and scrotum, from lymphatic obstruction by a tiny worm spread by the bite of an infected mosquito, in the Far East. Similar parasites spread by certain flies, cause infestations of the skin, subcutaneous tissues, and even the eyes (causing blindness) in parts of Africa.

TYPHUS

There are several varieties of typhus, due to infections with tiny bacteria of the Rickettsial group.

Classical TYPHUS FEVER was spread by the bites of infected lice, was the killing disease of beleaguered armies, and still occurs in refugees. There is high fever, rash, headache and delirium. Treatment is with tetracycline or chloramphenicol, and louse-infested clothing should be burned.

Less serious Rickettsial infections include scrub typhus in the Far East, transmitted by mites, and Q-fever (from Queensland) transmitted by ticks from infected cattle. Q-fever sometimes occurs in Britain as a lung infection with cough and sputum.

PLAGUE is caused by a bacillus spread by a rat flea, which only bites man if its preferred rat host is not available. Epidemics of plague were the scourge of the Middle Ages. In bubonic plague there were lymph gland swellings, and in the pneumonic form the lungs were infected. Rats should be exterminated, and precautions are taken at docks and airports to prevent importing the species of rat liable to carry the infection.

SCHISTOSOMIASIS (BILHARZIASIS)

This infestation causes an immense amount of illness in Egypt and East Africa. It is caused by a tiny parasite which develops in a water snail found in lakes and irrigation schemes. The parasite penetrates human skin (so one should not go barefoot) and ultimately reaches the bladder, causing haematuria, or the liver and lungs causing fibrosis. Niridazole (Ambilhar) is of some value in treatment, but the best measures are preventive ones.

TETANUS*

Cause: A bacillus, Clostridium tetani, which inhabits the intestine of horses and sheep, forming spores found in manure, soil and dust—rare in Britain as the diesel engine has replaced the horse, but common in the tropics where animal excreta may actually be used to dress wounds. The bacillus, like that causing gas gangrene, grows in the absence of oxygen in deep punctured wounds and injuries—but these may be trivial ones, or apparently healed. The bacilli produce a toxin which travels up the peripheral nerves to the central nervous system.

Symptoms and signs: Discomfort and stiffness at the wound, followed by spasm of the jaw muscles (hence the name lockjaw)—within a few days, or a few weeks, the latter giving a better prognosis. This is followed by painful general spasms of muscle, precipitated by stimuli such as movement or even a loud noise. These spasms may cause ultimate exhaustion and death.

Treatment: Tetanus antitoxin intravenously, and intramuscular penicillin. Surgical wound toilet. Sedation and the use of muscle relaxants such as the preparations of curare used by anaesthetists, with endotracheal intubation and artificial ventilation.

*Tetanus should not be confused with tetany, which is muscle spasm from nerve irritability in states of low blood calcium.

Prevention: Tetanus toxoid provides active immunization—given with diphtheria and pertussis vaccine in infancy, with booster doses at school, and to those at risk such as farmers and soldiers. After sustaining a deep wound, a patient should receive tetanus toxoid rather than antitoxin, which carries a risk of severe serum reaction. This risk may be justified if there has been heavy wound contamination in a non-immunized subject.

LEPROSY

This disease is now confined to parts of Asia, Central Africa and South America. It is caused by a bacillus with some similarities to the tubercle bacillus, being 'acid-fast' on staining. Leprosy is not, however, highly infectious, occurring only on close or family contact with a case of the disease. The bacillus invades the skin, causing nodulation and thickening especially of the face, with involvement of the eye and later destruction of deeper tissues. The nerves become palpably thickened, and there is loss of sensation and motor weakness, often with severe deformity. Sufferers used to be ostracized and confined to leper colonies, but leprosy responds to dapsone and newer drugs. The best method of control is to find and treat all patients with the disease as early as possible, thus preventing spread and reducing deformity. B.C.G. vaccination gives protection to those at risk, and is being tried in children under fifteen in endemic areas.

Worms

THREADWORMS

These are tiny worms $\frac{1}{2}$/1 centimetre long which inhabit the colon and crawl out from the anus at night laying their eggs and causing irritation. Re-infection occurs from hands and finger nails transferring the eggs to the mouth.

Treatment is with piperazine (Antepar, Entacyl and Pripsen are suitable preparations) or with a single dose of viprynium (Vanquin) 50–300 mg depending on age of patient. The whole family must be treated.

ROUNDWORMS (ASCARIS INFESTATION)

Roundworms live in the intestine, their eggs are excreted in the faeces and may contaminate foods especially vegetables. After ingestion the developing egg is absorbed from the stomach, reaches the lungs where it develops further (and may cause transient bronchitis or wheeze), crawls up the trachea then down the oesophagus into the stomach again, and becomes an adult worm in the intestine. It may be passed in the faeces, or vomited, otherwise causing little trouble to its host; but it is unpleasant to pass one or more wriggling creatures like small earthworms, and infestation is common in the tropics.

Treatment is with piperazine as for threadworms.

HOOKWORMS

Eggs pass in the faeces, develop into larvae which invade intact skin, then like roundworms, reach the lungs then the stomach, and live in the duodenum, drawing blood from the host and causing anaemia if present in sufficient number—thus hookworm infestation is a very common cause of anaemia in the tropics.

Treatment—bephenium (Alcopar), sachet of 5 G.

TAPEWORMS

The larvae are consumed in infested beef (Africa, and sometimes Britain) or pork (less common, found in Central Europe and India), the tapeworms (multiple in the case of beef tapeworm, single if pork) developing in the intestine. They may reach a length of several feet and white segments of worm appear in the stools.

Treatment—niclosamide (Yomesan), 2 tablets of 500 mg, repeated in an hour. This kills the worm, it is not thereafter identifiable in the faeces, and the test of cure is to check the stools for absence of tapeworm segments after a month or two.

Cysticercosis: This is the occurrence of the larval stage of the pork tapeworm in man (instead of, or following gut infestation with the adult worm). Cysts are formed in the muscles and brain, if calcified may be seen on x-rays, and epilepsy is a complication—rare.

Hydatid disease: This is the occurrence of the cystic stage of a dog tapeworm in man, causing orange-sized 'hydatid cysts' in liver, lung or brain—surgical removal may be possible. Hydatid disease occurs where man has close contact with dogs, as in sheep rearing countries such as Iceland, Tasmania and the Shetland Isles of Scotland.

TRICHINOSIS

Trichinosis is infestation by the larval stage of the worm from eating infested pork or sausages, the pig having been affected from having eaten an infected rat. There is acute abdominal pain followed by invasion of the muscles by the parasite, with a severe allergic reaction, e.g. oedema of the face and eyes. Thiobendazole (Mintezol) is used in treatment, with steroids to suppress the allergic reaction. The chronic stage of trichinosis may present as muscular weakness, and treatment is often unsatisfactory.

TOXOCARA

Toxocara worms are found in the faeces of puppies and kittens (if not 'de-wormed') and children become infected if they ingest the eggs. The larvae penetrate into many tissues and there was evidence of previous infection in 2 per cent of a population sample in London. Usually the infection dies out, but larvae may reach the brain and eye, causing tumour-like masses.

Worm infestation is usually accompanied by 'eosinophilia'—an increase in the number of cells with red-staining granules in the leucocyte count of the blood.

Pyrexia of unknown origin (P.U.O.)

Causes

Common infections	urinary tract chest— usually purulent sputum	often 'silent' in the elderly.
Rarer infections	glandular fever brucellosis typhoid—paratyphoid	white cell count and bacteriological (agglutination) tests, and blood culture may be necessary.
	subacute bacterial endocarditis (associated heart disease) malaria	
Septicaemias (Bloodstream infection)	occult collection of pus 'Gram-negative' in debilitated, or patients on steroids or cytotoxic drugs as in leukaemia	
Neoplasms	carcinoma of the kidney (hypernephroma) leukaemia and Hodgkin's disease	
Auto-immune diseases	rheumatoid arthritis, systemic lupus erythematosus and polyarteritis nodosa	
Severe anaemia	pernicious anaemia	

A high swinging temperature may indicate 'pus somewhere' but classification of the type of fever is not usually helpful. Fevers such as 'undulant' fever and malaria need not follow a cyclical pattern.

Where it is not obvious which organ or system of the body is involved, we are dependent on blood tests to elucidate the diagnosis. In such cases of obscure fever therapy is not urgently required, and can generally be delayed at least until blood samples have been taken. Measures directed to the patients comfort, such as tepid sponging, and adequate fluids, can proceed. 'Blind' antibiotic therapy should be avoided—it is best to make an accurate diagnosis, bearing in mind the sensitivity of the organism, before embarking on the appropriate drug therapy.

4

The cardiovascular system

The action of the heart

The heart is a muscular pump with four chambers—the right atrium which receives venous blood from the systemic veins, the right ventricle which pumps the blood through the pulmonary artery to the lungs to be oxygenated, the left atrium, which receives this blood from the lungs, and the left ventricle which pumps blood through the aorta to reach arteries and capillaries throughout the body.

At each beat the ventricles contract simultaneously to expel their blood, the heart valves (tricuspid and pulmonary on the right side, mitral and aortic valves on the left) preventing backward flow. The heart beat causes a wave palpable as the pulse in a peripheral artery such as the radial artery at the wrist. The heart sounds, audible with the stethoscope over the 'apex' medial to the left nipple, are two in number, 'lup-dup'. They are due to the valves closing at the beginning and end of the contraction phase, which is called systole, and this is followed by the resting and filling phase, or diastole.

Cardiac contraction is 'fired' by an electrical stimulus, arising at the pacemaker in the sino-atrial node, spreading through the right atrium to reach the atrio-ventricular node, then down an electrical 'bundle' between the ventricles; this bundle divides into two branches and the stimulus thence passes out into the ventricular muscle (myocardium). This tiny electric current can be detected by applying plates or 'electrodes' to the chest and limbs, and recorded on paper or displayed on an oscilloscope (monitor)—the electrocardiogram (E.C.G.).

Disturbances of rate and rhythm may arise anywhere in the electrical conducting system. While they may be detectable by feeling the pulse or by listening to the heart, an E.C.G. is essential for accurate diagnosis and treatment.

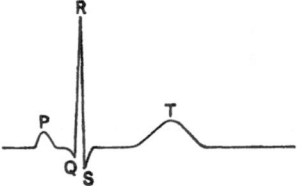

The P wave denotes atrial activity, the Q.R.S. complex and the T wave ventricular activity.

The pulse

Consider the *rate, rhythm* and *force* of the pulse. The normal rate is 60–80 per minute.

Rate: A rapid pulse, *tachycardia*, results from increased metabolism (exercise, emotion, fevers, thyrotoxicosis), blood loss, and some cardiac disorders—see below.

A slow pulse, *bradycardia*, occurs in simple faint (syncope, vasovagal attack), heart block, digoxin overdosage and raised intracranial pressure.

Rhythm: Note whether the pulse is regular or irregular—causes of irregularity are discussed below.

Force: Recognition of the normal force is largely a matter of experience: a soft weak pulse indicates poor cardiac output following blood loss or cardiac failure.

The blood pressure

The blood pressure is measured with the sphygmomanometer. The cuff is applied to the upper arm, inflated until the mercury is above the level where the pulse is no longer palpable, then deflated while the nurse listens with the stethoscope over the brachial artery. The level at which pulse sounds become audible is called the systolic blood pressure. As the cuff is deflated further, the sounds become faint and then inaudible—where they become faint is called the diastolic pressure. The systolic pressure depends on the force of the cardiac contraction and the state of the walls of the large vessels, being higher in the elderly whose vessels are harder and less elastic than those in young people. The diastolic pressure corresponds to the resting pressure in the artery between heart beats. The intensity of the blood pressure sounds may be diminished if the cardiac output is poor, when it may be difficult to be sure of the systolic and diastolic readings. They should be recorded to the nearest 5 mm. A fat arm causes a falsely high reading. The normal blood pressure is

$$\frac{100-140 \text{ (systolic)}}{70-90 \text{ (diastolic)}}.$$

A falling blood pressure indicates haemorrhage or deteriorating cardiac function, but cardiac disease may exist with a normal blood pressure. Hypertension—high blood pressure—is considered later.

Some general signs of heart disease

Breathlessness (dyspnoea, difficulty in breathing) from congested lungs, occurs on exertion and when lying flat.

Cyanosis is a blue discoloration of the face and lips, and fingertips. It is due to a sluggish peripheral circulation as a weak heart uses its limited output for the supply of more vital organs such as the brain and kidneys. The extremities are also cold.

Oedema—increased fluid in the tissues—may present as ankle swelling, the skin pitting on pressure. The neck veins may be distended from raised jugular venous pressure.

Confusion and restlessness may indicate a poor blood supply to the brain, and urinary output may be diminished from impaired renal blood flow.

Disorders of heart rate and rhythm

A patient may complain of *palpitations* (feelings of rapid or irregular heart beat)—these commonly occur in emotion or excitement in a healthy heart. Patients with serious heart disease seldom complain of palpitations and they may or may not be aware of any disturbance of rhythm.

SINUS ARRHYTHMIA—normal in youth, the pulse rate increases with inspiration, and decreases on expiration.

PAROXYSMAL TACHYCARDIA—sudden bursts of regular beating, rate 150–200—not usually a sign of heart disease, but heart failure may occur if the attack is prolonged. Manoeuvres such as breath-holding, eyeball pressure or massage of one carotid artery (all these cause vagal stimulation) may cut short the attack, or simple sedation may suffice. Digoxin 0·5 mg injected slowly intravenously, practolol

(Eraldin) 5 mg or oxprenolol (Trasicor) 2 mg, may be effective in resistant cases.

ATRIAL FIBRILLATION—3 causes:
(1) rheumatic heart disease involving the mitral valve,
(2) ischaemic (coronary) heart disease,
(3) thyrotoxicosis.

The atria are twitching rapidly and irregularly at around 300–400 'beats' per minute. The conducting bundle cannot respond to such a high rate, and the ventricles beat at an irregular 100–200 per minute. There may be a 'pulse deficit' as not all the heart beats are strong enough to produce a radial pulse. Treatment is with digoxin 0·5–1·0 mg slowly intravenously in urgent cases, but usually gradual digitalization using 2 tablets of 0·25 mg digoxin orally 6- or 8-hourly suffices. The action of digoxin here is to increase the block between the atria and ventricles, so that the ventricles respond to fewer atrial impulses thus beating more slowly and effectively. Digoxin also increases the strength of ventricular contraction. Dosage is adjusted to maintain a ventricular rate of 70–80 per minute, and varies from 0·0625 mg to 0·5 mg daily.

Digoxin overdose causes nausea and vomiting, visual upset, coupled beats from ventricular extrasystoles, undue slowing or sometimes rapidity of heart rate with E.C.G. changes. If such signs occur, digoxin should be stopped for a few days and resumed on modified dosage.

Where atrial fibrillation has a correctable cause (e.g. thyrotoxicosis), electrical conversion using direct current shock under light anaesthesia may be indicated.

ATRIAL FLUTTER—This is relatively rare and may be caused by the same heart diseases as atrial fibrillation. The atrium is 'fluttering' at a regular 200–400 beats per minute, again there is a block (which may be variable) in the conducting tissues, and the ventricular rate is less than 150, generally regular. Digoxin may convert flutter to fibrillation or to normal (sinus) rhythm.

EXTRASYSTOLES (ECTOPIC BEATS)—These arise from an abnormal focus in the atria (supraventricular extrasystoles) or in the ventricles. They may be unimportant, with no associated heart disease, or important in digoxin poisoning (coupled beats) and after myocardial infarction. The abnormal rhythm may be detectable at the pulse or on auscultation of the heart, but for early and precise diagnosis, E.C.G. monitoring is essential. Supraventricular extrasystoles may be treated with practolol or oxprenolol as described for paroxysmal tachycardia, or by direct current shock. Ventricular extrasystoles may occur when the basic heart rate is too slow, when atropine may be used as in heart block. The importance of multiple ventricular extrasystoles is in presaging more dangerous ventricular arrhythmias—ventricular tachycardia and ventricular fibrillation. Ventricular extrasystoles and tachycardia are treated with lignocaine 50–100 mg slowly intravenously, followed by an intravenous drip containing 1 mg per minute. Procainamide, practolol and oxprenolol may also be used, with direct current shock in resistant cases.

In VENTRICULAR FIBRILLATION—which may occur in myocardial infarction, electric shock and drowning—the ventricles are twitching ineffectively, there is no heart beat and no pulse, but the E.C.G. is characteristic—this is the main cause of CARDIAC ARREST—see below.

HEART BLOCK—this occurs when some or all of the stimuli from the atrial pacemaker fail to reach the ventricular muscle. Thus the block may be incomplete with missed beats and irregular rhythm, or complete when the ventricle takes up its own rhythm at a regular 40 beats per minute or less. Heart block may occur in myocardial infarction, and atropine 0·5–1·0 mg intravenously may help by its anti-vagal effect, allowing increased conductivity of the cardiac stimulus. It may, however, be necessary to pass a special catheter along a vein into the heart and connect an electrical 'pacemaker' to produce an adequate stimulus for cardiac contraction.

Elderly people may have a chronic heart block, not necessarily associated with coronary disease. If the heart rate is very slow they become easily breathless or may faint on exertion. Should there be a momentary stoppage of the heart, they will suddenly collapse, pale and unconscious. Usually the ventricle restarts within a few seconds, when consciousness returns and there is facial flushing with return of the circulation. This is called a Stokes-Adams attack. A long-acting adrenaline-like drug Saventrine, up to 8 tablets of 30 mg daily may usefully increase the heart rate. Otherwise a permanent intra-cardiac electrical pacemaker may be inserted, powered by a battery or nuclear source affixed to the chest wall, and maintaining the normal heart rate of 70 per minute.

Cardiac arrest

Cardiac unrest is due to ventricular fibrillation (the ventricular muscle twitching but failing to give a proper contraction) or to asystole (stoppage). In both cases there is a sudden failure of the circulation. In such circumstances the brain can survive for only three or four minutes. Recognition and management of cardiac arrest are therefore of the greatest urgency.

Causes:

Myocardial infarction—arrest may occur immediately, or in the first few hours from electrical irritability and arrhythmias.

Pulmonary embolism, when the pulmonary circulation is blocked by clots from the veins.

Severe haemorrhage and heart operations are other 'hospital' causes.

Electrocution and drowning.

Signs: Sudden collapse, loss of consciousness, absence of pulse and of heart beat, increasing cyanosis often with gasping respiratory efforts; pupils become dilated and patient will die if left untreated.

Treatment:

Summon help—alarm call in hospital.

Lay patient flat on a firm surface (bed boards or the floor) but elevate the legs.

Give a *sharp thump* on the chest—this may restart the heart. If not, proceed:

External cardiac massage—apply the heel of one hand to the lower sternum and with the other hand on top compress the sternum backwards some 3–4 centimetres about eighty times per minute.

Artificial ventilation—remove false teeth, clear the airway by supporting the chin well forward, insert plastic or Brook airway if available. Inflate the lungs by mouth-to-mouth breathing or Ambu bag once for every five chest compressions. With arrival of skilled help, endotracheal tube may be passed allowing better oxygenation but at first it is more important to *massage* and to *ventilate* than to rush for an oxygen cylinder.

Attach leads and record E.C.G.—the rhythm is usually ventricular fibrillation.

Defibrillation is performed with the D.C. defibrillator with an electric shock of 100–400 joules. Many doctors recommend defibrillation in all cases of sudden cardiac arrest, this taking precedence over cardiac massage, for the sooner the defibrillating shock is applied, the greater the chance of restoring sinus rhythm. Several shocks may be necessary.

A state of acidosis follows circulatory failure, and 100 ml 8·4 per cent sodium bicarbonate may be given intravenously. 5–10 ml of 1 in 10,000 adrenaline, and 5–10 ml of 20 per cent calcium chloride may be required if fibrillation persists, given into an intravenous drip.

Asystole is a rarer cause of cardiac arrest—the E.C.G. shows no tracing. Attempts with an external pacemaker are rarely successful but an intracardiac pacemaker may be effective and is passed in anticipation in some cases of myocardial infarction with heart block.

Successful treatment of cardiac arrest should be followed by management of the underlying disorder, with use of anti-arrhythmic drugs as lignocaine, and procainamide if indicated.

Ischaemic heart disease

Coronary heart disease is the commonest single cause of death amongst middle-aged men.

Cause: The heart muscle receives its blood supply from the coronary arteries. In middle-aged men, and the elderly of both sexes these arteries are often affected by the process of arteriosclerosis. Plaques of fatty material are laid down in the arterial lining, the condition called atheroma. Calcium may be deposited in the plaques. Minute clots (thrombi) tend to form on the irregular surface, further narrowing the lumen (bore) of the artery so that the heart receives insufficient blood for its own needs, i.e. there is myocardial ischaemia.

The cause or causes of coronary arteriosclerosis are uncertain but disturbance of fat and carbohydrate metabolism has been invoked, and some cases have a high blood fat, measurable as the serum cholesterol level—high animal fat intake has been blamed. A disturbance of the blood clotting mechanism, or of the normal fibrinolytic mechanism (which dissolves clots) has been postulated, but abnormalities are not usually demonstrable. Male sex, and oestrogen-containing contraceptive pills, are adverse factors in coronary disease.

There is a definite association with heavy cigarette smoking, and lack of exercise. The stresses and strains of modern life (e.g. motor car driving) may have some effect through the sympathetic nervous system, as adrenaline-release affects the blood fats. Raised blood pressure and obesity aggravate the condition.

Effects: If only a small segment of one coronary artery is affected, the collateral blood supply may be adequate; usually the involvement is more extensive, and myocardial ischaemia produces the following clinical conditions:

Angina pectoris

Myocardial Infarction (*Coronary Thrombosis*)

Congestive Cardiac Failure—usually preceded by angina or infarction, but these processes may be relatively silent in the elderly, who present with failure.

Such effects may be precipitated by anaemia or an episode of arrhythmia.

Angina pectoris

The blood supply through the narrowed coronaries is inadequate during effort and the impaired metabolism results in the formation of substances that cause pain.

Symptoms and signs: There is a constricting central chest pain brought on by exercise, especially hill-climbing, or emotional excitement (watching a football match), and relieved by rest. The pain may radiate to the arms, especially the left arm, and the lower jaw. The patient may describe the tight feeling as one of difficulty in getting his breath. There are no consistent pulse or blood pressure changes, but patients generally have an abnormal E.C.G.

Treatment: There is no cure—the patient must learn to live within his exercise tolerance, avoiding activities which provoke pain—thus stair-climbing can be obviated by having the toilet on the same floor as living room or bedroom, and the latter should be warm, as cold air is sometimes sufficient to cause an anginal attack.

Obesity should be treated, and cigarette smoking stopped.

Treatment: Drugs—Glyceryl trinitrate (trinitrin)—one tablet of 0·5 mg allowed to dissolve slowly under the tongue is used prophylactically—that is, taken before some essential activity which usually provokes angina, it will prevent the pain. It may also relieve an attack if taken early. Patients take comfort simply from having trinitrin tablets with them, and requirements vary from one every few weeks to several per day.

Propranolol (Inderal), practolol (Eraldin) and oxprenolol (Trasicor) are anti-adrenergic ('beta-blocking') drugs—80–200 mg daily may be effective in intractable angina. Propranolol may however cause cardiac failure, and it worsens bronchospasm in asthmatic subjects. The newer drugs practolol and oxprenolol may have fewer side-effects.

Clofibrate (Atromid S) lowers the serum cholesterol and two capsules of 500 mg twice daily may be used in cases with high cholesterol. There is however no proof as yet that lowering the cholesterol improves the condition. The substitution of vegetable oils for animal fats, and the avoidance of refined sugar have been recommended, but there is insufficient evidence to justify sweeping dietary changes in the population at large—it is more important to avoid obesity.

Prognosis: Patients may have angina over many years without deterioration, but some develop myocardial infarction or heart failure.

Myocardial infarction

Cause: Myocardial infarction is associated with arteriosclerosis of the coronary arteries. It is due to a sudden blockage of a narrowed artery by clot, hence the term Coronary Thrombosis; sometimes there may be no clot, only extreme narrowing of the vessels, and the precipitating factor is uncertain.

A part of the heart's blood supply is suddenly cut off, causing 'infarction' which means death of an area of tissue. If a vital part of the electrical conducting tissue is involved, even a small infarct may cause arrhythmia and sudden death from cardiac arrest—yet the rest of the myocardium is intact. Such a heart is 'too good to die' and immediate resuscitative measures, as already described, must be instituted. Usually, however the myocardial infarction involves the heart muscle mainly, though the conducting system may be affected. The infarct goes through processes of healing similar to those in a wound, scar tissue ultimately replacing the damaged area of myocardium.

Symptoms and signs: There is chest pain, similar in site and distribution to angina, but more severe and prolonged, and not necessarily related to exertion—symptoms may arise when the patient is in bed. There may or may not be warning, milder pains, or a previous history of angina. Severe pain is accompanied by sweating, nausea and vomiting, and by restlessness. There may be a feeling of extreme breathlessness and of impending doom.

Severe cases have pallor, cyanosis with cold extremities, irregularities of the pulse (which may be rapid or slow) and hypotension, and rapidly developing pulmonary oedema and congestive heart failure—

a picture called 'cardiogenic shock'—from failure of the heart to act as an effective pump.

Diagnosis: is confirmed by E.C.G.

There is a rise in the cardiac enzymes, S.G.O.T. and S.L.D.H., released from the damaged heart muscle, and measured by blood tests. The white cell count and erythrocyte sedimentation rate (E.S.R.) also rise after myocardial infarction, and raised temperature may be noted.

Complications:

Arrhythmias occur in most cases in the early stages, but may be transient. Serious arrhythmias are discussed below.

Cardiac failure may occur acutely, or gradually over some days, and indicates that the infarct is large.

Thrombo-embolism. It is rare for arterial embolism to occur from a thrombus forming on the damaged heart lining. Venous thrombo-embolism is a greater risk from enforced bed rest with venous stasis in the legs, from which a clot may travel to the lungs (causing pulmonary infarction).

Pericarditis may occur if the infarct involves the pericardial sac covering the heart, and there may be localized pain.

Rupture of part of the wall of the heart is rare, but a cause of death.

Management—Coronary Care: The risk of death from arrhythmias, cardiac arrest and failure is highest in the first few minutes, but remains very high during the few hours after myocardial infarction. It has therefore been recommended that patients should be treated by a coronary care team and admitted to hospital. There is some doubt, however, whether the stress and anxiety caused by transporting the patient to hospital from a comfortable bed in a good home may not itself provoke arrhythmias. But again, there is no way of separating the 'good risk' from the 'bad risk' case as the 'good risk' may suddenly develop a dangerous arrhythmia. Thus, once in hospital, all patients suspected of having a myocardial infarction should be nursed in a coronary care unit or area of the medical ward where close surveillance and E.C.G. monitoring are available. Many patients will feel reassured that such facilities and skilled attention are to hand but their simpler comforts and needs must not be neglected.

Treatment:

1. *Relieve Pain*—diamorphine (heroin) 10–15 mg by intramuscular injection. Heroin is less liable to provoke vomiting than morphine, though the latter is often used combined with the

anti-emetic cyclizine in Cyclimorph. Such drugs tend to cause hypotension, but this is not usually serious if the patient is in bed. Heroin and morphine are useful sedatives, and may ensure a good night's sleep used in the first few days after admission. There is little risk of addiction with such short term use, and these remain the best drugs in this situation.

2. *Management of arrhythmias*—sinus tachycardia is not amenable to drugs; supraventricular arrhythmias are often transient, but if they threaten cardiac efficiency, adrenergic blockers such as practolol or oxprenolol can be given slowly intravenously; atrial fibrillation may be treated with digoxin.

Sinus bradycardia and heart block may improve on atropine 0·5–1·0 mg intravenously. The insertion of an intravenous pacemaker may occasionally be indicated.

Ventricular extrasystoles are common, but if frequent, lignocaine 50 mg intravenously, followed by a drip containing 1 mg per minute is indicated, though practolol or oxprenolol have recently been suggested. Procainamide has been recommended prophylactically. Multiple ventricular extrasystoles may presage ventricular tachycardia, which may respond to similar treatment, but there is also a risk of ventricular fibrillation, producing cardiac arrest, and requiring immediate defibrillation with D.C. shock of 100–400 joules and resuscitative measures as already described.

D.C. shock is sometimes used when other arrhythmias prove refractory to drugs and may be carried out under sedation with diazepam (Valium) 10 mg intravenously.

3. *Oxygen*—oxygen is generally helpful, and is essential if the patient is cyanosed. Provided there is no history of chronic respiratory disease, oxygen in myocardial infarction should be given with a plastic face mask such as the Polymask at a flow rate of 4–6 litres per minute to give high oxygen concentration. (High concentration is dangerous if there is respiratory failure.) If the patient does not tolerate the mask, oxygen given by nasal catheters ('prongs') at 2 litres per minute will give useful slight oxygen enrichment of the inspired air.

4. *Bed rest*—clearly the damaged heart should be subjected to as little strain as possible until the part heals. Rest in bed is necessary, the patients position in bed being that which is most comfortable for him—usually fairly flat with one or two pillows, but if he is breathless from pulmonary oedema, he will breathe more easily if propped up.

The patient should be disturbed as little as possible in the first few hours, and not subjected to routine procedures such as washing and bed making. Male patients should use a urinal, and the urinary output noted. For bowel movements, it is probably best to allow the patient up to use a bedside commode if he so wishes, as the strain of getting out of bed may be less than that of using a bed pan. Bowel regularity can be attended to later. Again, it may be less strain if the patient feeds and shaves himself but of course he will need assistance if he remains too weak to do so.

Usually there is marked improvement within a few days. Most patients can be allowed gradually to be up and about if there are no complications and they are afebrile, within a week or ten days— there are no fixed rules, each case is decided on its merits.

5. Apart from E.C.G. monitoring, it is important to chart blood pressure, and the urine output which indicates if renal blood flow is satisfactory.

6. Heart failure—Early signs include breathlessness and 'moist sounds' heard on auscultation at the lung bases, and portable chest x-ray is helpful.

Treatment includes diuretics such as frusemide (Lasix) 40–80 mg orally, or 20 mg intravenously in acute cases, or bendrofluazide, and digoxin, as discussed later. Potassium chloride supplements are essential, for heart failure is associated with low body potassium, diuretics cause further loss, with increased risk of arrhythmias and digoxin toxicity.

The place of anticoagulants. These drugs are not of proven value in limiting established coronary thrombosis or myocardial infarction. Indeed, they may worsen any bleeding into the pericardium, and there is some evidence that heparin by its effect on blood fats, may increase the tendency to arrhythmia. Anticoagulants are contraindicated if there is a history of peptic ulcer, where there is a risk of haemorrhage.

Anticoagulants are, however, of value in preventing *venous* thrombosis with its risk of pulmonary embolism. Venous thrombosis is liable to occur after a period of enforced bed rest, especially if the circulation is already sluggish from cardiac failure. Anticoagulants may be used to diminish this risk—warfarin, phenindione (Dindevan) and nicoumalone (Sinthrome) are suitable oral drugs, the dose being controlled by estimation of the 'prothrombin time' of venous blood or 'Thrombotest' of capillary blood obtained by finger prick.

Anticoagulants are tailed off to zero when the patient has become ambulant. There has been some evidence that long term anticoagulant treatment lessens the likelihood of further myocardial infarction in men under sixty, but it is now felt that any benefit is marginal, and it is doubtful if such use is justified.

Fibrynolitic drugs. Trials are proceeding on the value of streptokinase, an enzyme which activates the body's clot-dissolving mechanism, and of Arvin, a substance obtained from snake venom, which acts on fibrinogen to render the blood less coagulable.

Subsequent management. Patients can usually be discharged from hospital in about three weeks, provided home circumstances are good. Proper periods of rest and the avoidance of sudden bursts of activity are important, but gentle and increasing exercise can be encouraged over the weeks, provided the patient is not having pain, and there is no evidence of heart failure.

The management follows the lines of that of angina pectoris, obesity should be controlled and cigarette smoking stopped.

Light work may be resumed a month after discharge, and a symptom-free patient should be encouraged to return to full employment. Heavy transport drivers and airline pilots are among the few exceptions to this recommendation.

Hypertension (high blood pressure)

The normal blood pressure ranges from $\frac{120}{80}$ for a person in his twenties to about $\frac{160}{90}$ in the sixties. The diastolic level is raised from narrowing of small arteries and arterioles, but the precise factors causing this are often unknown—renal and adrenal factors are referred to below. A raised diastolic pressure is usually accompanied by a raised systolic pressure. The effects of hypertension on the heart, kidneys and retinae of the eyes are more important than arbitrary blood pressure readings, which may be influenced by emotion. The finding of a raised blood pressure in a symptomless patient should direct attention to these organs, and treatment will prevent further damage to them.

Causes: Coarctation of the aorta—a congenital narrowing of the aorta just beyond its origin at the heart; occurs in the young; radial pulses normal, but femoral pulses diminished or absent.

Adrenal gland causes:

Phaeochromocytoma—tumour of medulla, produces adrenaline-like substances excreted in the urine as vanilmandelic acid (V.M.A., H.M.M.A., measured in 24-hour specimen) and causes hypertension, often paroxysmal, accompanied by sweating.

Cushing's syndrome—over-activity of adrenal cortex, trunk obesity with thin skin from excess cortisol production, measurable in the urine.

Aldosterone-producing tumour of adrenal cortex—polyuria, weakness and low serum potassium.

The above are rare, and the treatment is surgical,

Renal disease: Chronic glomerulonephritis

            chronic pyelonephritis

            renal artery stenosis

These may cause the kidney to produce renin, a substance which raises the blood pressure, and which also stimulates the adrenals to produce aldosterone, further raising the blood pressure.

Toxaemia of pregnancy—placental hormones may play a part, and there is accompanying albuminuria and oedema, and fits (eclampsia) in severe cases.

No definite cause can be found in the vast majority of cases, when the term *Essential Hypertension* is used. There may be a family history, suggesting a hereditary basis in some cases.

Symptoms and signs: The finding of a raised blood pressure is common, especially in women after the menopause, the condition may be symptomless and in the elderly it is often harmless. The symptoms and signs of hypertension are in fact due to its effects on the heart and blood vessels, especially the cerebral arteries and smaller vessels in the retina of the eye, and effects on the kidneys. Headache is not a common complaint except in severe hypertension, nor is epistaxis (nose bleeding) a usual mode of presentation.

Effects on the heart: the left ventricle must pump against the increased pressure in the arteries, gradually enlarges, shows signs of strain detectable on E.C.G. and eventually fails; the resultant pulmonary oedema causes breathlessness on exertion, and on lying flat in bed—nocturnal dyspnoea.

Pre-existing coronary artery disease may be made worse.

Effects on the cerebral circulation: Arteriosclerotic disease affecting the internal carotid artery and the intracerebral vessels is worsened and a vessel may break down causing cerebral haemorrhage (and often death); there is also an increased risk of cerebral thrombosis. The smaller intracranial arteries may be affected causing cerebral oedema, and the condition hypertensive encephalopathy, with headaches, fits, disturbance of consciousness and transient episodes of paralysis.

The retinal arteries may be affected and severe cases have retinal haemorrhages and papilloedema (blurring of the optic discs), visible with the ophthalmoscope, and visual upset.

The kidney: Not only may kidney disease cause hypertension, but hypertension from any cause will in turn damage the kidneys. The renal units (nephrons) are gradually destroyed, and remaining nephrons work at maximum level, but the kidneys are no longer able to produce concentrated urine. They can only eliminate the body's waste products, such as urea, in large quantities of dilute urine (polyuria). The patient may admit to having to rise at night to pass urine, and may complain of thirst. The blood urea gradually rises, and if the condition is untreated, the patient passes into renal failure with dehydration, vomiting, coma and death.

These effects of hypertension may be very gradual, with progressive deterioration over many years. In some younger patients, however, the process is much more rapid, and is called *Malignant or Accelerated Hypertension*—with very high diastolic pressure (over 140 mm), retinal haemorrhages and papilloedema, and progressive renal failure.

Investigations in hypertension
1. Charting of the blood pressure.
2. Urine: specific gravity—fixed at 1010 with renal involvement.
   may contain albumin.
   lab. examination may show red cells and casts, and superadded renal infection causes pus cells and positive bacteriological culture (colony count).
   24-hour specimens sent for V.M.A. assay (and 11-hydroxycorticosteroids in suspected Cushing's syndrome).
3. E.C.G. shows left ventricular enlargement or strain.
4. Chest x-ray—shows enlarged heart, and early pulmonary oedema.
5. Intravenous pyelogram x-ray (I.V.P.)—assesses size and function of kidneys.
6. Serum 'electrolytes' (sodium and potassium) and the blood urea level.
7. Special investigations such as arteriography (the demonstration

of arteries by injecting an x-ray-opaque substance into them) are only justified in the rare cases in which surgical treatment is contemplated.

Treatment: Coarctation of the aorta and the adrenal gland causes of hypertension are treated surgically.

In a few cases of unilateral kidney disease, where the kidney is acting as an endocrine organ secreting blood pressure-raising substances such as renin, nephrectomy (removal of the kidney) may be indicated.

A severe urinary tract infection and pyelonephritis occasionally exacerbates hypertension, and chemotherapy is indicated here.

In most cases of hypertension, there is no curable cause, and treatment is 'medical', the object being to reduce the blood pressure to nearly normal levels without producing undue side-effects in the patient.

As far as possible, the patient's activity should not be restricted, but heaving or humping heavy weights should be discouraged. He should have reasonable hours of work, sleep and recreation. Cigarette smoking should stop. Obesity should be controlled, but except in renal failure, there need be no other special dietary restrictions.

Drugs: Phenobarbitone 30 mg 2 or 3 times daily may be helpful in mild cases.

Oral diuretics such as bendrofluazide 2·5–5·0 mg, or chlorthalidone (Hygroton) 50 mg daily are mild hypotensives, and with the drug reserpine (central sedative hypotensive) 0·1 mg, may be adequate in many cases, especially the elderly in whom sudden lowering of the blood pressure is undesirable.

The action of the following drugs may be augmented and 'smoothed' by the oral diuretics; though diuretics lower the serum potassium, there is doubt whether potassium supplements are always necessary; fresh oranges may be an adequate dietary source.

Methyldopa (Aldomet), tablets of 250 mg, dosage up to 8 daily, blocks the formation or action of adrenaline and lowers the blood pressure without causing marked postural changes, so that very close control is not necessary. Side-effects include fluid retention, and haemolytic anaemia, detectable early by a positive Coombs' test in the blood.

Guanethidine (Ismelin), bethanidine (Esbatal) and debrisoquine (Declinax) are more powerful adrenergic-blocking drugs indicated especially in younger patients with severe hypertension. They have a marked postural effect, causing fall in blood pressure in the erect posture. Blood pressure readings are therefore taken with the patient standing, and dosage carefully adjusted over the weeks until optimal control is achieved. Patients should sleep with the head of the bed propped, and should avoid sudden change of posture, especially in the mornings when the hypotensive effect of drugs is often marked.

Treatment of hypertensive crises (acute left ventricular failure and hypertensive encephalopathy): Intravenous frusemide (Lasix) 40 mg may relieve pulmonary oedema, but urgent lowering of the blood pressure is necessary. Hexamethonium or pentolinium (Ansolysen) (the older ganglion-blocking drugs) 1–3 mg by subcutaneous injection, repeated depending on the B.P. response, checked every 15 minutes; or diazoxide, 300 mg intravenously—produce rapid lowering of the B.P., and the above drugs are introduced later.

Prognosis and follow-up: Proper management of hypertension will allow the patient to return to work. He must be kept under surveillance, with checks on the blood pressure reading, cardiac and renal function (E.C.G., chest x-ray, blood urea and electrolytes) and retinal examination with the ophthalmoscope, so that suitable adjustments in treatment may be made. Good control prevents hypertensive heart failure, previously the most common cause of death. Used judiciously in hypertensive patients with cerebro-vascular disease, hypotensive drugs lower the incidence of cerebral haemorrhage and thrombosis. In patients with normal renal function, treatment prevents kidney damage and even in those with mildly raised blood urea, the prognosis is improved; where renal damage is already severe, treatment is usually unsatisfactory and the outlook remains poor.

Thus the importance of hypertension is in the early recognition of its adverse effects on the heart, cerebral circulation and eyes, and kidneys. Treatment will prevent deterioration and allow the patient to continue his normal life.

Congenital heart disease

Congenital heart disease results from defects in the development of the heart during foetal life—german measles (rubella) in the mother is one cause. The baby may be stillborn. There may be an abnormality such as a heart murmur, heard with the stethoscope, or cyanosis, and the earlier this is recognized, at birth or in infancy, the better—

surgical correction may allow normal growth of the child. Cases may however, pass unrecognized until medical examination later, or until there is a complaint such as breathlessness in adult life.

Defects include pulmonary valve stenosis, coarctation of the aorta (already mentioned as a cause of hypertension), and patent ductus arteriosus (blood here passes from aorta to pulmonary artery and one sign is a loud murmur). Or there may be a 'hole in the heart' from patency of the septum (wall) between the atria or the ventricles. Thus atrial septal defect is not uncommon in young adults, presenting with breathlessness from lung engorgement with typical heart sounds and x-ray appearances.

Some cases are cyanosed, as venous blood is 'shunted' from the right side of the heart to the left side, without first going through the lungs, and the defects in Fallot's tetralogy cause such a state of affairs. Rarely an adult may develop a similar condition from abnormal rise in pressure in the right ventricle and shunting of blood through a pre-existing congenital communication between the two sides of the heart. Cyanosis of heart origin, central cyanosis, is often accompanied by clubbing of the fingers.

Investigations include angiocardiography (injection of radio-opaque material to outline the chambers of the heart on x-ray) and cardiac catheterization (insertion of a fine catheter into the heart to measure pressures and blood oxygen content).

Surgical correction may be possible.

There is an increased risk of subacute bacterial endocarditis in patients with congenital heart disease.

Rheumatic heart disease

RHEUMATIC FEVER (ACUTE RHEUMATISM) has been considered above. Rheumatic fever is an allergic reaction to streptococcal throat infection, commonest in children and young adults. There is fever and joint pains and swelling, the pain 'flitting from joint to joint'. Severe cases have tachycardia and heart involvement—acute rheumatic carditis. Treatment is rest (till E.S.R. settles), aspirin and steroids in severe cases, and penicillin. The joints return to normal. A very few cases develop acute heart failure. The real danger, however, is that of residual heart damage. The myocardium recovers, but the heart valves may be permanently affected.

Thus CHRONIC RHEUMATIC HEART DISEASE may follow in adult life, especially if there have been repeated attacks of rheumatic fever.

The mitral and aortic valves are especially liable to scarring and deformity, causing conditions such as mitral stenosis and incompetence and aortic incompetence, considered under Valvular Disease of the heart.

Penicillin prophylaxis prevents recurrences of rheumatic fever.

Subacute bacterial endocarditis is a complication of chronic rheumatic heart disease.

Pulmonary heart disease

A. COMPLICATING CHRONIC LUNG DISEASE

B. PULMONARY EMBOLISM

A. PULMONARY HEART DISEASE COMPLICATING LUNG DISEASE (COR PULMONALE)

Chronic lung diseases, especially chronic bronchitis and emphysema, throw a strain on the right ventricle. Superadded lung infections may precipitate right sided heart failure. *Symptoms and signs* are those of the lung disease, such as cough, sputum and breathlessness, and heart failure causes increasing cyanosis, raised jugular venous pressure, liver swelling and peripheral oedema. The pulse may be full and the extremities warm in pulmonary heart failure.

Treatment is unsatisfactory because there is much irreversible lung damage, but antibiotics may be helpful. Oxygen should be given only at low concentration here. The treatment of heart failure is discussed later.

B. PULMONARY EMBOLISM

Cause: A pulmonary embolus usually arises from deep vein thrombosis in the leg. Venous thrombosis is a complication of bed rest, especially in those with cardiac failure, obesity, following abdominal operations and it may also occur in those on the contraceptive 'pill'.

Symptoms and signs: In about half the cases, there is evidence of leg vein thrombosis such as calf pain and oedema, but often the clot has arisen silently from upper parts of the vein in the thigh, and the first sign of trouble is in the lungs or heart:

Pulmonary infarction—pain on breathing, from pleural involvement, breathlessness, haemoptysis (blood in the sputum) and rise in pulse rate. A pleural rub may be heard with the stethoscope, and there may be x-ray changes.

Recurrent emboli—there may be none of the above signs, but the diagnosis should be suspected if the patient has episodes of breathlessness, tachycardia and evidence of right heart strain on E.C.G., with progression to right ventricular failure.

Massive pulmonary embolus—a large clot may completely obstruct the pulmonary artery, with sudden collapse, severe breathlessness and cyanosis, chest pain, raised jugular venous pressure, and rapid thready pulse with low or immeasurable blood pressure. Death will follow unless the clot breaks up or can be speedily removed surgically.

Special investigations include pulmonary angiography and lung scanning with radio-active isotopes but there may be no time for these in severe cases.

Treatment: The best treatment is preventive—heparin 10,000 units 6–8 hourly intravenously followed by oral anticoagulants such as warfarin or phenindione. Anticoagulants are also indicated in established pulmonary infarction, to limit spread and prevent recurrence.

Fibrinolytic therapy with intravenous streptokinase may prove useful in dissolving venous thrombi and in some cases of pulmonary embolism, but the effect is not immediate. Thus, in life-threatening cases, in addition to heparin and oxygen therapy, the patient may require urgent transfer to a thoracic unit. Here, using a heart-lung machine to maintain the circulation, thoracotomy (opening of the chest) and surgical removal of the clot may be carried out.

In view of the high incidence and silent nature of venous thrombosis, increasing attention is being given to early methods of detection. These include the use of ultra-sound with the portable Sonicaid instrument, radio-isotope labelled fibrinogen, and venography. Surgical removal of thrombus in the femoral vein in the thigh may also be indicated.

Syphilitic heart disease

This is now uncommon. In late syphilis, up to fifteen years after the primary infection, the ascending aorta, just where it arises beyond the left ventricle, may be involved by syphilitic aortitis. This has three effects:

1. Weakening of the vessel wall, causing a dilatation or aneurysm of the ascending part of the aorta. There may be pain, rupture of the vessel, and death.

2. The dilatation affects the aortic valve ring, causing aortic incompetence and left ventricular failure.

3. Puckering of the orifices of the coronary arteries, a rare cause of coronary artery disease and angina.

The diagnosis is confirmed by the history, other signs of late syphilis (such as the Argyll-Robertson pupils, failing to react to light, described under Neurosyphilis), and positive blood V.D.R.L. or W.R. test.

Treatment is with penicillin, though a severe reaction may occur at this stage.

Thyroid disorders and the heart

THYROTOXICOSIS—Overactivity of the thyroid gland—increases metabolism causing tachycardia, and in the elderly the risk of atrial fibrillation and heart failure. Treatment is that of the cause; digoxin, and adrenergic blocking drugs such as practolol and oxprenolol (which control the sympathetic overactivity associated with thyrotoxicosis) may also be indicated.

MYXOEDEMA—underactivity of the thyroid—here the heart is slow and sluggish, there may be a pericardial effusion. Treatment is with thyroxine, building up the dose very gradually to avoid precipitating heart failure.

Valvular disease of the heart

Causes:

1. Congenital valve defects, e.g. pulmonary stenosis, which may present as weakness and breathlessness.

2. Rheumatic heart disease—the valves are scarred as the result of rheumatic fever, especially repeated attacks. The mitral and aortic valves are most commonly affected. There may not be a clear history of acute rheumatism, the patient simply presenting with symptoms due to the valve affection.

3. Arteriosclerotic valve thickening—affecting the aortic valve in the elderly causing a murmur and sometimes signs of stenosis.

4. Syphilitic aortitis with aortic valve incompetence.

5. Subacute bacterial endocarditis may complicate any of these, and is considered below.

Rheumatic heart disease is the most important cause, and its effects are as follows:

MITRAL VALVE DISEASE—STENOSIS (NARROWING) AND INCOMPETENCE

Mitral valve disease is commoner in women.

Symptoms and signs: MITRAL STENOSIS—fatigue, breathlessness on exertion and winter bronchitis may be admitted to, rather than complained of, in the early case; here the pulse is regular but of small force and there are characteristic heart sounds with a murmur. It is important to make the diagnosis at this stage. Later there are episodes of breathlessness from pulmonary oedema, and there may be haemoptysis. In some cases there is constriction of the blood vessels in the lung, causing strain on the *right* ventricle, and the patient may present with right ventricular failure and peripheral oedema rather than with initial breathlessness.

MITRAL INCOMPETENCE—this causes regurgitation of blood into the left atrium when the left ventricle contracts, so that the left side of the heart is always overloaded and backpressure on the lungs causes pulmonary oedema and breathlessness—left heart failure. Then the right ventricle feels the strain and fails, causing peripheral oedema. There is a characteristic murmur with enlarged heart on x-ray.

Mitral stenosis and incompetence often co-exist. *Atrial fibrillation* may complicate either, further impairs cardiac output and carries risk of embolus (to a cerebral, renal or peripheral artery) from clot accumulating in the left atrium behind the diseased mitral valve—a 'stroke' may be the first sign of the heart disease.

Treatment: Mitral stenosis should be detected early and its severity assessed by special investigations such as cardiac catheterization, so that the operation called *mitral valvotomy* can be carried out in suitable cases. This allows relief of the obstruction at the mitral valve, and cardiac function returns to normal without the need for drugs or restrictions of activity. Where there is mitral incompetence surgical valve repair or replacement (by grafting, or by Starr ball-valve prosthesis) may improve function, but results are not entirely satisfactory. Thus medical measures such as diuretics and digoxin, as for heart failure, are indicated, plus anticoagulants if there has been a history of embolic episodes, to prevent their recurrence.

Mitral valve disease in pregnancy—the valve disorder should be recognized and treated before-hand if possible; close surveillance is necessary because of the extra strain the heart is carrying; proper rest is essential, and any deterioration of cardiac function may indicate the need for drug therapy, or even emergency valvotomy. Young women with known mitral disease should have their babies early, and some family limitation may be desirable to allow patients to cope with their household chores.

AORTIC VALVE DISEASE—STENOSIS AND INCOMPETENCE

The aortic valve may be affected alone or in combination with the mitral valve in rheumatic heart disease. (In syphilitic heart disease only the aortic valve is affected and the lesion is usually aortic incompetence.)

Aortic valve disease is commonest in middle-aged men.

Symptoms and signs: AORTIC STENOSIS—the reduced cardiac output causes weakness and fainting, and there may be anginal pain from poor coronary filling. The pulse is small and of 'plateau' character due to sustained ejection of blood through the narrowed valve. The blood pressure is low, and the 'pulse pressure', the difference between the systolic and diastolic readings, also low. At the heart, a systolic 'thrill' or vibration is palpable over the aortic valve near the upper sternum, and a loud murmur is heard with the stethoscope.

AORTIC INCOMPETENCE—The pulse is 'collapsing' in character, with wide pulse pressure from raised systolic and lowered diastolic blood pressure as the column of blood regurgitates through the leaking valve into the left ventricle. A diastolic murmur is audible with the stethoscope. E.C.G. and x-ray show left ventricular enlargement.

The lesions are commonly combined. Patients may remain symptomless for many years, then develop breathlessness on exertion and on lying flat in bed (nocturnal dyspnoea) from left ventricular failure. When deterioration occurs, it does so relatively rapidly over a period of months (rather than years, as in mitral disease), and death may occur within two years of the onset of symptoms. Atrial fibrillation is rare in pure aortic valve disease.

Treatment: Early diagnosis is essential, and if the patient's general condition allows, the best treatment is surgical repair or replacement of the diseased aortic valve, using a graft or Starr ball-valve prosthesis, the results being generally better than in mitral valve surgery.

Otherwise, the treatment is that of heart failure.

The *Pulmonary Valve* is rarely involved in rheumatic heart disease, and the *Tricuspid Valve* is rarely involved in the absence of mitral or aortic disease. The dilatation of the heart following mitral or aortic disease may, however, affect the tricuspid valve, causing tricuspid incompetence with back-pressure effects—raised venous pressure, swollen tender liver, and peripheral oedema.

Subacute bacterial endocarditis

Cause and prevention: Subacute bacterial endocarditis is due to bacterial invasion of a deformed or diseased heart valve, usually the aortic or mitral valve. A healthy valve is resistant to such invasion. Thus the condition occurs in those with congenital or acquired usually rheumatic, valvular disease which may in itself be quite mild. The bacterial invasion of the valve follows a bloodstream infection, the commonest cause of which is a dental extraction or deep filling. Streptococcus viridans, normally living harmlessly in the mouth is the usual organism. A rarer cause of bloodstream infection follows trauma with instruments during pelvic or urinary investigations, and here the invading organism may be a 'coliform' one from the bowel.

Prevention: Patients with valvular disease should have 1 mega unit of penicillin by intramuscular injection, not more than an hour before dental extractions, the injection to be repeated 12 hourly over the next 48 hours. If the patient is already receiving penicillin (e.g. for rheumatic fever prophylaxis), his mouth organisms may be resistant to it, and erythromycin or cephaloridine should be given to cover the dental treatment.

Symptoms and signs: Subacute bacterial endocarditis is now most common in elderly patients, and diagnosis may be difficult if the condition is not borne in mind.

There is fever, malaise, loss of weight, anaemia and raised E.S.R. There is evidence of heart valve disease, and heart failure may worsen. Little vegetations are formed on the affected valve and these may break off as small emboli causing tender little nodes or tiny haemorrhages at the finger-tips and under the nails; there may be haematuria (blood in the urine), detectable only microscopically. Cerebral emboli cause strokes which may be transient. Advanced cases may have brownish (cafe-au-lait) skin and finger clubbing. The patient may die of toxaemia or from cardiac or renal failure.

Diagnosis is confirmed by a positive blood culture of the responsible organism. Several blood specimens may be necessary, but if the patient is dangerously ill, treatment may be started after one blood culture has been taken.

Treatment: Proper therapy requires knowledge of the organism, and of its antibiotic sensitivity. Penicillin is usually effective against the streptococcus viridans, and is given in dosage sufficient to maintain a serum penicillin level four times that which kills the organism in laboratory cultures. 4–20 mega units penicillin daily is required and as therapy is necessary for six weeks to eradicate the organism from the valve, intravenous therapy by infusion in dextrose or normal saline, using a fine plastic cannula is preferable to repeated intramuscular injections. A resistant organism may demand the use of streptomycin in addition, with probenecid to block renal excretion and boost blood levels of penicillin. If the organism is not streptococcus viridans, alternative antibiotics may be required. In the usual case, penicillin is the sheet-anchor of treatment and clinical improvement usually occurs in a few days, temperature and E.S.R. settling to normal.

Bed rest is indicated in the early stages, with treatment of heart failure as necessary. Gradual ambulation is allowed when the temperature settles, and the intravenous drip can be made suitably portable.

Pericarditis

Pericarditis is inflammation of the pericardial sac covering the heart. Pericarditis may be 'dry', or there may be a pericardial effusion.

Causes:

1. Occurs as a complication of rheumatic fever (part of the 'carditis' of severe cases), or of myocardial infarction, and in the late stages of renal failure.

2. Acute benign pericarditis—cause unknown, possibly viral.

3. Rheumatoid arthritis and collagen diseases.

4. Pericarditis with effusion—cause often uncertain, sometimes myxoedema.

5. Spread of infection from lung or pleura—rare.

6. Chronic constrictive pericarditis—often tuberculous.

Symptoms and signs: In rheumatic fever and myocardial infarction, the symptoms are mainly those of the underlying condition, with more superficial chest pain and a pericardial 'friction rub' heard with the stethoscope. The presence of pericarditis contra-indicates the use of anticoagulant drugs, for these may provoke bleeding into the inflamed pericardium. Sometimes pericarditis occurs a few weeks after myocardial infarction or operations on the heart, and an auto-immune reaction may be responsible.

Acute Benign Pericarditis

This occurs in young adults and Coxsackie virus infection may be a cause, with associated symptoms such as cough, sore throat and muscular pains. There is fever and retrosternal pain which may be suggestive of myocardial infarction. There is a friction rub and typical E.C.G. changes of pericarditis, but the myocardium is not involved to any extent and the cardiac enzymes (S.G.O.T. and S.L.D.H.) are not raised.

Pericarditis with effusion, if large, and *Constrictive Pericarditis.*

These prevent the proper pumping action of the heart, especially the right ventricle, causing right ventricular failure—distended neck veins, enlarged liver and peripheral oedema. These signs are out of proportion to breathlessness, and the patient may lie flat without dyspnoea as the lungs are not engorged. There may be complaint of weakness, from poor cardiac output, with small pulse and low blood pressure. In pericardial effusion the cardiac shadow is grossly enlarged on x-ray, in constrictive pericarditis the heart is small and calcification may be seen in the pericardium.

Treatment: With treatment of underlying rheumatic fever and myocardial infarction, the pericarditis usually settles in a few days.

Acute benign pericarditis may require analgesics to relieve pain, and steroids may be helpful in severe cases.

Where pericardial effusion is embarrassing the heart and where there is no treatable cause such as myxoedema, aspiration through a needle inserted under local anaesthesia may be required.

Tuberculous pericarditis requires anti-tuberculous chemotherapy, and constrictive pericarditis requires surgical removal of the densely adherent tissue, which allows dramatic relief of symptoms.

Myocarditis and cardiomyopathy

Myocarditis is an old term indicating inflammation of the heart muscle, which may occur as part of the carditis of rheumatic fever. Such a myocarditis may cause acute heart failure, but this is rare and we have seen that the heart valve involvement is the important aspect in later years. Myocarditis may complicate infections such as measles and glandular fever, but it is seldom serious. Occasionally viruses of the Coxsackie group cause a myocarditis with symptoms similar to those of ischaemic heart disease and heart failure, but full recovery usually occurs.

The term cardiomyopathy is used to describe several conditions involving the heart muscle, without definite evidence of infection or inflammation. In *alcoholic cardiomyopathy*, there is disturbance of rhythm and heart failure—the patient may also have cirrhosis of the liver and peripheral neuritis. In '*wet beri-beri*' from vitamin B_1 deficiency, there is cardiomyopathy with right heart failure. In tropical Africa there occurs a curious fibrosis of the heart muscle, and nutritional factors and malaria have been suggested as causes.

Cardiomyopathy of unknown cause may produce disturbances of left ventricular function and heart failure, with cardiac enlargement on x-ray and E.C.G. changes. Cases occur in young adults, and adrenergic blocking drugs may be of value; disturbance of the nerve supply to the heart muscle has been postulated. Treatment is however generally unsatisfactory.

Heart failure

It is impossible to overstrain the healthy heart. Heart failure is considered here near the end of the section on cardiovascular disease, for it is the end result of the diseases already considered. Heart failure may occur acutely, for example after massive myocardial infarction, but usually it is a gradual process over months or years. Often the heart muscle has enlarged despite ischaemia, or in the attempt to maintain cardiac output with diseased valves, but ultimately the myocardium fails.

Thus heart failure is pump failure.

Pump failure is associated with salt and water retention. The reasons for this are not clear, but are related to impaired circulation to the kidneys. The kidneys produce factors causing salt (sodium) retention—one of the these may be the hormone renin which in turn stimulates the adrenal cortex to secrete aldersterone which acts on the renal tubule to prevent sodium excretion. Salt retention causes water retention, itself provoked by other circulatory factors. The result is an excessive blood volume, so that the circulation becomes overloaded, further embarrassing the heart.

It may be helpful to think in terms of conditions causing left heart failure, and those causing right heart failure, but the distinction between the two types is often artificial, for left heart failure is often associated with or followed by right heart failure. In each case, there is fluid retention and 'congestion' but the term *congestive heart failure* tends to be applied descriptively to signs such as raised venous pressure and peripheral oedema, seen following failure of the right side of the heart.

Causes:
Main   *Less common*
Ischaemic (coronary)
    heart disease   Congenital heart disease
Hypertension   Syphilitic aortic incompetence
Rheumatic valvular disease   Thyrotoxicosis
Chronic lung disease   Multiple pulmonary emboli ⎫ *These cause*
    (bronchitis and   Pericardial effusion or   ⎬ *pure Right*
    emphysema)   constriction   ⎪ *Ventricular*
                                                          ⎭ *Failure*

Left Ventricular Failure results from ischaemic, hypertensive, and aortic valve disease, for in these conditions, the brunt of the trouble is borne by the left ventricle. Mitral incompetence also causes left ventricular overload. Symptoms result from back-pressure on the vessels in the lungs, causing pulmonary oedema.

Pulmonary oedema may occur in tight mitral stenosis, again from back-pressure, though the left ventricle is not involved.

Right Ventricular Failure follows left ventricular failure, but may occur first in some cases of mitral stenosis where there is constriction of the blood vessels in the lung producing right ventricular strain.

Chronic bronchitis and emphysema also throws a strain on the right side of the heart, and right ventricular failure may be added to the pulmonary signs such as cough and sputum.

Right ventricular failure results in systemic congestion—raised venous pressure, swollen liver and peripheral oedema—signs which may be added to those of pulmonary congestion in left ventricular failure, or occur in isolation in 'pure' right ventricular failure.

Precipitating factors: In patients with known heart disease, heart failure may be precipitated by a fresh cardiac insult such as further myocardial infarction or an episode of arrythmia—thus the onset of atrial fibrillation may cause heart failure in mitral valve disease.

Intercurrent infection, especially respiratory infection, and anaemia are non-cardiac precipitating factors.

Symptoms and signs

There are three cardinal ones—*breathlessness, cyanosis*, and *oedema*.

Breathlessness (dyspnoea, difficulty in breathing) may be noted first on exertion or stair climbing. In left ventricular failure and pulmonary oedema, breathlessness waking the patient from sleep is characteristic—paroxysmal nocturnal dyspnoea. This occurs from increased lung congestion when the patient lies flat and is relieved by sitting up in bed. In heart failure generally, patients feel less dyspnoeic when propped up—the condition called orthopnoea. Severe pulmonary oedema causes extreme breathlessness and the production of frothy red sputum.

Cyanosis—a blue discoloration of lips, cheeks and fingertips from sluggish peripheral circulation and reduced oxygen content of the blood in the capillaries. The skin is usually cold, except in heart failure following pulmonary disease, when the extremities may be warm. Very severe cyanosis involving the tongue suggests a 'central' cause such as a right-to-left shunting of blood in congenital heart disease.

Oedema is fluid retention in tissues, and in heart failure is gravitational—thus there is oedema pitting with finger pressure over the ankles and legs, or above the sacrum if the patient has been confined to bed. Swelling of the abdomen may be due to ascites, fluid exudation into the peritoneal cavity.

In right heart failure the jugular venous pressure is raised and pulsation is visible in the neck. The liver may be tender and swollen.

Restlessness and *confusion* are due to cerebral anoxia, and there may be Cheyne-Stokes breathing from affection of the respiratory centre in the medulla. This is a form of periodic breathing—depression of the respiratory centre causes apnoea (no breathing) followed by carbon dioxide retention which stimulates the centre into causing deep sighing respirations.

The pulse rate is usually raised, and may be regular or irregular. The commonest irregularity is atrial fibrillation with a rapid ventricular rate. Not all the beats of the heart may be strong enough to reach the periphery so that the apical rate may be higher than the pulse rate—pulse deficit.

The *blood pressure* may be normal, raised (e.g. in hypertensive failure) or low; a low blood pressure associated with cold, blue extremities indicates poor cardiac output and carries a bad prognosis.

Lack of appetite, nausea and vomiting occur from congestion of the stomach, and impaired circulation to the large bowel causes constipation or occasionally diarrhoea.

Urinary output may be lowered from poor circulation to the kidneys, and there may be albuminuria. However, in patients with hypertensive heart failure, previous renal damage may have been associated with polyuria, which may persist. Disturbances of electrolyte (sodium and potassium) balance are part of the picture of cardiac failure. Not only is there sodium and water retention, but there is also potassium loss rendering the heart more irritable and liable to arrhythmias. In very advanced cases of failure, although the total body sodium content is high, blood tests may show a low serum sodium concentration. This indicates a severe disturbance of mineral metabolism in the cells, is accompanied by a rising blood urea, and the prognosis in such cases is poor.

Venous thrombosis in the legs, with risk of pulmonary embolism, may occur from circulatory slowing, and is an important complication of cardiac failure.

Treatment

1. *Rest*. Rest in bed is indicated in severe cardiac failure. The patient should be nursed propped up, with the legs horizontal, with a bed-cage to take the weight of the bedclothes off oedematous limbs. If however, the patient has been most comfortable sitting in a chair, with the legs dependent, it may be wise to continue treatment in this position initially, for sudden transfer of fluid from the legs to the lungs is undesirable. The patient should be allowed to use a bedside commode, or may be wheeled to an adjacent toilet.

Urine output should be measured.

Daily weighing (using a chair) will indicate if oedema is improving.

Prolonged bed rest is undesirable, for there is risk of venous thrombosis, muscle wasting and pressure sores especially in the elderly. Gradual ambulation is usually possible within two weeks.

2. *Diet*. A light diet is allowed, and it is more important to serve something which the patient finds palatable than to insist on a rigid scheme. Added salt should be avoided but there is no need for rigid salt restriction as modern diuretics are so effective. A reasonable fluid intake is generally allowable. Fresh oranges provide a pleasant source of extra potassium.

3. *Oxygen*. In heart failure the blood oxygen content is lowered and can be improved by oxygen inhalation. Provided the patient does not have chronic respiratory disease, oxygen should be given by plastic face mask (e.g. the Polymask or M.C. mask) at a flow rate of 6 litres per minute—this gives an oxygen concentration of 40 per cent instead of the normal air concentration of 20 per cent. If a mask is not tolerated, oxygen may be given by nasal catheters at 2 litres per minute, giving about 30 per cent oxygen content of inspired 'air'. Patients with chronic respiratory disease must not be given high concentration of oxygen, for their respiratory centre requires the stimulus of relative anoxia to continue to function, and if

they are given too much oxygen, they will stop breathing. This must be borne in mind in patients whose heart failure follows lung disease.

Smoking and naked lights are banned when oxygen is in use, to avoid the risk of fire or explosion.

4. *Drugs in heart failure*

A. MORPHINE AND DIAMORPHINE. These drugs, 10–15 mg subcutaneously, are the best sedatives, and have a unique effect in relieving dyspnoea in pulmonary oedema. They allow the patient a good night's sleep and should be used in the first few days of treatment, except in heart failure complicating lung disease, where respiratory depression is undesirable.

B. DIURETICS. These increase renal salt and water loss, the increased urine output being termed diuresis. Pulmonary congestion is relieved, and systemic oedema mobilized.

Frusemide (Lasix). 40–80 mg orally produces diuresis within two hours, or 20–40 mg intravenously has immediate effect in severe cases, e.g. in pulmonary oedema.

Ethacrynic acid (Edecrin) is also rapidly effective.

Bendrofluazide (Neo-Naclex, Centyl) 5 mg tablet, is one of many thiazide diuretics which are slower in action than frusemide, but a less abrupt action may have some advantages when the acute stage is over, so bendrofluazide is often substituted after a few days, given daily, or alternate days when oedema has cleared.

These diuretics cause potassium loss, and potassium chloride supplements, such as Slow-K tablets, or one of the effervescent potassium chloride preparations, must be given.

Spironolactone (Aldactone-A), 25 mg 4 times daily may be added to the standard diuretics in resistant oedema. It helps to increase sodium loss by antagonizing the action of the salt-retaining hormone aldosterone on the renal tubules.

Aminophylline, 250 mg slowly intravenously, may be tried in resistant cases, to improve renal blood flow sufficiently to allow the above diuretics to be effective.

C. DIGOXIN is especially useful if there is atrial fibrillation, for it has a blocking effect on the conducting tissue, thus slowing the ventricular rate and allowing more effective contraction. As the ventricular beats may not all be strong enough to be perceptible at the pulse in atrial fibrillation, an apical rate chart should be kept. Digoxin has a further effect of increasing the strength of ventricular contraction (apart from the rate) and may help in cardiac failure even unassociated with atrial fibrillation. Dosage is 0·25–0·5 mg orally 6- or 8-hourly; 0·5–1·0 mg slowly intravenously may be used initially, provided the patient has not recently received the drug by mouth, if a rapid effect is desired. Generally, however, oral treatment is adequate and the dose is adjusted when the ventricular rate or the cardiac failure has improved, to a maintenance dose of 0·25–0·5 mg daily. The drug is cumulative, and is sometimes given only five days weekly to avoid toxic effects. These include loss of appetite, nausea and vomiting and slow heart rate with coupled beats (pulsus bigeminus), but sometimes there is atrial tachycardia and rapid pulse. The E.C.G. may give advanced warning of such toxic effects. They occur more readily if the patient is potassium deficient—a risk that has increased since the availability of the potent oral diuretics, which demand potassium supplements as explained above.

D. ANTICOAGULANTS. Warfarin, phenindione (Dindevan) or nicoumalone (Sinthrome) are indicated prophylactically in patients with severe heart failure necessitating prolonged bed rest, with its risk of venous thrombosis. Dosage is controlled by 'prothrombin time' (venous blood) or 'Thrombotest' (capillary blood from finger prick) estimations. In patients whose heart failure is due to recurrent pulmonary emboli from leg vein thrombosis, prolonged anticoagulant therapy is necessary.

In atrial fibrillation and mitral stenosis, anticoagulants may diminish the risk of systemic embolism from clot in the left atrium.

Where cardiac failure has been precipitated by arrhythmia, treatment may include anti-arrhythmic measures already discussed.

Respiratory infection is an important cause of heart failure in pulmonary disease, and appropriate chemotherapy or antibiotics are indicated.

Anaemia should be treated with appropriate drugs, and blood transfusion should generally be avoided for fear of precipitating circulatory overload.

Results of treatment

It is now rarely necessary to resort to paracentesis, needle aspiration of fluid from the pleural and peritoneal cavities. In a few cases of severe heart failure, treatment proves ineffective and attempts with further diuretics merely worsen the biochemical abnormalities. Occasionally restriction of water intake may be justified in such cases, but usually such a condition is terminal, and denotes irreversible pump failure.

Many patients can, however, return to useful activity, avoiding sudden unaccustomed exertion, and being maintained on diuretics, potassium and digoxin with suitable surveillance. Curative surgery may be possible in those with heart valve lesions.

Heart transplantation. Remarkable technical success has been achieved, and patients have survived for up to two years after operation. It is, however, difficult to decide which cases are suitable, for early cases may benefit from less drastic measures, and late cases have involvement of lungs and liver, lessening the changes of success. There are problems too, of transplant rejection, immunosuppression and of the ethics of obtaining donor hearts. There may be a greater place for the use of plastic pumps, which are being developed for use as temporary supports to the circulation, e.g. in myocardial infarction, until the heart function improves.

Prevention of cardiac disease; a summary

Congenital heart disease should be recognized early, for cure is often possible.

Rheumatic heart disease has diminished with the conquest of the streptococcus, but where it has occurred, early recognition and treatment of valvular complications will prevent heart failure. Hypertension and its effects can be remedied before the stage of heart failure.

We are left with arteriosclerotic heart disease, and while alleviation of its effects is possible, prevention awaits understanding of the arteriosclerotic process. Meantime, we can advise the control of obesity and the cessation of cigarette smoking.

Aneurysm of the aorta

Aneurysm (dilatation from weakening of the vessel wall) of the ascending arch of the aorta may be syphilitic, but this is now uncommon. Aortic aneurysm is usually due to arteriosclerosis and occurs in the elderly. The thoracic aorta may be involved, and more frequently the abdominal aorta. The patient usually has no complaint, but there is a pulsatile swelling in the abdomen, and on x-ray calcium may be seen in the dilated walls of the vessels. In fit younger patients, operation (using a plastic graft) may be advised, for the aneurysm may leak, causing abdominal, lumbar or groin pains, often the prelude to rupture with catastrophic haemorrhage.

Peripheral arterial disease

Just as arteriosclerosis commonly involves the coronary arteries, so it may involve the carotid and intracerebral arteries (discussed under Cerebro-vascular disease), sometimes the renal arteries and the mesenteric arteries supplying the intestine, and often the branches of the aorta that supply the legs. Arm vessels are rarely affected.

The victims again are middle-aged men, and the elderly of both sexes. Cigarette smoking and obesity are predisposing factors, and arteriosclerosis of the distal leg arteries, and those in the feet, is commoner in diabetics.

CHRONIC ARTERIOSCLEROSIS OF LOWER LIMB VESSELS

Cause: There is arteriosclerotic narrowing and varying degrees of obstruction, involving the iliac arteries in the pelvis, and femoral vessels (and their branches) in the thigh. The condition may spread to involve distant arteries, but in diabetics vessels in the feet may be involved before there is gross disease proximally.

Symptoms and signs: The term 'intermittent claudication' is used to describe the characteristic pain in the limbs on exertion. Like coronary pain, it is due to poor oxygenation and accumulation of metabolites in the muscles, and is felt in the calf (or rarely the buttocks) after walking a fixed distance. The pain is immediately relieved on stopping. Symptoms may improve over some months as collateral channels open up to supply blood, or the condition may advance. The patient may complain that his feet are always cold. The popliteal pulse behind the knee, and the foot pulses are impalpable, the leg loses its hairs, the skin is pale and may have a shiny appearance and is cool to the touch. Wounds heal poorly and are liable to infection. Signs are usually bilateral though one leg may be more markedly affected.

Severe cases develop 'rest pain', occurring characteristically during the night, the patient putting his feet on a cold floor in an attempt to gain relief. This indicates extensive disease, with risk of skin breakdown and gangrene.

Management: In patients with intermittent claudication and evidence of arterial disease elsewhere, it may be sufficient to advise general measures such as weight reduction, and the prevention of undue heating and cooling, and of trauma to the legs. The feet should be carefully washed and dried daily, socks should be changed frequently, and the services of a chiropodist enlisted to attend to the care of the nails.

Search should be made for conditions such as heart failure, anaemia, and diabetes, treatment of which may improve the circulation to the legs.

In younger patients in whom there is no evidence of generalized arterial disease, arteriography should be carried out to ascertain if there is a localized segment of arterial narrowing amenable to surgery. Such surgery involves patch grafting or reconstruction, and is more successful in the large arteries above the groin.

In severe cases with rest pain, surgery may occasionally be helpful in improving the blood supply, but usually no cure is possible because of the extensive arterial involvement. The limb should be kept cool, for heating it increases its metabolic demand, and the circulation is unable to cope, worsening the threat of gangrene. It may be of some value to apply heat to other areas of the body to cause reflex vasodilatation and increased skin blood supply. The operation of sympathectomy may help by abolishing vasoconstrictive reflexes. Reflex heating, and vasodilator drugs may, however open up the blood vessels in healthy arteries rather than diseased ones, thus in fact depriving the ischaemic limb of blood and doing more harm than good.

Should the skin have broken and infection occurred, appropriate antibiotic treatment may allow healing, but persistent sepsis means an increased metabolic demand for which the blood supply is inadequate, and gangrene—death of tissue, with putrefaction, occurs.

Pain may require morphine for its relief, but where pain persists and there is gangrene with toxaemia, surgical amputation of the limb should not be delayed.

ACUTE ARTERIAL OBSTRUCTION

Cause: This is usually an embolus from the left side of the heart, from thrombus in the left atrium in mitral stenosis, or from mural thrombus under a myocardial infarction. Clot may also become detached from a large arteriosclerotic vessel, or form over an existing arteriosclerotic plaque, causing occlusion in a vessel such as the femoral.

Symptoms and signs: There is sudden severe pain, pallor (or cyanosis from associated venospasm), coldness, loss of senation and muscular weakness in the affected limb, with absent arterial pulses. Patients usually have a history of arterial disease, or may be in heart failure, but the condition may occur without previous symptoms.

Treatment: This has been revolutionized by use of the Fogarty catheter. This is a long slender catheter with a balloon tip which is distended with fluid after the catheter has been inserted into the obstructed artery, between the clot and the vessel wall. The catheter is then withdrawn, allowing removal of the clot. Even in frail and ill patients, this small operation can be performed under local anaesthesia.

Where there is doubt as to the site and extent of the obstruction, arteriography may be necessary. It may be justified to observe the patient for a few hours, during which time treatment of arrhythmia or heart failure can proceed. If there is persisting pallor and sensory loss in the limb, surgery as above, or a more extensive operation may be required. With these new techniques, the place of anti-coagulants and fibrinolytic drugs in treatment is in some doubt preoperatively, but they may be of value in preventing spread or recurrence of the thrombus.

THROMBO-ANGIITIS OBLITERANS (BUERGER'S DISEASE)

There is some doubt as to whether this condition is a separate entity, or simply the occurrence of severe arteriosclerosis with occlusion of arteries in the legs and feet, but the veins may also be involved. It occurs in men under forty who are heavy cigarette smokers. Symptoms and management are as in arteriosclerotic disease.

RAYNAUD'S SYNDROME

This is due to spasm of the small arteries of the fingers and hands. It is commonest in young women, who complain of pallor and numbness of the fingers on exposure to cold. Avoidance of this precipitating factor may be all that is necessary, but drugs such as reserpine and griseofulvin (which is used also for fungal infections of the skin) may be helpful. Sympathectomy, which abolishes the vasoconstrictive stimuli, may be considered in severe cases.

Similar symptoms may occur in men using vibrating tools, and in auto-immune disorders such as scleroderma, where destruction of the small vessels, and gangrene, may follow.

Venous thrombosis and embolism

DEEP VEIN THROMBOSIS

This is the presence of thrombus (clot) in the deep veins of the calf, but the femoral vein in the thigh may also be involved.

Precipitating factors:

Bed rest, especially if circulatory slowing as in congestive cardiac failure.

Surgical operations; thrombus often develops at the time of operation, but spreads in the following days due to alterations in coagulability of the blood.

Pregnancy, and contraceptive tablets of high oestrogen content.

Neoplasm, often hidden, e.g. carcinoma of pancreas.

Symptoms and signs: There is calf pain and tenderness, and ankle oedema, and sometimes slight rise of temperature.

However, it is important to note that at least half the patients with thrombosis have no complaint or physical signs in the legs, and it has been estimated that up to one third of all patients who have had an operation have leg vein thrombosis, often silent.

The first evidence may be the occurrence of pulmonary embolism, already described—presenting as pleural pain, haemoptysis or complete obstruction of the pulmonary circulation, with collapse.

Early diagnosis is therefore essential. Clinical scrutiny is necessary, but is not accurate enough to allow diagnosis in many cases where thrombosis is suspected. Special methods of investigation include the use of ultra-sound with the portable Sonicaid detector, which fails to emit its characteristic flow-noise if the circulation is obstructed. Injected radioactive fibrinogen may be detected at the site of thrombosis by using a special counter. X-ray venography may be necessary to localize the site and extent accurately. Large emboli may arise from the femoral vein just below the groin, rather than from peripheral veins.

Prevention and treatment: It may be possible to avoid some of the precipitating factors described. Elevation and massage of the legs during operations may help to prevent stasis of the circulation, and constrictions and pressures on the calves avoided. Patients in bed should have leg exercises. Early ambulation is encouraged—but it is wrong to have patients squeezed into an uncomfortable chair with their legs dependent.

Heparin intravenously (10,000 units 8-hourly) followed by an oral anticoagulant such as warfarin, phenindione or nicoumalone, is indicated prophylactically in high risk cases, and in established thrombosis, to prevent spread.

Streptokinase, given by intravenous infusion, activates the fibrinolytic system and dissolves thrombi, and the place of such *thrombolytic therapy* is under study.

Where deep vein thrombosis has occurred, the patient should rest in bed until anticoagulants have time to be effective, when mobilization is allowed with a firm crepe bandage or elastic stocking on the leg, to provide support and prevent oedema.

Surgical removal of thrombus in the femoral vein, or ligation, may be indicated to prevent pulmonary emboli—treatment of which has already been considered.

SUPERFICIAL VEIN THROMBOSIS (PHLEBITIS)

Thrombosis in a superficial vein may occur after injury or use of indwelling cannulae for intravenous infusions. The condition may occur spontaneously in the legs, especially in relation to varicose veins. Episodes of superficial thrombosis may occur as a complication of neoplasm, as in deep vein thrombosis.

There is pain, and a red tender area along the line of the vein, which may be palpable as a thrombus-containing cord. Though the thrombus is usually well-attached, in extensive cases there is risk of embolism, and anticoagulants are indicated, with analgesics to relieve pain. Phenylbutazone is very effective, but carries risk of bone-marrow depression. A supporting bandage or elastic stocking may be helpful.

MASSIVE VENOUS THROMBOSIS

This is rare. There is severe pain and swelling of the leg, with purplish-blue discoloration. The engorgement may be so severe that the arterial blood supply is compressed, with risk of gangrene, and the condition may be difficult to distinguish from a primary arterial occlusion. It usually occurs in association with some systemic disease, often carcinoma with involvement of the iliac veins in the pelvis. Anticoagulant and fibrinolytic drugs may be of value.

5

Diseases of the respiratory system

The object of breathing, respiration, is to take air into the lungs, where it gives up its oxygen to the blood and receives the waste product carbon dioxide, which is exhaled.

Anatomy and physiology

In the upper respiratory tract, which includes the nose and mouth, the sinuses, and the throat or pharynx, inspired air is warmed and moistened. The pharynx leads into the voice-box or larynx, containing the vocal chords. Beyond the larynx is the lower respiratory tract—the windpipe or trachea, dividing into a main bronchus to each lung. The bronchi divide further, ultimately becoming the very small air passages called bronchioles, which terminate in the air sacs or alveoli in the substance of the lung. The very fine alveolar membrane separates the air from the blood in the capillaries of the lung, and it is here that the gaseous exchange occurs.

The lungs are covered by the pleura, separating them from the chest wall, and from the diaphragm, the muscular sheet between the thorax and the abdomen.

The lungs can be regarded as a pair of 'bellows'—during inspiration the chest wall expands and the diaphragm descends, increasing the capacity of the lungs so that air is drawn into them; in expiration there is elastic collapse of the lungs, expelling the air.

Control of respiration. We are not normally conscious of our respiratory movements. They are controlled by the respiratory centre in the medulla of the brain. The respiratory centre is sensitive to carbon dioxide in the blood, excess of which stimulates respiration, and to the blood oxygen level, lack of which (anoxia) again stimulates breathing. However, it is important to note that in chronic respiratory disease with carbon dioxide retention, the respiratory centre no longer responds to the raised CO_2 level, and the stimulus of some anoxia is necessary for respiration to continue.

The respiratory centre acts on the nerves controlling the muscles of the chest wall, and the diaphragm (phrenic nerves).

Causes of respiratory disease

Infection. The air passages are lined by mucous membrane. In the nose and throat, the mucous membrane is susceptible to virus infections such as the common cold and influenza. Harmless 'commensal' bacteria may be found in the healthy throat, but the bronchi are sterile. Bacterial infection may however follow virus infection, or occur from the start in those with existing respiratory disease. Droplet spray in sneezes and coughs, and infected handkerchiefs and dust transmit respiratory infections.

Cigarette smoking and *atmospheric pollution* predispose to respiratory disease.

Disorders of the air passages—narrowing in asthma from bronchospasm, and obstruction in chronic bronchitis; the latter leads to CO_2 retention.

Disturbed 'bellows' function—occurs in emphysema from destruction of alveoli.

Disturbance of gaseous exchange—from thickened alveolar septa in lung fibrosis, or presence of fluid in heart failure, or lung destruction or consolidation—associated with anoxia.

In addition, disorders affecting the *Respiratory centre* may affect breathing, discussed below, under Dyspnoea.

Symptoms and signs in respiratory disease

COUGH

Cough is caused by a forced expiration against a closed glottis (the space between the vocal chords), which is suddenly released allowing the spitting-up or expectoration of irritant foreign particles or mucus from the air passages. Thus a cough is a protective device which comes into action if normal cleansing methods involving the cilia of the mucous membrane fail.

Cough may be acute in the common cold, or recurrent in chronic bronchitis and carcinoma of the lung, and may be dry or productive of sputum.

SPUTUM (PHLEGM)

Mucoid sputum is clear and gelatinous, indicates irritation of the air passages or chronic bronchitis, and may contain soot particles from the atmosphere.

Purulent sputum is yellow or green from the presence of pus cells, and it indicates infection. Thus purulent sputum is found in bronchitis, bronchopneumonia and tuberculosis, and copious amounts occur in bronchiectasis and lung abscess.

A response of respiratory infection to antibiotic treatment is indicated by reduction in quantity, and change from purulent to mucoid sputum.

HAEMOPTYSIS

Haemoptysis is the coughing up of blood, with or without sputum. The blood is usually a definite red colour, and should be distinguished from that in haematemesis or vomiting of blood which is often brown from the effect of stomach acid. The patient's description of the episode, and his history may help to distinguish haemoptysis from haematemesis, but where there is doubt, specimens should be preserved.

Causes:

Carcinoma of lung.

Tuberculosis.

Pulmonary Infarction—may be accompanied by pleural pain.

Bronchiectasis—may be large amounts of blood.

Pulmonary oedema from heart failure—frothy pink sputum rather than frank blood.

Lobar pneumonia—'rusty' sputum rather than frank blood.

Treatment includes that of the causative condition, and in mild cases this is all that is required.

Severe haemoptysis is alarming to the patient. Morphine or diamorphine 10–15 mg intramuscularly calms the patient, and may be helpful by its depressant action on the respiratory centre. Continued blood loss is rare, but may demand surgery, x-ray therapy, and blood transfusion.

PAIN

Pleurisy—inflammation of the pleura—is associated with pain, worsened when the inflamed surfaces rub together on deep breathing; causes include lobar pneumonia and pulmonary infarction.

DYSPNOEA (BREATHLESSNESS)

Dyspnoea means difficult breathing, an unpleasant awareness of the act of breathing.

Dyspnoea is usually due to oxygen-lack, which stimulates the respiratory centre to increase the rate of breathing in an attempt to improve oxygenation. Thus in acute respiratory disease such as pneumonia there may be rapid shallow breathing.

In chronic bronchitis and emphysema the mechanics of respiration, the bellows function of the lungs, has suffered and the patient is dyspnoeic and distressed. His rib-cage lifts instead of expanding properly, and his respiratory efforts involve the use of the neck muscles rather than the diaphragm.

In left heart failure, there is dyspnoea from congested stiff lungs and pulmonary oedema, worse lying flat and relieved when propped up, the condition called orthopnoea. The patient with purely respiratory disease is usually, but not necessarily more comfortable sitting up—sometimes he prefers to lie flat.

In lung fibrosis the patient is breathless on slight exertion, but not necessarily dyspnoeic at rest.

Dyspnoea may be due to the pain of pleurisy, the patient being afraid to take a deep breath.

Wheezing due to bronchospasm and narrowing accompanies the breathlessness of asthma, and the patient has especial difficulty in expiration.

Stridor is noisy inspiration from inflammation of obstruction of larynx, trachea or large bronchi.

Disturbances of breathing distinguishable from dyspnoea include:

Periodic breathing or Cheyne-Stokes breathing—anoxia, uraemia and drugs such as morphine depress the respiratory centre. There follows a period of apnoea (no breathing) then, as carbon dioxide builds up in the blood, stimulation of the respiratory centre occurs and deep sighing respirations, followed again by apnoea.

Air hunger is continuous deep breathing due to stimulation of the respiratory centre by acidosis in diabetic coma (where the breath may smell of acetone) and some cases of uraemia (renal failure), and in aspirin poisoning.

CYANOSIS

Cyanosis in respiratory disease is due to deficient oxygenation of blood in the lungs, and unlike the peripheral cyanosis of heart failure, may be accompanied by warm extremities. Respiratory cyanosis indicates severe lung disease.

Restlessness and *Twitching* indicate cerebral anoxia, and are common accompaniments of cyanosis.

CLUBBING OF THE FINGER TIPS

Finger clubbing may occur in bronchiectasis and carcinoma of the lung, and rarely in other lung diseases. Congenital heart disease, subacute bacterial endocarditis and intestinal malabsorption are also causes of finger clubbing.

Further investigations

Sputum examination:

Purulent sputum denotes infection.

Bacteriology (staining and culture). Reports should be considered in the light of the clinical findings, and response to treatment.

A knowledge of the infecting organism and its sensitivity allows adjustment of treatment if necessary.

Cytology for malignant cells in suspicious cases—especially useful if the sputum is blood-stained.

Peak expiratory flow rate (P.E.F.R.):

Measured by rapid exhalation into Wright Peak Flow meter.

Indicates 'bellows' efficiency of the lungs and is impaired in airways obstruction in chronic bronchitis and asthma.

Normal is 500 litres per minute.

Chest x-ray:

Essential addition to clinical examination of the chest.

Portable film in ward if patient too ill to move to x-ray dept.

Tomogram is special view focused on lesion.

Bronchogram is x-ray following injection of radio-opaque iodized oil through mouth or larynx to outline bronchi.

Laryngoscopy:

Passage of instrument into throat to allow visualization of larynx and vocal chords.

Bronchoscopy:

Passage of tube (metal or glass-fibre) via throat and larynx into trachea and large bronchi, allowing visualization and biopsy, and suction of retained secretions.

Blood-gas analysis:

Blood specimens, preferably arterial, are examined for their oxygen and carbon dioxide content, expressed as pO_2 and pCO_2 respectively. The effect of changes in these on the acidity of the blood is measured as the pH.

The common cold

Cause: A virus infection of the upper respiratory tract. There are several causative viruses, the commonest being those of Rhinovirus group.

Symptoms and signs: Stuffy, streaming nose (catarrh), cough and sometimes sore throat.

Feverish cold causes rise in temperature and more systemic upset.

Complications are superadded bacterial infection with purulent catarrh, sputum, laryngitis, tracheitis and bronchitis from spread to lower respiratory tract.

Treatment: No treatment is of proven value in the uncomplicated cold; aspirin lowers the temperature, but its effects are not necessarily beneficial. A person suffering from a streaming cold should stay indoors and away from work for a few days to avoid infecting others. The infection usually subsides in a few days.

Antibiotics may be indicated for complications.

Prevention: Immunization is unlikely to be effective due to the number of causative viruses, and even specific immunity appears to be short-lived.

Influenza

Cause: One of the influenza viruses, which have recently spread in epidemics from the Far East. Thus influenza virus A2, Hong Kong strain caused epidemics in Britain in 1968 and 1970. The diagnosis is relatively easy during such recognized epidemics. In non-epidemic years, the term 'influenza' is often vaguely applied to any febrile illness of uncertain cause.

Symptoms and signs: Fever, headache, cough, sore throat and catarrh, often of sudden onset and associated with limb pains and prostration.

Influenza-like illness, not necessarily due to the same virus, may be associated with conjunctivitis and running eyes, and sore throat,

Complications include bronchitis and pneumonia; occasionally this is a true virus pneumonia but more commonly it is a bacterial infection with pneumococci or staphylococci, and is a serious hazard in those with existing respiratory disease.

Treatment: Amantadine is a drug of possible value, but in most cases it suffices for the patient to go to bed with hot drinks for a few days.

Watch should be kept for complications in young children, those with respiratory disease, and the elderly.

Prevention: Vaccination against the current strain of virus offers protection for a few months. It should be carried out in the autumn in patients with respiratory disease or cardiac failure, persons at risk such as doctors and nurses, and key workers.

During an epidemic it is reasonable to avoid crowded places but though 'droplet spread' is postulated, the exact way of acquiring infection is not quite clear.

Hay Fever

Cause: Allergic response to hay or pollens.

Symptoms and signs: Streaming nose and eyes plus variable fever.

Treatment: Antihistamine drugs such as chlorpheniramine (Piriton) and triprolidine (Actidil), which are available in long-acting form.

Steroids in 'depot' form may rarely be justified.

Prevention: Where skin or inhalation tests show pollen allergy, a course of desensitizing injections before the pollen season may be helpful.

Sinusitis and otitis media

Sinusitis is inflammation of the nasal sinuses. Otitis media is inflammation of the middle ear, usually from spread of infection along the Eustachian tube from the throat. Sinusitis and otitis media may complicate colds and upper respiratory tract infections, and antibiotics may be indicated.

Sore throat

Causes: Infection with haemolytic streptocci, viruses, and in glandular fever.

Diphtheria is now a rare cause.

Agranulocytosis (lack of white cells in the blood, often drug-induced) may present as sore throat, as the patient is prone to infection.

Symptoms and signs: There is pain, sometimes worse on swallowing.

The tonsils, if present, are inflamed and often purulent, and the surrounding pharynx is involved, especially in streptococcal cases, but there is no certain clinical distinction. The tonsillar glands are swollen and tender. There is fever.

Diagnosis is confirmed by throat swab, and white cell count and antistreptolysin (A.S.O.) titre; Paul Bunnell test may be positive in glandular fever.

Treatment is that of the cause, where possible, e.g. penicillin for haemolytic streptococcal infection. Antibiotics are of no value if the cause is viral, or in glandular fever—indeed ampicillin may cause a rash in the latter.

Disorders of the larynx

Acute laryngitis may complicate a cold or respiratory infection, and presents as hoarseness, with cough and sputum. Steam inhalations may be soothing, plus antibiotics if there is purulent sputum indicating bacterial infection.

Croup in children is due to laryngotracheobronchitis, is caused by a virus, but superadded bacterial infection may be serious, requiring antibiotics.

Angioneurotic oedema, an allergic reaction to something inhaled, ingested, or injected, may be so severe as to cause laryngeal oedema and obstruction, requiring immediate adrenaline 0·5 ml of 1/1,000 solution by injection, plus hydrocortisone 100 mg.

Diphtheria may occasionally present as laryngitis with hoarseness.

Chronic laryngitis occurs in auctioneers and those who over-use the voice, especially if working in dusty atmospheres. It causes hoarseness and chronic cough.

Carcinoma of the larynx may also present with hoarseness, so it is important to perform a laryngoscopy plus biopsy in suspected cases. Treatment is surgery or x-ray therapy.

Tuberculosis of the larynx is now rare.

Acute tracheitis and bronchitis

Cause: Spread of infection, usually bacterial from the upper respiratory tract after a cold or influenza.

The inflammation of the mucous membrane may involve the smallest bronchi, and spread into the alveoli and surrounding lung, when the condition becomes a bronchopneumonia.

Symptoms and signs: There is fever, cough with moderate mucoid or purulent sputum, and substernal discomfort.

Treatment: Bed rest in a warm atmosphere.

Copious fluids may help to loosen cough and sputum, plus steam inhalations. So called expectorants are not of value, with the possible exception of bromhexine (Bisolvon) tablets, which may liquefy tenacious sputum.

Cough suppressants such as linctus codeine (5–10 ml) should be used only if useless cough is disturbing sleep.

Antibacterial drugs are indicated if the sputum is purulent, especially in patients with existing respiratory disease. Trimethoprim-sulphamethoxazole (Septrin, Bactrim) tablets, penicillin injections, ampicillin or tetracycline can be used, as in pneumonia.

Chronic bronchitis and emphysema (chronic obstructive airways disease)

In Britain, chronic bronchitis is a common and disabling disease, a frequent cause of hospital admission, and it results in some 30,000 deaths annually.

Chronic bronchitis is an inflammation of the small bronchi and bronchioles resulting in chronic cough and sputum.

The swelling of the bronchial mucous membrane causes narrowing and obstruction of the airflow, especially on expiration.

Emphysema is due to distention and destruction of the lung alveoli from the air-trapping in chronic bronchitis. Emphysema less commonly occurs in the absence of bronchitis, from a primary degenerative change. The lungs become distended, and their bellows efficiency is impaired.

Causes

Cigarette smoking is by far the most important cause. Atmospheric pollution with smoke and sulphur dioxide, especially in damp foggy climates plays a part. Thus hospital admissions for bronchitis are high in large towns subject to 'smog', and the Clean Air Act is helping to reduce the incidence. Bronchitis is more common in certain occupations, e.g. coal mining from the effects of the inhaled dust.

Heredity factors contribute, for a family history is common.

Infection causes flare-ups of the condition. While infection may initially be viral, bacterial infection follows, the organisms being commonly Haemophilus influenzae and the Pheumococcus (Streptococcus pneumoniae). (H. influenzae is a bacterium, so named because it was thought, wrongly, to be the cause of influenza which is of course a virus infection).

Symptoms and signs

Chronic bronchitis causes chronic cough and sputum.

Emphysema causes breathlessness.

Chronic bronchitis and emphysema occurs mainly in middle-aged men, usually heavy cigarette smokers. They complain at first of 'smoker's cough' with production of mucoid sputum. Symptoms worsen over months or years with exacerbations in winter and cold, foggy conditions, with increasing cough and often wheezy breathlessness.

The mechanics of breathing are disturbed, the patient lifting his chest instead of expanding it on inspiration, and a 'barrel-shaped' chest may occur in emphysema.

Relapses are usually due to superadded infection, with increased cough, the sputum becoming purulent and increased in volume, and fever.

Severe relapses are characterized by cough, sputum, dyspnoea and cyanosis, and the condition is really a pneumonia from spread of the infection into the lungs.

Patients have been divided into two groups—the 'pink-puffers' who pant and wheeze but remain of good colour, and the 'blue-bloaters' who become cyanosed and go on to right heart strain and failure, with raised venous pressure and peripheral oedema; the former group have emphysema, the latter chronic bronchitis, but there is usually a mixed clinical picture, just as there is a combined pathological basis for bronchitis and emphysema.

Further investigations

The *Peak Expiratory Flow Rate* is impaired early, and in exacerbations is a guide to progress.

Chest x-ray may show emphysema, but is not necessarily helpful in chronic bronchitis. It may, however, show a complicating pneumonia.

Sputum if purulent indicates infection. Routine bacteriology is not essential, but culture and sensitivity of the organisms is indicated in severe cases.

Blood gas analysis—the blood carbon dioxide content (pCO_2) is raised, and a rising level with lowered oxygen content (pO_2) indicates respiratory failure—manifest clinically by cyanosis, restlessness and disturbance of consciousness, twitching and collapse and death if the condition is unrelieved.

Treatment

General measures:
Stop cigarette smoking.
Avoid atmospheric pollution and fog.
Sleep in warm bedroom, with window closed if night air cold.
Treat obesity.

Prophylaxis:
Chronic bronchitics should be vaccinated against influenza, as infection may cause a flare-up of their condition.

Breathing exercises:
Attempts to 'retrain' patients to breathe properly using the diaphragm rather than accessory chest and neck muscles are not usually successful, but may help psychologically. Deep breathing is helpful in promoting coughing and expectoration of sputum, however, and exercises are desirable in bronchitics before and after surgical operations.

Treatment of flare-ups

Treat infection—antibacterial drugs:
Tetracycline—500 mg 6-hourly.
Ampicillin (Penbritin)—500 mg—1 G 6-hourly.
Trimethoprim-sulphamethoxazole—2 tablets twice daily (Septrin, Bactrim).
One of these three drugs should be given if the sputum is purulent. It is best to select a drug different from one previously used in the patient, in case his organisms have become resistant. If clinical and

sputum improvement (change from purulent to mucoid) does not occur within three days, the antibiotic should be changed depending on bacteriology.

More severe cases should have penicillin and streptomycin by injection, e.g. Crystamycin or Crystamycin Forte twice or three times daily. Resistant organisms may demand the use of cloxacillin (Orbenin) or cephaloridine in addition.

Bronchodilators;

Aminophylline may be given orally as Choledyl or Silbephylline tablets, by suppository, or 250–500 mg slowly intravenously.

Ephedrine tablets and isoprenaline tablets or inhalations may help bronchospasm, but cause tachycardia, so newer drugs such as salbutamol (Ventolin) and orciprenaline (Alupent) without this cardiac effect, are preferable.

Clearing of secretions—coughing to clear secretions must be encouraged, not suppressed. Warm drinks may help to loosen phlegm. Aspiration of pharyngeal secretions using a plastic catheter and suction may be required.

Oxygen—slight oxygen enrichment of the inspired air is helpful. Too much oxygen removes the stimulus of the slight anoxia on which the chronic bronchitic patient is dependent to maintain respiration, his respiratory centre having become unresponsive to carbon dioxide. Thus oxygen should be given at a flow rate of 2 litres per minute using nasal catheters, the Edinburgh mask (with open end) or the Ventimask—*not* by a closed plastic mask; if too much oxygen is given, the patient will become pink, but he will stop breathing.

Respiratory stimulants such as nikethamide are useful in emergency, but their action is short. Respiratory depressants such as morphine must never be given to bronchitic patients. If sedation is required, chlorpromazine (Largactil) 50 mg may suffice.

Steroids such as prednisone are occasionally helpful in combating the bronchospasm and bronchial swelling in severe cases.

Treatment of cardiac failure—diuretics such as Frusemide (Lasix), and digoxin may be indicated.

Treatment of respiratory failure—see below, page 97.

Prognosis and follow up

Many patients with chronic bronchitis and emphysema have only minor disablement, with occasional exacerbations, but the condition deteriorates little over the years and they are able to continue at work. They may be given a supply of an antibacterial drug such as tetracycline, ampicillin or trimethoprim-sulphamethoxazole to take at the first sign of flare-up such as the development of purulent sputum. This has proved more successful than continuous antibacterial drugs in prophylaxis.

Other patients become increasingly breathless and are forced to give up work and to lead a sedentary existence. The availability of oxygen in the home may enable them to perform tasks that they could not manage without oxygen—its dangers in excess in respiratory failure must be re-emphasized and of course naked lights must not be used near an oxygen supply.

The outlook is poor in patients with severe breathlessness, cyanosis and right heart failure.

It is therefore of great importance to *prevent* chronic bronchitis, and this will be largely achieved when the social evils of cigarette smoking and atmospheric pollution are eliminated.

Bronchiectasis

Cause

Bronchiectasis is a dilatation with some destruction of the bronchial walls, associated with chronic infection. Localized dilatations occur which may be filled with pus.

Bronchiectasis may follow childhood whooping cough and conditions where mucus plugs or an inhaled foreign body cause bronchial obstruction. The air is absorbed in the alveoli beyond the obstruction, causing areas of lung collapse. The surrounding healthy and elastic lung causes traction on the affected part, resulting in bronchial dilatation. Some cases follow chronic bronchitis, and pneumonia.

Symptoms and signs

Bronchiectasis may occur in young adults, but due to the lowered incidence and better treatment of childhood respiratory infection, the condition is now more commonly seen in the middle-aged.

The commonest symptoms are cough and the production of large quantities of purulent sputum.

'Dry' bronchiectasis may present as haemoptysis, sometimes massive.

Signs include 'moist sounds' heard with the stethoscope over the affected part of the lung. Finger clubbing occurs.

Diagnosis may be confirmed by bronchogram, the radio-opaque oil outlining the affected bronchi on x-ray.

Complications

Pneumonia.

Lung abscess.

Cerebral abscess (septic emboli having travelled to the brain).

Treatment

Postural drainage:

The patient is taught to cough and clear his purulent sputum in the position causing best drainage of secretions. Usually the lower lobes of the lungs are affected, and to clear them the patient leans downwards over the side of the bed. Clearing may be aided by percussion over the affected lobes by the physiotherapist.

Postural drainage should be performed twice daily.

Antibacterial drugs:

Tetracycline, ampicillin or trimethoprim-sulphamethoxazole may be used in courses of 1–2 weeks in an attempt to clear the sputum of infection, but this is not always effective. These and other drugs may be required for pneumonia.

The haemoptysis of dry bronchiectasis usually settles with rest and sedation, but respiratory depressant sedatives such as morphine should not be used if there is associated chronic bronchitis or pneumonia. Blood transfusion is rarely required.

Surgical removal of the affected lung lobe is indicated where the above measures fail and the disease is localized; the remaining lung lobes must be healthy and tests must show good respiratory function.

Pneumonia

Cause

Pneumonia is an infection and inflammation of the alveoli of the lung. The infection is usually bacterial, but virus invasion of the respiratory tract may be a predisposing factor.

Pneumonia results in impaired oxygenation of the blood and various degrees of toxaemia.

Types

1. LOBAR PNEUMONIA—a whole lobe becomes solid—consolidation usually caused by pneumococcus, sometimes by staphylococcus.
2. BRONCHOPNEUMONIA—scattered areas of consolidation in one or both lungs.

When there is infection and retained secretions in the smallest bronchi, the air in the related alveoli becomes absorbed causing patchy collapse (atelectasis) and infection of the lung substance.

Thus bronchopneumonia includes:

pneumonia following spread of respiratory tract infection.

aspiration pneumonia, where it is assumed infected matter has been inhaled.

hypostatic pneumonia—a complication of bed rest in elderly patients with cardiac failure or cerebro-vascular disease, often a terminal event.

postoperative pneumonia—from failure to clear secretions (but some cases are really pulmonary infarction).

Such attempts at classification are not necessarily helpful, for treatment depends more on the mode of onset, history, and on the infecting organism.

3. TUBERCULOUS PNEUMONIA
4. 'VIRUS' PNEUMONIA—pure virus pneumonia without secondary bacterial infection is rare, but may occur in influenza.

The organism mycoplasma pneumoniae, not a true virus may cause outbreaks of mild pneumonia in young adults. Organisms such as that causing ornithosis in birds may also, rarely, cause pneumonia.

Symptoms and signs

Classical lobar pneumonia is now rare, but occurs at any age. The onset is sudden with shivering and rigor followed by fever. There is a harsh cough productive of a little rusty sputum, later purulent, with breathlessness and often pleuritic pain.

In influenza epidemics a fulminating staphylococcal pneumonia may occur quite suddenly without gross preceding upper respiratory symptoms. Young adults may be affected, and there is high fever, cough and breathlessness with local or diffuse signs in the chest and on x-ray. Toxaemia may be severe with delirium, hypotension and circulatory collapse.

Most cases of pneumonia develop relatively slowly following an upper respiratory infection, often in a subject with existing respiratory disease such as chronic bronchitis and emphysema, bronchiectasis, and bronchogenic carcinoma. There is fever, cough with purulent sputum, breathlessness and in severe cases cyanosis. The pulse is rapid.

Chest examination may reveal dullness on percussion over the affected part and changes in the breath sounds.

The evolution of these symptoms and signs may be prevented by modern treatment with antibacterial drugs, but where treatment has been ineffective, the patient may pass into a state of *Respiratory Failure*, due to anoxia, with increasing dyspnoea and cyanosis. restlessness, delirium and coma.

Further investigations

Chest x-ray—shows the consolidated areas, and is essential for accurate diagnosis.

Sputum—bacteriological culture and antibacterial drugs sensitivity tests especially helpful in resistant cases.

Blood gas analysis—lowered oxygen content, and sometimes raised carbon dioxide content—may warn of impending respiratory failure.

Complications

Empyema is a collection of pus in the pleural cavity following pneumococcal pneumonia and pleurisy.

Lung abscess may follow a staphylococcal pneumonia.

Such complications are now rare, with early effective treatment of pneumonia.

Treatment

General measures

Bed rest is indicated until the febrile stage is over.

Hot drinks—orange or lemon squash, tea or coffee—are comforting, and a high fluid intake helps to loosen sputum, as well as being indicated in fever. The patient may have a light diet—there need be no rigid restrictions.

Antibacterial drugs

These are now the most important aspect of treatment.

Penicillin 1-mega unit intramuscularly 6-hourly (or penicillin and streptomycin combined as in Crystamycin), is the drug of first choice, especially in patients infected outside hospital. The pneumococcus is always penicillin-sensitive.

In the patient with previous respiratory disease, or a patient who has developed his pneumonia in hospital, it may be wise to use or add other drugs in case of penicillin resistance. The drug chosen should be different from one that may have been used recently.

Trimethoprim-sulphamethoxazole (Septrin, Bactrim) 2 tablets 3-times daily appears to be very effective.

Tetracycline 500 mg 6-hourly is used in less severe cases, and tetracycline or demethylchlortetracycline (Ledermycin) in some so-called virus pneumonias.

Ampicillin 500 mg–1·0 G 6-hourly may be used alone or with penicillin, and ampicillin and cloxacillin are available as a combined injection—Ampliclox, for the seriously ill.

Cloxacillin (Orbenin) is effective against penicillin-resistant staphylococci, and given in doses of 500 mg 6-hourly along with 1–2 mega units of penicillin, may be the treatment of choice in fulminating post-influenzal staphylococcal pneumonia. Its new derivative, Flucloxacillin (Floxapen), may be equally effective in smaller doses—and is tending to displace it.

Cephaloridine, a broad-spectrum antibiotic, and fusidic acid (Fucidin), an anti-staphylococcal drug, may sometimes be used.

Thus one cannot state an antibacterial drug regime applicable to all cases of pneumonia. The circumstances of onset of the infection and the clinical and x-ray findings give the doctor a guide to the probable infecting organism. Sputum is sent for culture, and antibacterial drug treatment is initiated. Penicillin, ampicillin and cloxacillin are at present the most widely used drugs. If the patient shows clinical improvement in the first 24-hours, then the selected drugs should be continued, in modified dosage, for about a week or 10 days, when cure will have been effected. If, on the other hand, the patient shows no improvement or deteriorates in 24-hours despite therapy, then the antibacterial regime should be modified in the light of bacteriological and drug sensitivity reports from the laboratory.

Clearing of secretions—coughing is helpful if productive of sputum, for this clears the airway and allows aeration and re-expansion of the lung.

Deep breathing exercises are similarly useful, and should be practised whenever the patient is strong enough to co-operate.

Cough suppression is generally undesirable, but linctus codeine 5–10 ml is permissible where useless cough disturbs sleep.

Oxygen—a previously-healthy patient who develops pneumonia may be helped by oxygen, given at 4–6 litres per minute by plastic mask such as Polymask or M.C. mask. A water-bottle on the flow tubing allows slight humidification. This method allows inspiration of 'air' containing 40–60 per cent oxygen. (Room air contains 20 per cent oxygen and 80 per cent nitrogen.)

Such a high concentration of oxygen is dangerous in chronic bronchitics, or where the respiratory centre has become depressed, as may occur from toxaemia or misuse of sedative drugs. In these situations, the respiratory centre is dependent on the stimulus of a degree of anoxia to maintain respiration, and if too much oxygen is given, the patient will stop breathing.

Steroids—in fulminating pneumonia with severe toxaemia and hypotension, large doses of hydrocortisone may be tried intravenously—500 mg–1·0 G 6-hourly, or by continuous infusion by intravenous drip—the fluid itself may be helpful, its quantity being determined by monitoring the venous pressure by a manometer connected to a cannula in the great veins or right atrium.

Treatment of respiratory failure—involving endotracheal intubation or tracheostomy and artificial ventilation is discussed on page 98.

Prognosis and follow up

With early and appropriate antibacterial treatment most previously healthy patients with pneumonia improve rapidly, the lungs return to normal, and the patient can resume his usual activities within a few weeks, during which deep breathing exercises in the fresh air are helpful.

In those with existing lung disease, the prognosis is more guarded, and some deterioration of lung function may result.

'Unresolved' pneumonia should raise suspicion of underlying carcinoma, tuberculosis, bronchiectasis and lung abscess, or rarely, fungus infection.

Pulmonary tuberculosis

Cause

Infection of the lung with Mycobacterium (Bacillus) tuberculosis.

Infection is acquired from inhalation of droplets or dust from the sputum of a person suffering from the disease. In Britain, the source of infection is usually a neglected elderly person, or a vagrant or alcoholic, or an immigrant from an underdeveloped country where tuberculosis may be rampant.

Primary infection may cause few symptoms (malaise, erythema nodosum) or pass unnoticed. Failure to heal may cause miliary spread. There may be healing with post-primary reactivation or reinfection involving a small part of the lung, or spreading to cause tuberculosis pneumonia, or the infection may become chronic; there is lung destruction with caseation (formation of cheesy material) and calcification, cavitation and fibrosis-chronic fibro-caseous tuberculosis.

Persons with chronic fibro-caseous tuberculosis form the important reservoir of infection and x-ray campaigns are directed towards detecting them. It is a wise precaution to have a chest x-ray of a patient with chest symptoms and living in poor circumstances, before admitting him to the general medical ward. A patient with a history of pulmonary tuberculosis who develops a chest infection should also be assumed to have a recrudescence of tuberculous infection until proved otherwise.

Symptoms and signs

There may be none in the early stages, the diagnosis being made on chest x-ray.

Cough, sputum which may be mucoid or purulent, haemoptysis, fever and night sweats, and weight-loss occur. Only in late stages are there physical signs in the chest, such as consolidation in pneumonia, or altered breath sounds over a cavity in fibro-caseous tuberculosis.

Further investigations

Chest x-ray.

Sputum—direct staining, culture, or guinea-pig inoculation for tubercle bacilli.

Gastric washings if sputum unobtainable.

Sputum cytology if differentiation from lung cancer, which may co-exist, is required.

Treatment

Where direct sputum staining shows tubercle bacilli, the patient should be isolated, and have his own crockery. Ill and neglected patients should also be treated in tuberculosis units, which have the further advantage of ensuring that the patient gets his drugs. In non-infective cases, outpatient management is satisfactory.

Streptomycin 1 G daily intramuscularly, plus sachets containing isoniazid 300 mg with para-aminosalicylic acid (P.A.S.) 12 G daily are the three standard drugs given initially, followed by isoniazid and P.A.S. for 1–2 years. Ethambutol and rifampicin are used if there is drug allergy or resistance.

Contacts should be traced and examined for infection. Tuberculin testing and B.C.G. in *prevention* are discussed later.

Asthma

Cause

Bronchial asthma is a condition characterized by recurrent attacks of wheeze and breathlessness. Attacks are due to airways obstruction from bronchial muscle spasm, and mucosal swelling and secretions.

Types

Asthma has recently been classified into two clinical groups, *extrinsic asthma* and *intrinsic asthma*.

EXTRINSIC ASTHMA. Onset is in childhood and there is often a family history of atopy, a predisposition to allergic disorders including asthma, hay fever, eczema and skin sensitivity. The term extrinsic is used because an external allergen often precipitates an attack. The child or adolescent is symptom-free between attacks, which often become less frequent in adult life.

Precipitating factors include:

(a) *Allergy*—an allergic reaction to a substance following inhalation, ingestion or skin contact.

House-dust is a common allergen, probably due to the presence of a mite which feeds on the scales shed from human skin, and is found in mattresses and bedding. Feathers, and the hairs from cats, dogs and horses, and moulds may also provoke asthma attacks.

Pollens are important in the spring and early summer. Simple contact with plants such as certain primulas and foods such as shellfish affect some subjects.

(b) *Infection*—such as a cold or other respiratory infection.

(c) *Exposure* to cold air.

(d) *Psychological* factors—emotional upset such as anger, a broken love affair or domestic crisis (sometimes added to the above factors) precipitates many an attack of asthma. The attack may serve to gain sympathy. Nevertheless, asthma can be a serious condition requiring urgent treatment followed by psychological support and understanding.

INTRINSIC ASTHMA. This affects those over forty, wheeze persisting after a chest infection, and allergic factors may be less obvious. The patient may never be free of wheeze, and attacks tend to become more frequent and severe.

Symptoms and signs

The patient becomes acutely wheezy and distressed with dyspnoea and tightness of the chest. The chest tends to become fixed in inspiration, for the obstruction mainly affects expiration. The patient feels he cannot get his breath out, and he may be anxious with a fear of death. There may be cough, with the difficult expectoration of viscid sputum, but the sputum may be purulent if there is an infective basis for the attack.

Most cases improve with treatment, but where this fails the patient goes into *Status Asthmaticus* with extreme dyspnoea, cyanosis, confusion and exhaustion—the picture of respiratory failure; in such cases the bronchioles may be plugged with viscid, rubbery secretions, and there is danger of death.

Blood gas analysis is the most important further investigation, for it reveals oxygen-lack or carbon dioxide disturbance in advance of clinical signs of anoxia.

Prevention of asthma attacks

Avoidance of precipitating factors: Those allergic to pollens should avoid flowers and plants and possibly stay indoors when the pollen count in the atmosphere is high.

House-mite dust can be decreased by enclosing mattresses in plastic, bed clothes should be changed frequently and bedrooms should be vacuum cleaned. Feather or horse-hair bedding may be replaced by plastic or latex foam material, and domestic pets should be borne in mind as sources of allergen in some cases.

Desensitization: A course of desensitizing injections may be helpful if a specific allergen such as a pollen can be incriminated. Where there is doubt as to the allergen, skin tests may reveal sensitivity, but these do not necessarily reflect lung allergy. Desensitization may prove more successful with the isolation and understanding of the house-mite factor.

Disodium cromoglycate (Intal): Inhalations of this drug from a special 'Spinhaler' suppress the allergic reaction in the lung and are useful in prophylaxis, and sometimes in treatment of an attack.

Relief of anxiety with drugs as diazepam (Valium) 5–10 mg may help in times of stress but sedative drugs should be used cautiously in attacks.

Infection in asthmatics should be treated early with appropriate antibacterial drugs.

Treatment

Antispasmodic drugs: Isoprenaline is rapidly effective, but over-use of inhalers causes dangerous tachycardia, so that salbutamol (Ventolin) and orciprenaline (Alupent) are now preferred. Although adrenaline-like, they have less cardiac-stimulant effect. These drugs are given by metered-dose aerosol inhaler (carefully following the instructions on the label) or as tablets.

Ephedrine 30 mg is an older drug with a prolonged adrenaline-like effect, and tablets or suppositories containing aminophylline are also used.

Steroids: These suppress the inflammatory swelling in the bronchial walls, relieving obstruction. Hydrocortisone by injection or prednisone tablets may be required in severe asthma, but prolonged dosage is undesirable, because of side-effects (see under Cushing's syndrome). In older subjects with intrinsic-type asthma, continued prednisone (e.g. 5–20 mg daily) may, however, prove necessary.

Treatment of Status Asthmaticus: This is a medical emergency. While adrenaline injections were formerly recommended, most patients will already have attempted self-treatment with inhalers of adrenaline-like drugs, often used to excess. Such patients have rapid pulse and worsening anoxia, and further adrenaline may be dangerous. Aminophylline 500 mg may be given slowly intravenously, but steroids are now advised.

Hydrocortisone 100–200 mg intravenously, repeated or given by drip infusion is used in the first 24-hours and prednisone 15–20 mg is given by mouth 6-hourly, the dose being decreased with the improvement that occurs over a few days.

Oxygen is given usually by plastic face mask at flow rate of 4–6 litres per minute. However, high concentration oxygen is unsafe in a few asthmatics who develop carbon dioxide retention, and blood gas studies are advisable. Deterioration may require endotracheal intubation and artificial ventilation—see Respiratory Failure.

Pulmonary embolism and infarction

These important conditions have been considered on page 45.

It should be noted that while they are complications of leg vein thrombosis associated with bed rest or operation, there are often no signs in the legs, the first symptoms being chest ones from pulmonary infarction. Thus there may be pleural pain, breathlessness and haemoptysis, but sometimes simply a rise in pulse rate or temperature, and the condition may be mis-diagnosed as pneumonia. Such symptoms may also be the forerunners of massive pulmonary embolism with extreme breathlessness and collapse.

Thus in unexplained chest illnesses, it is wise to examine the legs for calf tenderness and oedema, and special diagnostic aids such as the Sonicaid detector should be used in patients at risk from venous thrombosis. Anticoagulants such as heparin are used in prophylaxis and treatment.

Pulmonary heart failure (cor pulmonale)

This has been considered on page 55.

The commonest cause is chronic bronchitis and emphysema, which throws a strain on the right ventricle. Heart failure may develop slowly, or more quickly if there is superadded chest infection and pneumonia.

Obesity, by causing difficulty of movement of respiratory muscles and diaphragm may produce a similar effect.

Other causes are pulmonary fibrosis, as in coal-workers' pneumoconiosis and recurrent pulmonary infarction or embolism.

Respiratory failure. Intensive respiratory care

This is defined as a failure of the respiratory system to maintain a normal oxygen and/or carbon dioxide content in the blood.

Causes

Depression of the respiratory centre—this may follow head injury, complicate cerebral haemorrhage, or occur with anoxia and in poisoning such as barbiturate poisoning, and in diabetic ketosis and uraemia.

Paralysis of the respiratory muscles—poliomyelitis, ascending neuritis and tetanus. *Crushed chest injury* has the same effect.

Lung disorders—severe pneumonia, lung collapse and drowning may cause anoxia and respiratory failure. However, chronic bronchitis and emphysema, usually with superadded infection and often pulmonary heart failure, is the commonest cause in clinical practice, and here there is carbon dioxide retention as well as oxygen-lack. Very severe asthma is associated with anoxia, and occasionally there is carbon dioxide retention.

Symptoms and signs

The symptoms are those of the underlying condition, and there is dyspnoea, cyanosis, poor respiratory movements, restlessness and in severe cases, coma.

Blood gas analysis confirms the diagnosis, and is essential in management: arterial blood samples are preferred, though capillary samples by finger prick may be used.

Treatment

Infection should be vigorously treated with appropriate antibacterial drugs, such as penicillin, cloxacillin, ampicillin or trimethoprim-sulphamethoxazole.

Clear the airway: aspirate secretions with plastic catheter and encourage coughing.

Bronchodilators such as salbutamol aerosol or aminophylline may help.

Oxygen—should be given at high concentration (40–60 per cent) by Polymask or M.C. mask with a flow rate of 4–6 L/min (with water bottle to humidify) provided the blood CO_2 level is not raised. In chronic bronchitis, the CO_2 is raised and high concentration oxygen is dangerous. Thus, where there is doubt, and until blood gas results are available, it is better to give oxygen at low concentration (30 per cent) using nasal catheters, or Edinburgh mask at a flow rate of 2 L/min. The Ventimask can also be used.

Stimulation of ventilation with nikethamide 2 ml i.v. may be temporarily helpful.

Circulatory measures—diuretics such as frusemide (Lasix), and digoxin are indicated in associated heart failure. On the other hand, fluid depletion with low blood volume occurs in prolonged asthma and fulminating pneumonia. Intravenous fluids are indicated, guided by the central venous pressure measured by a cannula passed intravenously. Hydrocortisone in massive doses such as 5·0 G i.v. in 24-hours is indicated in states of hypotension and circulatory collapse.

Intubation and Artificial Ventilation (Artificial Respiration). These measures may be indicated when blood reports show worsening anoxia and the clinical state is deteriorating, with impending coma.

An *Endotracheal tube* is passed through the mouth using a laryngoscope, the patient being sedated with diazepam (Valium). This tube allows aspiration of secretions and use of a mechanical ventilator and may be left in place for up to 48 hours.

Tracheostomy (insertion of tube through incision in trachea) is required beyond that time or in patients not tolerating the endotracheal tube.

Artificial Ventilation can be given temporarily with the Ambu bag, but is maintained by coupling the endotracheal tube, or the tracheostomy tube, to a mechanical ventilator such as the Cape or East-Radcliffe machine. This method is called 'Intermittent Positive Pressure Ventilation'.

As the patient improves, he is gradually weaned from the respirator, and the tracheostomy tube may be removed in about a week, depending on the cause of respiratory failure.

Nursing care

Attention to the patient's comfort, changing his position in bed, care of the mouth and tracheostomy toilet are important aspects of treatment. Adequate fluids, a palatable light diet or feeds with Complan, plus moral support and encouragement help the patient through a trying time. Skilled nursing is essential in the management of respiratory failure.

Cancer of the lung (bronchogenic carcinoma)

Lung cancer is an important disease causing some 30,000 deaths annually in Great Britain. Over two thirds of patients die within a year of the diagnosis being made, and the overall five year survival rate is only 5 per cent.

Causes

The malignant growth arises in a bronchus, and spreads to involve the lung, lymph glands and distant organs by metastatic spread by lymphatics or bloodstream.

Most cases are caused by heavy cigarette smoking (twenty-five or more daily). Irritant and 'carcinogenic' substances in tobacco smoke may act by promoting malignant change in predisposed individuals. The incidence of lung cancer declines in those who stop smoking.

Atmospheric pollution plays a minor part.

Symptoms and signs

There are none in the early stages, the diagnosis being made on chest x-ray.

Middle-aged men are chiefly affected, there is dry cough and sometimes haemoptysis. Sputum may become purulent from infection, and bronchial obstruction causes breathlessness and partial collapse of the lung, pneumonia or lung abscess. There may be finger clubbing. Weakness and weight-loss are late signs.

The initial growth may be silent and presentation may be as complications.

Complications

Pneumonia, lung abscess, pleural effusion.

Obstruction of the superior vena cava from spread to the mediastinum, causing pain, plethora and swelling of the face and neck; the recurrent laryngeal nerve may be involved, causing hoarseness. Metastases in liver with jaundice, brain, or in the skin.

Metabolic effects, including neuropathy with sensory loss and weakness in the limbs, and ataxia (balance disturbance). Endocrine effects include a low salt state and hypotension, and the opposite state from salt-retention, with Cushingoid features, the tumour producing an A.C.T.H.-like hormone.

Further investigations

Chest x-ray.
Sputum for cytology.
Bronchoscopy.

Treatment

Surgical removal of the affected lobe or lung offers the best chance of cure, but in many cases the growth is too extensive.

Radiotherapy (x-ray therapy) should be used for the inoperable case (and post-operatively). It may be urgently required for superior vena caval obstruction, where it produces relief for weeks or months. Radiotherapy may also relieve pain, cough and haemoptysis.

Chemotherapy with a cytotoxic drug such as cyclophosphamide may afford temporary benefit, and mustine intrapleurally may delay recurrence of a pleural effusion.

In late stages, chlorpromazine (Largactil) and morphine should be given to allay pain and suffering and properly used these drugs ensure comfort and tranquillity in terminal cases.

Prevention

Lung cancer would be largely prevented if cigarette smoking were stopped. Doctors and nurses have a duty to make this fact clear, and to show a proper example to patients under their care.

Lung abscess

With early antibacterial drug treatment for lung infections, lung abscess is now rare.

Causes:

Bronchial obstruction: following inhalation of foreign body (e.g. a peanut) or septic material from the throat after an operation.
Carcinoma of lung.
Pneumonia: abscess may follow staphylococcal pneumonia.
Septic embolism to lungs in septicaemia, e.g. following illegal abortion.
Symptoms and signs: Swinging fever, cough with foul purulent sputum.

Chest x-ray will show the abscess cavity. Sputum is sent for bacteriology and drug sensitivity.
Treatment: Bronchoscopy is required to remove a foreign body. Postural drainage is carried out, and appropriate antibacterial drugs given. Surgical removal of the affected lobe is now rarely required.

Collapse of the lung (atelectasis)

The term atelectasis is used to describe lung collapse following blockage of a bronchus. Lung collapse also occurs when air enters the pleural cavity (pneumothorax) and may rarely be caused by a massive pleural effusion.

Causes of atelectasis: A large bronchus may be blocked by an inhaled foreign body or retained secretion post-operatively. The air distal to the obstruction is absorbed, and the affected lobe or lung collapses. The same process may occur less acutely when carcinoma obstructs a bronchus. Patchy atelectasis affecting smaller segments of lung again occurs post-operatively or in states of coma from retained mucus due to inadequate depth of respiration, and failure to cough effectively. Superadded infection causes pneumonia.

Symptoms and signs: If a lobe, or a whole lung is involved, there is sudden dyspnoea and cyanosis. In the more common and lesser lung atelectases, there may be only slight breathlessness and the symptoms and signs are those of pneumonia. There is dullness to percussion and diminished breath sounds over the affected part, with x-ray changes including raising of the diaphragm from shrinkage of the lung.

Pulmonary embolism and infarction may cause a similar picture, sometimes with pleural pain and haemoptysis.

Prevention: Stopping smoking, and breathing exercises pre-operatively are important in those with existing respiratory disease. Breathing exercises and adequate coughing are advisable in all patients post-operatively; similar encouragement. and frequent turning is necessary for patients confined to bed.

Treatment: Deep breathing, coughing, and postural drainage aided by percussion by the physiotherapist may clear an obstructing mucus plug and allow re-expansion of the lung.

Oxygen may be required to relieve breathlessness.

Bronchoscopy is required to remove a foreign body, and will also be indicated to remove an obstructing plug of mucus when the above measures over a few hours have failed to prove effective.

Pneumonia following patchy atelectasis should be treated with antibacterial drugs as already described.

Spontaneous pneumothorax

Pneumothorax is the presence of air in the pleural cavity, causing partial or complete collapse of the underlying lung.

Causes: Spontaneous pneumothorax follows rupture of a lung alveolus. While a distended area of lung in emphysema, an emphysematous 'bulla', may be responsible, in most cases the underlying lung is normal and the reason for the occurrence of pneumothorax obscure.

Symptoms and signs: The condition is commonest in young men, and may occur when quietly at rest or on respiratory effort in running or blowing a wind instrument. There is sudden severe pain or discomfort as something is 'felt to give' and breathlessness. Breathlessness usually improves in a few minutes, except in the rare occasions when the opening between lung and pleural cavity is valvular, allowing air in but not out, and causing 'tension' pneumothorax.

Most cases are relatively mild and the patient may delay seeking medical advice. Examination reveals poor expansion on the affected side, and hyper-resonance on percussion.

Sometimes, myocardial infarction, pulmonary infarction, pleurisy or pneumonia may have been wrongly suspected as the cause of symptoms.

Diagnosis is confirmed by chest x-ray, which shows air between the lung and the rib-cage.

Treatment: In young adults with no history of respiratory disease, a period of rest, not necessarily bed rest, is all that is required, the lung re-expanding within a week or ten days—x-ray should be taken to confirm this.

Tension pneumothorax is an emergency and in extreme cases with dyspnoea and cyanosis a hypodermic needle should be plunged into the pleural cavity to release the air.

In cases of pneumothorax with dyspnoea and underlying lung disease, and where no re-expansion of the lung is occurring, the insertion of a plastic cannula (through the second rib interspace), attached to a simple one-way ball-valve (or a bicycle valve) will allow air out and speed re-expansion. This is less cumbersome than attachment to a water-seal drain, and allows the patient to be ambulant. Suction is rarely required.

In recurrent pneumothorax, surgical treatment of an emphysematous bulla may be required, or attempts made to seal the two surfaces of the pleura by causing an inflammatory reaction by the insertion of talc.

Fungus disease of the lung

Fungal infection is rare. Monilia (Candida) mouth or throat infection (thrush) may spread to the lungs in debilitated patients who have received multiple antibiotics or steroid drugs. Aspergillus fungus may grow in lung cavities. Inhalations of natamycin or systemic treatment with amphotericin may be tried, but results are disappointing.

Other fungal infections such as histoplasmosis occur in North America.

Allergic reaction to fungi may present as bronchospasm, and some cases of asthma are an allergic reaction to aspergillus.

A rather different type of fungal allergy presents as a somewhat delayed inflammatory and destructive reaction, analagous to the serum sickness reaction, with alveolar involvement and breathlessness. Farmer's Lung, described below, is an example.

Lung fibrosis

Local fibrosis: This is a scarring of the lung following damage from pneumonia, bronchiectasis, tuberculosis or lung abscess.

Generalized fibrosis.

Causes:

Dust diseases of the lung such as coal-workers' pneumoconiosis and silicosis see below.

Sarcoidosis.

'*Fibrosing Alveolitis*'—from extrinsic causes, e.g. Farmer's lung.

Intrinsic; the cause may be a collagen disease such as Rheumatoid arthritis or scleroderma. There is also an 'idiopathic' group of unknown cause. The symptom is breathlessness on slight exertion from stiff lungs and lack of oxygen. X-rays and special lung function tests are required. Steroid drugs may cause some improvement.

Occupational diseases of the lungs

Pneumoconiosis is a term covering several lung diseases produced by dust, but the pathology varies and it is better to consider some important dust diseases separately.

COAL-WORKERS' PNEUMOCONIOSIS

Cause: Gradual accumulation of fine dust in the lungs after many years inhalation at work.

Symptoms and signs: None in the early stages, the disorder being seen on chest x-ray as multiple minute opacities. Breathlessness, morning cough with dark sputum follow. In severe cases there is increasing lung fibrosis and disability and tuberculosis may be associated.

Management: Dust suppression in coal mines decreases the incidence. Severely affected men should be re-employed above ground. The disease is compensatable under the Industrial Injuries Act.

SILICOSIS

This is due to inhalation of silica dust and occurs in workers in industries such as stone crushing and sand blasting where dust suppression precautions are inadequate. Masks afford only limited protection. The symptom is breathlessness from lung fibrosis, and there is increased risk of pulmonary tuberculosis.

ASBESTOSIS

Asbestos has many industrial uses for it is a good insulator and is fire-proof thus it is used to line boilers. It is resistant to friction hence its use in brake-linings. There is a high concentration of asbestos fibres in the atmosphere in factories using it, and in large towns from motor traffic. 'Blue' asbestos causes lung fibrosis and cancer in the lung, pleura, peritoneum and abdomen, often years after exposure. Blue asbestos has been largely replaced by white asbestos, which appears safe.

BYSSINOSIS

Byssinosis occurs in cotton and flax workers and presents as 'Monday morning fever' with chest tightness and wheeze on the resumption of work after the weekend break. Repeated inhalation of the dust in the mills if accompanied by smoking and atmospheric pollution generally, results in chronic wheezy bronchitis.

FARMER'S LUNG AND RELATED DISEASES

Cause: Farmer's lung is an allergic reaction to the spores of a fungus that grows in mouldy hay. Baled hay from a damp season stored in a hay loft is the common source of infection. The reaction is an inflammatory and destructive one in the alveoli, an allergic alveolitis, though there may be a bronchospastic element in some cases.

Symptoms and signs: The patient, usually a farmer, complains of tight breathlessness and chest oppression, cough and fever, and may have a little mucoid or blood tinged sputum, 6–8 hours after exposure to hay. Thus symptoms often occur in the evening. There need not be bronchospasm or wheeze (as there is in asthma). Recurrent exposure results in episodes of severe breathlessness from patchy pneumonia and ultimate lung fibrosis. A 'precipitin' test in the blood is positive.

Treatment: Prevention is important—hay should not be baled when wet, nor should it be kept for long periods before use. The wearing of a mask when handling hay may be helpful but once diagnosed, it is probably advisable for the patient to avoid hay altogether, exchanging his employment if necessary. Steroids such as prednisone 10 mg 6-hourly may be indicated in severe cases, tailing off the dose to zero over a few weeks.

Barley workers' lung, Bagassosis from sugar cane, and Bird-breeders' lung are similar lung reactions to different spores and fungi. The lung disease following inhalation of enzyme washing powders has a similar basis.

Disorders of the pleura

PLEURISY AND PLEURAL EFFUSION

Pleurisy is inflammation of the pleural membrane and may be 'dry' or accompanied by *Pleural Effusion*—fluid in the pleural cavity.

Causes: Usually there is underlying lung disease:

Lobar pneumonia.
Pulmonary infarction.
Lung cancer or pleural metastases.
Tuberculosis.

Rarer causes are virus infection of the chest wall (see below) and collagen diseases such as rheumatoid arthritis.

In effusion, the fluid may be an inflammatory exudate, containing cells and protein, or a transudate, a watery fluid formed as a reaction to the underlying disease.

Pleural effusion is sometimes called *Hydrothorax* and may accompany oedematous states such as heart failure, nephrotic syndrome, and cirrhosis of the liver.

Empyema is a collection of pus in the pleural cavity; it may complicate lobar pneumonia from spread of pneumococcal infection, but is rare with effective antibacterial therapy.

Symptoms and signs: Symptoms are those of the underlying condition.

Pain, worse on deep breathing, occurs in dry pleurisy due to the rubbing-together of the inflamed surfaces and a 'pleural rub' may be heard with the stethoscope. As fluid forms, pain disappears. Large effusions cause breathlessness, and there is dullness on percussion over the effusion. In empyema, the patient is usually toxic and ill, with swinging fever.

Further investigations:

Chest x-ray confirms the presence of fluid.
Diagnostic aspiration of fluid—clear and straw coloured if transudate.

May be cloudy if infected, or pus with empyema.

Blood-stained often in carcinoma and sometimes in pulmonary infarction.

Fluid is sent for bacteriology, antibacterial drug sensitivity, and cytology for malignant cells.

Treatment: Pleurisy generally settles with treatment of the underlying condition. Analgesics such as aspirin or paracetamol, or the more powerful drug pentazocine (Fortral) may be required for the pain of dry pleurisy, but the pain subsides usually over a few days. Diuretics such as frusemide (Lasix) are often effective in pleural effusion in heart failure, nephrotic syndrome and cirrhosis, but rarely in malignant effusions.

Paracentesis (aspiration of the fluid) is indicated where these measures fail, and for large effusions embarrassing respiration. This is performed with local anaesthetic, the needle being inserted below the scapula. Suction is applied by syringe or using a vacuum bottle with reversed-valve Higginson's syringe. Quantities up to a litre may be aspirated; with larger effusions it is wiser to repeat the procedure in a day or two.

Where the fluid is purulent, an appropriate antibacterial drug, usually penicillin 500,000 units, is instilled into the pleural cavity.

In malignant effusion, instillation of a cytoxic drug such as mustine may delay or prevent recurrence.

Chest wall pain

Pleurodynia is the name given to pains in the chest muscles. The pain, like that of pleurisy, is related to respiration. There may be tenderness of the affected muscles. An epidemic occurred in the Danish island of Bornholm, hence the term Bornholm disease. The cause is uncertain, but infection with a virus of Coxsackie group is sometimes responsible, there is a mild febrile illness and sometimes associated pleurisy and pericarditis. Some cases of chest wall pain in young adults may be due to an inflammation at the junction of rib and costal cartilage, Tietze's syndrome.

It is important to differentiate these types of pain in the chest wall from more serious conditions such as myocardial infarction, pulmonary infarction, pneumonia and pleurisy, and pneumothorax.

Treatment is with analgesics such as aspirin or paracetamol, and local heat from a hot water bottle, electric pad or infra-red lamp may be comforting. The condition usually settles within about a week.

6

Disorders of the alimentary system

The mouth

The inspection of the tongue and the mouth is as important as the examination of the pulse. The mouth reveals local pathology and the effects of many general conditions. Many bacteria live harmlessly in the mouth. Adequate fluids, the flow of saliva and the mechanical cleansing action of mastication, plus sound teeth and gums, contribute to a healthy mouth. It is an important part of the nurse's duty to encourage and maintain proper oral hygiene.

Before the patient opens his mouth, conditions of the lips such as cold sores, from herpes simplex virus infection and accompanying febrile conditions such as pneumonia, may be noted. Cracks at the corners of the mouth (angular cheilitis) are as likely to be due to ill fitting dentures as to poor nutrition or vitamin B deficiency.

THE TONGUE

The normal tongue is moist with somewhat rough surface from the papillae on it. A *dry tongue* implies mouth breathing or dehydration. A light coating is normal, fur being normally removed by food and saliva. A *furred tongue* may simply indicate that the tongue is not being used much; marked furring occurs in heavy smokers, and in uraemia (renal failure), and does not necessarily signify constipation.

A *smooth tongue* has been called 'glossitis' but it is an atrophy of the papillae rather than an inflammation. A smooth pale tongue suggests anaemia, and in pernicious anaemia (vitamin B_{12} deficiency) the tongue may be sore. A fiery red or magenta tongue occurs in other B vitamin deficiencies, sometimes due to intestinal malabsorption.

The tongue may show a *tremor* in alcoholism or Parkinson's disease, may be bitten in an epileptic fit, and following a stroke may be protruded towards the paralysed side of the body (being pushed over by the healthy side).

The tongue may be affected in stomatitis—see below. Carcinoma of the tongue may present as a painful, non-healing hard ulcer.

TEETH AND GUMS

Dental decay (caries) is very common in Britain. Bacterial action on sugary foods and sweets produces acids which destroy the enamel, especially if sweets are eaten between meals and brushing of the teeth is neglected. Fluoride in the water supply is protective. In adults, periodontal disease with inflammation at the gum margins (gingivitis) is common, and there may be a mixed bacterial infection. Even when there is no obvious sepsis, bacteria such as streptococcus viridans enter the blood stream at dental extractions or deep fillings. In a healthy person this may be of no consequence, but in those with congenital or rheumatic heart disease such bacteriaemia can cause subacute bacterial endocarditis. Severe bleeding after dental extraction suggests a disorder of blood clotting such as haemophilia.

Bleeding of the gums occurs in scurvy (vitamin C deficiency) and in purpura and blood disorders such as leukaemia (excessive white cells) and agranulocytosis (lack of white cells), where there may also be ulceration.

Long term treatment with phenytoin in epileptic patients may lead to swollen, hypertrophic gums. In lead poisoning, a blue line forms on the gums.

STOMATITIS

Stomatitis is inflammation of the mucous membrane of the mouth. There are many causes; prolonged fever and generalized illnesses with poor nutrition and lack of oral hygiene contribute to its development.

Thrush is an infection with the fungus Candida (Monilia) albicans and occurs where immunity is lowered, often in patients who have had steroids or broad-spectrum antibiotics such as tetracycline which destroy bacteria but allow monilia to flourish.

There are white patches on a sore inflamed mucous membrane; removal of these fungal patches leaves a raw bleeding surface. The tongue, gums and throat may be involved.

Treatment is with amphotericin (Fungilin) lozenges, nystatin suspension, or gentian violet.

Vincent's infection is due to a bacillus and a spirochaetal organism and is severe ulcerative stomatitis with involvement of the gums. Metronidazole (Flagyl) 200 mg thrice daily for three days, or penicillin can be used in treatment.

Aphthous ulceration is recurrent crops of shallow ulcers of uncertain cause, often related to emotional stress. Tincture of benzoin may help, but local or systemic steroids are given in severe cases.

Mouth ulceration occurs in skin diseases such as lichen planus and in blood diseases such as leukaemia and angranulocytosis.

Transient white spots, Koplik's spots may be seen in the cheeks or gums near the molar teeth in measles. Petechiae (tiny red spots) on the palate occur in glandular fever.

Sore throat has been described on page 20.

SALIVARY GLANDS

Mumps (parotitis) is a virus infection with swelling, usually bilateral, of the parotid glands at the angle of the jaw. Parotid swelling sometimes occurs in diabetes and pancreatic disease and with some drugs, e.g. phenylbutazone.

Swelling of parotid or submandibular glands may be due to bacterial infection in patients with prolonged, debilitating conditions such as carcinoma of any part of the body. Proper care of the mouth helps to prevent such infection.

A *stone* may obstruct a salivary gland duct, causing pain and swelling. Surgical removal of the stone may be necessary.

The oesophagus

The oesophagus (gullet) is a muscular tube about 250 cm (10 inches) long connecting the pharynx with the stomach and lying for much of its course in the mediastinum behind the root of the lung and the heart. It ends just below the diaphragm at the 'cardia', the name given to the junction of oesophagus and stomach.

DYSPHAGIA—difficulty in swallowing
Causes:
Painful conditions of the mouth and throat.
Swallowed foreign body.
Carcinoma of the oesophagus, or involvement by extrinsic growths.

Stricture from corrosive fluids or following reflux oesophagitis and hiatus hernia.

Achalasia of the cardia (cardiospasm)—failure of relaxation of the muscle at the lower end of oesophagus from atrophy of nerve endings here.

Neurogenic causes, such as bulbar palsy, or after strokes.

Emotional, the 'lump in the throat' feeling at times of stress; hysteria (display of symptoms without obvious basis) is a risky diagnosis, and not now a common cause of dysphagia.

Myasthenia gravis, a rare condition with muscle weakness.

The Patterson-Kelly (Plummer-Vinson) syndrome, associated with smooth tongue and iron deficiency anaemia—now uncommon.

Symptoms and signs: Carcinoma of the oesophagus occurs in the middle-aged and elderly, achalasia in younger people. In any form of obstruction, the patient can usually point accurately to its site. Carcinoma at the lower end of the oesophagus may arise in fact from the stomach.

Where there is an obstruction, the swallowing of solids becomes progressively more difficult, ultimately only liquids can be passed and there is considerable loss of weight and emaciation. Attempts at swallowing are followed by regurgitation of the food.

With neurogenic causes, there are other signs. Following a stroke there may be transient dysphagia, but only after bilateral upper motor neurone involvement is there persistent disturbance of the swallowing mechanism, with risk of regurgitation of food into the lungs. Silent spill-over into the lungs may present as pneumonia. Where the swallowing mechanism is deranged, solids may pass more readily than liquids, the oesophageal muscle being stimulated sufficiently by distension to propel the food onwards.

Further investigations include barium swallow x-ray, oesophagoscopy and biopsy.

Treatment: Treatment is that of the cause, where possible. Hiatus hernia is considered below.

Carcinoma of the oesophagus may be treated by surgical resection, but often the growth is extensive and the patient elderly and frail. Here it may be possible for the surgeon to insert a plastic tube which allows passage of food. Usually the outlook is poor and in later stages only palliative therapy, with proper use of opiates to relieve discomfort, is possible.

Achalasia of the cardia is best treated by Heller's operation, which consists in cutting the muscular layers of the lower oesophagus, allowing food to pass along the previously narrowed segment. Results are usually gratifying.

'Indigestion', pain and vomiting

Patients may complain of indigestion or dyspepsia, meaning discomfort related to eating or to the alimentary tract. It is, however, important to define symptoms more precisely.

Pain is localized to the epigastrium (pit of the stomach) in peptic ulcer. Hollow viscera such as the intestine are insensitive to cutting, pain occurring from distention or muscular spasm related to obstruction of the lumen. *Colic* was originally applied to the colon but now means pain gradually increasing in severity, then passing off, and occurring in waves. In biliary and ureteric (renal) colic the pain increases to a maximum over minutes or even up to an hour, then subsides. Intestinal pain may be poorly localized and felt centrally in the abdomen. However, when the parietal peritoneum (the layer lining the abdominal wall) becomes involved, pain, tenderness and muscle guarding occur over the affected part. Thus the initial pain of appendicitis is felt at the umbilical region, but when the inflammation spreads to the parietal peritoneum there is localized pain and tenderness at the right iliac fossa. Generalized peritonitis may be associated with tenderness and rigidity of the entire abdomen.

Heartburn is a sharp pain felt behind the breast bone and may be due to oesophagitis from reflux of gastric contents; there may be associated *acid regurgitation*, but this may occur in otherwise normal people, when it is of no significance.

Waterbrash is the sudden filling of the mouth with tasteless watery fluid, possibly saliva and is an important indicator of duodenal ulcer.

Flatulence is 'wind' which is belched up (eructated) and the most common cause is air-swallowing. *Flatus* is wind passed by rectum.

Anorexia is lack of appetite and occurs in many illnesses apart from abdominal disorders, where if persistent and associated with weight loss, it suggests carcinoma. It should be noted that patients with peptic ulcer generally have a good appetite.

Nausea is a feeling of sickness and may precede vomiting.

Vomiting is the forcible ejection of stomach contents through a relaxed cardiac sphincter.

Causes:

Abdominal:	*irritation* of stomach, e.g. in poisoning and alcoholism. *infection* such as peritonitis. *obstruction:* pyloric stenosis, intestinal obstruction from hernia or neoplasm, appendicitis, biliary and renal colic (from stones).
Cerebral:	raised intracranial pressure: meningitis, tumour, haemorrhage, hypertensive encephalopathy. disturbance of vestibular system (ear and its brain connections): motion sickness, epidemic vertigo (dizziness), brain stem ischaemia.
Metabolic:	in pregnancy, and in diabetic ketosis (acidosis) and uraemia.
Emotional:	severe pain, or distressing sights; 'psychological' vomiting often settles after hospital admission.
Drugs and x-ray therapy:	morphine, and digoxin overdose; vomiting may also follow radiotherapy, possibly by effect on vomiting centre in medulla.

Vomiting of blood, haematemesis, may complicate peptic ulcer and cirrhosis of the liver with oesophageal varices and is considered with these disorders.

Treatment is that of the cause. Drugs used symptomatically include prochlorperazine (Stemetil) which acts on the vomiting centre, and hyoscine for motion sickness.

'*Biliousness*' is a lay term for upper abdominal discomfort, nausea and vomiting; the vomitus may contain bile. Such symptoms do not necessarily signify disease of the biliary tract. 'Bilious attacks' may in fact be due to migraine.

Hiccup (*Hiccough*). A hiccup is an involuntary contraction of the diaphragm causing an abupt intake of breath immediately followed by closure of the glottis (larynx) producing the 'hic'. Infection or neoplasm irritating the diaphragm, and cerebral disease and uraemia affecting the medulla may be responsible, but usually hiccup is an innocent symptom of unknown cause. Remedies include breathing into a paper bag and chlorpromazine (Largactil) 50 mg orally or intramuscularly, but a catheter passed through the mouth or nose to tickle the pharynx is often the most effective cure.

Hiatus hernia and reflux oesophagitis

A hiatus is an opening, and a hernia is a protrusion of a viscus known in lay terms as a 'rupture' when it occurs at the groin. In hiatus hernia, part of the stomach slides up through the diaphragmatic hiatus, or less commonly rolls up alongside the oesophagus, into the thorax. If the sphincter between stomach and oesophagus becomes incompetent, reflux of acid gastric juice has an irritant effect on the mucous membrane of the lower oesophagus causing oesophagitis, and stricture in severe cases. Such reflux does not always occur in hiatus hernia, and on the other hand reflux may occur in the absence of hernia if the cardiac sphincter is incompetent.

Symptoms and signs: Hiatus hernia is common in middle-aged women, especially if there has been recent gain in weight, pushing up the abdominal contents. The condition is often symptomless.

There is heartburn and retrosternal pain which may simulate cardiac pain, with feeling of fullness and flatulence, and symptoms are worse on lying down or stooping. Acid regurgitation, vomiting and dysphagia may occur. Anaemia may be due to oozing of blood from erosion or ulceration.

Hiatus hernia may be associated with duodenal ulcer, gall stones and diverticular disease of the colon and it may be difficult to decide how far symptoms are due to these conditions.

Barium meal x-ray shows the hernia, or allows demonstration of reflux.

Treatment: Weight loss, avoidance of stooping, and the use of pillows or raising the bed-head on 8-inch blocks may be all that is required. Small meals and antacids as for peptic ulcer may help. Surgical repair is indicated only if these measures fail, or if a fibrous stricture has formed.

The stomach

The stomach is a muscular organ which breaks up and mixes food; the mucous membrane contains cells secreting hydrochloric acid and pepsin which contribute to digestion. Intrinsic factor, necessary for the absorption of vitamin B_{12} in the ileum, is produced by the same cells.

Gastritis

Acute gastritis is an inflammation of the mucous membrane of the stomach from ingestion of irritant substances such as alcohol, aspirin or staphylococcal endotoxin in one form of food poisoning. There is discomfort or pain, nausea and vomiting usually settling in a day or two if further irritation is avoided—the stomach has remarkable healing powers.

Aspirin, whether plain or soluble, may however cause an erosive gastritis with multiple small ulcerations and haematemesis. Preparations containing aspirin should therefore not be used where the stomach has already been insulted with excessive alcohol.

Chronic gastritis is a term sometimes used to describe the loss of appetitite, morning nausea and vomiting (often of mucus) that occurs in alcoholism and heavy cigarette smoking.

Atrophic gastritis occurs in the middle-aged and elderly and may be associated with gastric ulcer and increased incidence of carcinoma. Some cases are due to auto-immune destruction of the mucosa, and antibodies may be detected in the blood. Atrophic gastritis results in achlorhydria (absence of hydrochloric acid) and pernicious anaemia from lack of intrinsic factor and failure of absorption of vitamin B_{12}.

Peptic ulcer

A peptic ulcer is a hole in the mucous membrane of a part of the gastro-intestinal tract to which gastric juice, hydrochloric acid-pepsin, has access.

Types

Gastric ulcer occurs in the stomach usually on the lsser (inner) curvature.

Duodenal ulcer occurs in the first part of the duodenum, just beyond the pyloric outlet of the stomach.

Stomal ulcer occurs at the site of the stoma (anastomosis) after gastric surgery.

Incidence

In Britain duodenal ulcer is much the commonest type, and predominantly affects young and middle-aged men of all social classes and occupations. Gastric ulcer is the type seen in Japan, but is not so common in Britain; it occurs in older persons, affecting men and women equally and the incidence is higher in the lower socio-economic groups.

Cause

The cause of peptic ulcer is uncertain. As duodenal and gastric ulcers have some factors in common (and may co-exist) they are considered here together. It must be stressed, however, that the causes and management may be different. Moreover, a duodenal ulcer is never malignant, whereas a gastric 'ulcer', while usually benign may turn out in fact to be a gastric carcinoma.

Peptic ulcer tends to run in families, suggesting a genetic predisposition. Ulcer is commoner in those of blood group O, and in persons who do not secrete their blood group substances into the alimentary tract, 'non-secretors'.

The mucous membrane is normally resistant to the action of hydrochloric acid and pepsin. Ulceration occurs when the acid-pepsin versus mucosal resistance balance is disturbed. In duodenal ulcer there is a high acid-pepsin production from excess secreting cells in the stomach. In gastric ulcer the acid secretion may be high or low, and decreased mucosal resistance may be more important. Mucosal resistance is lowered by heavy cigarette smoking, alcohol, and certain drugs. Thus aspirin may cause acute erosions and bleeding; phenylbutazone and indomethacin, used in the treatment of rheumatoid arthritis, cause gastric ulceration though persons with chronic diseases such as rheumatoid arthritis may have lowered mucosal resistance in any case. There is no proof that steroids such as prednisone cause ulceration, though high doses may prevent ulcer healing. Similarly, factors such as overwork and mental stress cannot be proved to be causative, but they may exacerbate ulcer symptoms.

Symptoms and signs

The chief symptom is pain, felt in the epigastrium, and the patient may be able to point with one finger at its site, where there may be tenderness and resistance to palpation, with muscle 'guarding'. With a posterior penetrating ulcer pain may be felt through to the back. The pain occurs between meals, is relieved by food and alkalis and often occurs in the middle of the night, around 2 a.m. waking the patient from sleep. In gastric ulcer the pain may not be so clearly defined and may come on after meals or certain foods, which the patient learns to avoid. Generally, however, the appetite remains good.

The pain has a characteristic periodicity, occurring over a few days or a week then the patient may remain symptom-free for weeks or months.

Vomiting is rare in uncomplicated duodenal ulcer and its occurrence suggests the development of pyloric spasm or stenosis. This and the other complications of peptic ulcer—haemorrhage and perforation, are described below.

Further investigations

Barium meal x-ray and screening shows an ulcer 'crater', or, in the duodenum, deformity, but duodenal abnormality is often difficult to visualize on x-ray; a patient with peptic ulcer may have a negative barium meal. Where barium shows a gastric ulcer, repeat investigation is indicated to ascertain healing.

Cytological examination of gastric washings (obtained by nasogastric tube) and techniques such as *gastroscopy* and use of gastric camera may be indicated in cases of gastric ulcer where malignancy is suspected.

Stool occult blood tests using a guaiac method such as 'Hemoccult' (orthotolidine having been withdrawn for carcinogenic risk) may be positive if there is an active ulcer with oozing of blood.

Test meals are not of value, and only rarely is it helpful to measure the overnight acid secretion or the maximum stimulation with pentagastrin (which replaces histamine) in dubious cases of duodenal ulceration.

Treatment

Ideally this should consist of relieving symptoms, aiding healing and preventing recurrence. As the cause of peptic ulcer is uncertain, we cannot always achieve these aims. The three important principles are rest, stopping smoking, and a small frequent meals regime.

Rest—a spell off work, with proper rest and sleep may allow rapid relief of symptoms. If the home environment is unsuitable, hospital admission is indicated; symptoms usually settle within a few days without any additional measures.

Stopping smoking—this speeds healing of a gastric ulcer, and probably of a duodenal ulcer. No ulcer patient should smoke.

Other irritating factors such as alcohol and aspirin must be avoided.

Frequent meals—peptic ulcer heals as quickly on a normal ward diet as on special 'gastric' or 'bland' diet. Meals should be taken at regular intervals with snacks such as milk and biscuits between the main meals, to help neutralize the acid responsible for the pain. Patients should avoid foods that they have discovered to upset them, and should take food that they like. Milk is usually acceptable to most, and in hospital should be available on the bedside locker to take liberally between meal times and during the night. If pain does not settle, an intragastric milk drip may be helpful.

'Diets' may be demanded, or imposed by patients or their relatives, but protein should not be restricted if the patient enjoys his meat, fried foods are not necessarily harmful, and fruit is not in effect 'acidic'—undue restriction of fruit and vegetables results in vitamin C deficiency and impaired ulcer healing.

Drugs used in treatment

Antacids—these neutralize or reduce the acidity of the gastric contents but their effect is very temporary and they are of value only in relieving pain.

Sodium bicarbonate (baking soda) 4–5 G (about a teaspoonful) mixed with water is rapidly effective and is contained in many proprietary remedies. It is, however, absorbed into the circulation and excessive use causes alkalosis.

Non-absorbed antacids include *magnesium trisilicate*, which is also mildly laxative, and *aluminium hydroxide*, which tends to be constipating. Aluminium hydroxide in liquid or gel form is given in 5–10 ml doses hourly between meals if pain is severe.

Nulacin is a tablet preparation containing milk solids and magnesium antacids. The tablets can be sucked between meals in the ward, and are convenient for patients when they return to work.

Anti-cholinergic drugs—theoretically these reduce vagus-mediated gastric acid secretion but in practice their effect in the short-term is slight and side-effects such as drying of the mouth and blurring of vision limit their use—poldine (Nacton) is one such drug tried long-term. These drugs delay gastric emptying and are contra-indicated in pyloric stenosis.

Liquorice derivatives

Carbenoxolone (Biogastrone) 100 mg three times daily after meals speeds the healing of *gastric* ulcers and may allow outpatient management. If the ulcer is not healed at four weeks, 100 mg twice daily is given for a further two to four weeks. Carbenoxolone may act by promoting mucus secretion, but it may also stimulate the adrenal cortex, and the cortisol or aldosterone-like effect causes salt and water retention with risk of hypertension, and potassium loss. Thiazide diuretics and potassium supplements may be given to counter these effects; the diuretic spironolactone (Aldactone-A) nullifies the beneficial effect of carbonoxolone on ulcer healing. It is still unknown if long-term use prevents recurrence.

Duogastrone is a capsule containing carbenoxolone, taken before meals and formulated to disintegrate in the duodenum. It is being tried in *duodenal* ulcer, but its value is as yet uncertain.

Caved-S is a proprietary preparation containing liquorice derivatives plus antacids recommended for treatment of gastric and duodenal ulcers. It does not have the fluid-retaining or potassium-losing side-effects of carbenoxolone but its value is unproven.

Sedatives and tranquillizers. Drugs such as phenobarbitone or diazepam (Valium) may be useful to allay anxiety, but have no direct effect on ulcer healing.

Prognosis and follow up

If symptoms can be controlled with the above measures, the patient who has a duodenal ulcer can continue to live with it. Stopping smoking and the avoidance of long spells without food may suffice to keep symptoms away, with a few days rest with milk feeds or antacids on the first sign of recurrence. Sometimes an ulcer may heal completely, but more often there is persistent deformity on barium meal examination. As duodenal ulcer is not malignant, the x-ray appearances do not matter in a symptomless patient. If, however, ulcer pain persists or recurs and the patient is having repeated periods off work on account of it, surgery is indicated.

With the advent of carbenoxolone, an increased proportion of gastric ulcers may be found to heal and remain healed. Failure to heal in twelve weeks does however, raise suspicions of malignancy and in this situation, surgery is indicated.

Complications of peptic ulcer

HAEMORRHAGE—HAEMATEMESIS AND MELAENA

A haematemesis is a vomiting of blood which may be fresh and red or dark brown and 'coffee-ground' in appearance if altered by stomach acid.

A melaena is a loose black tarry, glistening stool from blood altered by passage through the alimentary tract, but if the haemorrhage is severe the stool may contain dark red blood.

Causes

Gastric or duodenal ulcer eroding a blood vessel, and rarely gastric carcinoma.

Aspirin ingestion, often with another irritant such as alcohol, and possibly high doses of steroids. Aspirin provokes bleeding from an existing peptic ulcer and in addition causes acute erosions, often multiple with oozing of blood.

Cirrhosis of the liver with bleeding from oesophageal veins.

Bleeding states, caused by anticoagulants, or in purpura and leukaemia.

Haematemesis should be differentiated from haemoptysis (where the blood may be brighter and frothy), from a vomit of swallowed blood from a nose bleed, and from the vomiting of gastric contents in pyloric stenosis. If there is doubt, specimens must be preserved; their volume gives some indication of the severity of the haemorrhage.

Symptoms and signs

Bleeding may present as haematemesis, melaena or both, or may be 'silent' into the alimentary tract. The signs are those of blood loss (one cause of a state of 'shock', rather an unsatisfactory term)—pallor, cold and clammy skin, apprehension, restlessness, rapid pulse and low blood pressure, with fainting or collapse. There is circulatory compensation, and haemodilution later, causing improvement in the general state, but the patient is dehydrated from fluid loss and there is risk of continued or recurrent haemorrhage.

Usually there is no pain, but there may have been an exacerbation of ulcer symptoms a few days previously. In those without an ulcer history aspirin may have been taken for some aches or flu-like illness, followed by haematemesis though previously the drug had caused no ill-effect.

Treatment

Bed rest. Indicated in all but the mildest cases, with a low pillow.

Detailed observation—the important factor is the extent of the blood loss. Careful and repeated note is made of the patient's appearance, pulse and blood pressure. The haemoglobin is a further guide but may be falsely high before haemodilution takes place.

Blood transfusion—grouping and cross-matching is carried out in all cases. Transfusion is indicated with a pulse rising above 100 or a systolic blood pressure falling below 100 mm 3 or 4 units of 500 ml is required in the first few hours, the rate of transfusion and the need for further blood depending on the clinical response. Elderly patients stand blood-loss badly and should be transfused if there is any doubt, for there is seldom a real risk of circulatory overload.

Sedation—morphine or diamorphine 10–15 mg is best but is not always required; as morphine may cause vomiting it may be given combined with cyclizine (Cyclimorph), or chlorpromazine (Largactil) or diazepam (Valium) used instead.

Fluids should be given by mouth, for the patient is dehydrated and thirsty. Frequent sips of water and milk are suitable followed by light diet with milky foods such as Horlicks or Ovaltine, then normal diet with milk between meals.

The bleeding usually stops spontaneously with such measures. Occasionally it may be useful to pass a nasogastric tube as a guide to the occurrence of fresh haemorrhage, and aspiration may relieve discomfort from a stomach distended with blood. Barium meal and gastroscopy may be indicated as an emergency to ascertain the site of severe bleeding.

Surgery should be considered if bleeding continues. It is a good plan to have a combined medical-surgical unit so that the surgeon can share assessment. Following aspirin ingestion without ulcer history, it is generally better to transfuse further and continue conservative treatment. With continued severe bleeding, and in older patients with known ulceration and previous bleeds, surgery is indicated. Operation is directed to dealing with the bleeding point or local resection of the ulcer, radical gastrectomy being avoided if possible nowadays.

Follow-up includes stool-tests for blood, which become negative over a few days. There is also an improvement in the haemoglobin level. To make up for the iron deficiency following haemorrhage, ferrous sulphate 200 mg 3 times daily is indicated and is continued for a week or two after the haemoglobin has reached 100 per cent to replete iron stores. Possibly ascorbic acid (vitamin C) aids iron absorption, and some cases of aspirin haematemesis may be associated with ascorbic acid deficiency; ascorbic acid will aid healing only when there is such deficiency.

Aspirin should subsequently be avoided—this applies to plain and soluble aspirin, and to many proprietary pain remedies containing it. Peptic ulcer is treated as described above.

PERFORATION

Cause: The ulcer erodes through the wall of stomach or duodenum with escape of gastric contents into the peritoneal cavity, causing severe irritation and peritonitis.

Symptoms and signs: Sudden severe upper abdominal pain, with tenderness and board-like rigidity of the abdomen and rapidly rising pulse. Differential diagnosis includes pancreatitis and myocardial infarction; in perforation, x-ray shows gas below the diaphragm.

Treatment: A surgical emergency, demanding closure of the perforation. In elderly and debilitated patients conservative treatment—gastric aspiration, intravenous fluids and antibiotics—may be justified.

PYLORIC SPASM AND STENOSIS

These are complications of duodenal ulcer. Acute exacerbation of the ulcer may be associated with muscle spasm, so that the stomach does not empty properly and distends. In chronic ulceration there may be fibrous contraction at the duodenum beyond the pyloric outlet of the stomach, pyloric stenosis, with gross hold-up and distension.

Symptoms and signs: Pyloric spasm during ulcer exacerbation causes vomiting which settles as the ulcer becomes quiescent.

In pyloric stenosis, the ulcer pain changes its characteristics, now occurring after meals or in the evening when the stomach is distended. Vomiting becomes frequent and copious, the vomit containing food residues from many hours earlier and its appearance may be confused with a haematemesis. There is increasing weight loss, dehydration, salt and acid loss, and alkalosis on blood testing. Gastric aspiration shows residual volumes of $\frac{1}{2}$–1 litre, and barium meal confirms gastric distension.

Treatment: Pyloric spasm settles with ulcer treatment and a fluid diet in the acute stages. Anticholinergic drugs delay gastric emptying and should not be used. Evening gastric aspiration and lavage may be helpful, and may be tried also in pyloric stenosis, for some improvement in gastric emptying may occur when longstanding distension has been relieved. Intravenous fluid replacement may be necessary.

Surgery is however, usually necessary in pyloric stenosis. In a debilitated patient the surgeon may by-pass the obstruction with a gastro-jejunostomy, avoiding a more major procedure.

A note on the surgery of peptic ulceration

In duodenal ulceration, the principle of surgical therapy is to decrease or abolish the acid gastric secretion that bathes the ulcer, thus allowing it to heal. The ulcer itself need not be removed unless there is associated obstruction. Thus the currently favoured operation is vagotomy, which abolishes the vagal stimulus to gastric secretion. Partial gastrectomy, removing the acid-secreting part of the stomach, is an alternative procedure. With gastric ulcer, most surgeons prefer to remove the ulcer-bearing part of the stomach and this is indicated if there is any suspicion of malignancy; vagotomy may however be indicated for certain types of gastric ulcer.

In most cases, the results of surgery are good, the patient becomes symptom-free, can enjoy his meals and do his normal work. Short-term complications include a dumping feeling in the stomach during or at the end of meals, sometimes shakiness from hypoglycaemia from hyperinsulinism related to peaks of sugar absorption, and there may be mild looseness of the bowels.

Long term complications are, however, becoming increasingly recognized. They may be delayed for up to ten years after an apparently successful operation and are due to malabsorption of food (see below), really a form of malnutrition. The commonest finding is iron deficiency anaemia, but the serum B_{12} is lowered following lack of intrinsic factor and pernicious anaemia may ensue. There may also be deficiency of calcium (with raised serum alkaline phosphatase level) and osteomalacia (thinning of the bones).

The incidence of pulmonary tuberculosis is higher in patients who have had a partial gastrectomy.

Thus patients should be seen yearly after gastric surgery and blood tests carried out so that deficiencies can be remedied at an early stage. These effects should also be borne in mind in patients subsequently admitted with another condition.

Carcinoma of the stomach

This occurs in the middle-aged and elderly. It should be suspected in non-healing gastric ulcers.

Symptoms and signs: Carcinoma may remain silent until far advanced, with a fungating mass of tissue or a quiet infiltration and ulceration. There is upper abdominal pain or discomfort not clearly related to meals, loss of appetite, weight loss, nausea and vomiting. A mass may become palpable in the epigastrium, and there is anaemia from blood loss. The first signs may be of metastatic growths in the liver causing enlargement and jaundice, or in the peritoneal cavity causing ascites (fluid distention).

Gastric carcinoma may complicate atrophic gastritis and pernicious anaemia, but not all cases of carcinoma show achlorhydria.

Further investigations: Early diagnosis is essential and is aided by a high index of suspicion, barium meal, gastric cytology and gastroscopy. Stool tests for occult blood may be positive.

Treatment: Surgical exploration and removal of the growth where possible. It is however, often difficult to remove all the neoplastic tissue and glands, when treatment must be purely palliative, with proper use of opiates to relieve discomfort, and the prognosis is generally poor.

Small intestine

The small intestine consists of the duodenum, a C-shaped tube round the head of the pancreas, and the jejunum and ileum lying in coils attached to the posterior abdominal wall by the mesentery, a fold of peritoneum in which blood vessels and lymphatics run. The ileum ends in the caecum, the start of the large intestine (colon) at the right iliac fossa. The small intestine is concerned with digestion and absorption of foods minerals and vitamins, the mucosa being in folds and having finger-like projections or villi which greatly increase the absorptive area. Enzymes secreted by the mucosa split food protein into amino acids, carbohydrates and sugars into glucose, and these are absorbed into the blood vessels which join to form the portal vein to reach the liver. Fats are digested by the action of bile salts and pancreatic lipase, absorbed into lacteals in the villi to reach the lymphatics and are carried via the thoracic duct to join the general circulation in the great veins near the heart. Some fats with fewer carbon atoms in their molecule, the medium chain triglycerides, are, however, absorbed directly into the blood vessels of the portal system.

The terminal part of the ileum contains patches of lymphoid tissue, Peyer's patches, which become involved in typhoid infection. The lymphoid tissue may be concerned in the body's immunity mechanism and the production of antibodies, and viruses may colonize here before spreading to other tissues.

Inflammation (Enteritis) and infection

GASTROENTERITIS (FOOD POISONING)
This is caused by preformed staphylococcal enterotoxin, clostridium and salmonella infections (and atypical Esch. Coli in babies), symptoms are vomiting and diarrhoea—see page 26.

TYPHOID AND PARATYPHOID (ENTERIC FEVER)
Caused by invasive salmonellae—see page 26.

CROHN'S DISEASE (REGIONAL ILEITIS)
This is a relapsing inflammatory disorder of areas of the small intestine, usually the terminal ileum; the colon and anus may also be involved. The cause is unknown but there is a familial incidence, the disease affecting mainly young adults.

Symptoms and signs: These include bouts of abdominal pain and diarrhoea, lack of appetite, weight loss and fever. Acute episodes may simulate acute appendicitis with pain and tenderness at the right iliac fossa, and there may be intestinal obstruction with vomiting and a palpable mass or peritonitis.

The stools may contain blood or be fatty (steatorrhoea) with malabsorption of vitamin B_{12} from the lower ileum and anaemia.

Fistulae may occur from bowel to skin or urinary tract.

Diagnosis may be confirmed by narrowing of terminal ileum on barium 'follow-through'.

Treatment: Steroids such as prednisone 10 mg 6-hourly suppress the inflammatory flare-ups through broad spectrum antibiotics such as tetracycline may help if there is secondary infection. Long term steroids may reduce recurrent attacks.

Surgical resection is indicated in severe cases, but the condition may develop in another part of the intestine.

Malabsorption syndrome

This is a group of conditions in which absorption of foods through the small intestine is impaired. Fat absorption is especially impaired, but carbohydrates, proteins, minerals and vitamins are also poorly absorbed, in varying degree.

Steatorrhoea means frequent, pale, greasy, bulky and offensive stools which float in the w.c. and are difficult to flush away. While steatorrhoea is the hallmark of the malabsorption syndrome, it may not be gross—the patient may complain of diarrhoea or may deny that there is anything wrong with his stools.

Causes

A. LESIONS OF THE SMALL INTESTINE

Coeliac disease occurs in children (failure to thrive, 'pot-belly' and rickets).

Coeliac syndrome or *idiopathic steatorrhoea* is the adult equivalent.

These conditions are due to an intolerance to the protein fraction called gluten in wheat and rye flour. The mucosa of the intestine is damaged, the mechanism being uncertain. ('Gluten-induced enteropathy'.)

Tropical sprue occurs in certain zones especially in the Far East, but may persist on return to temperate climates, is confusable with coeliac syndrome but of unknown cause.

Crohn's disease and *infiltrations of the intestine* in conditions such as Hodgkin's disease and blood disorders, tuberculosis, and amyloidosis also cause malabsorption, and vascular insufficiency may do so.

B. LACK OF DIGESTIVE ENZYMES OR BILE SALTS

E.g. chronic pancreatitis and obstructive jaundice. Intestinal lactase deficiency is of importance in causing failure of digestion of lactose (milk-sugar) with resultant intolerance to milk; here, milk and milk products worsen the symptoms.

C. AFTER SURGICAL OPERATIONS

E.g. gastrectomy, massive resections of intestine, and with 'blind-loops' which often harbour bacteria which utilize nutrients and impair digestive action.

D. The parasite Giardia lamblia may cause malabsorption in children.

Symptoms and signs

These include steatorrhoea, weight-loss, anorexia and distended abdomen. Anaemia is a common presentation from deficiency of iron, folic acid and vitamin B_{12}. Other vitamin B deficiencies cause sore red tongue and peripheral neuritis.

Osteomalacia is the adult equivalent of rickets, is due to lack of vitamin D and calcium and causes bone thinning and fractures. Bleeding tendency is due to lack of vitamin K. Oedema and ascites are due to hypoproteinanaemia, and low blood potassium causes further general weakness.

There may be finger-clubbing and dermatitis.

Thus the coeliac syndrome may be present in many ways. The symptoms and signs may also be added to those of the other conditions causing malabsorption. It is noted that steatorrhoea may be marked in chronic pancreatitis, but anaemia is here unusual.

Further investigations

Faecal fat estimation—stools are collected for 3–5 days on a normal ward diet; with steatorrhoea, faecal fat output exceeds 6 G per 24-hours.

Glucose Tolerance Test—in malabsorption the blood sugar curve is 'flat' after 50 G oral glucose, but the test is not reliable in chronic pancreatitis where there may be associated diabetes.

Xylose absorption test—xylose is a sugar which in normal people is absorbed but not metabolized so it is excreted unchanged in the urine. In malabsorption, 25 G is given by mouth and less than 20 per cent appears in the urine in 5-hours.

Barium meal and follow through shows a 'clumping' pattern.

Intestinal biopsy—the Crosby capsule is a small metal capsule attached to a thin plastic tube; the capsule is swallowed, preferably in the evening so as to pass into the small intestine by the next morning, its position being verified on x-ray. A syringe is now attached to the tubing (which has been fixed at the mouth) and suction triggers off a tiny cutting edge in the capsule, into which a minute piece of intestinal mucosa is drawn. The device is now slowly withdrawn through the mouth, and the biopsy specimen examined under a hand-lens or microscope. In coeliac disease and some of the other conditions, the villi, instead of having their usual beautiful feathery appearance are deformed and flattened. Mucosal infiltrations causing malabsorption may also be detected on biopsy.

Other investigations are directed towards the anaemia and include serum levels of iron, folic acid and B_{12}, and the Dicopac (Schilling) test of B_{12} absorption which uses radio-active isotopes.

Mineral-lack may be detected by serum calcium, phosphorus and alkaline phosphatase tests, and by x-rays of bones. The serum potassium may be low. Protein deficiency results in a low serum albumin.

The estimation of pancreatic enzymes and bicarbonate, obtained by duodenal aspirate, is difficult and not carried out as a routine.

Treatment

A. SPECIFIC

Coeliac syndrome is treated by a gluten-free diet; the exclusion of wheat and rye gluten must be absolute; special flour and bread are available. Until the diet takes effect (about 3 weeks in children and 3 months in adults) the undernoted treatment must be given. If the diagnosis is correct, a gluten-free diet will alone suffice subsequently, but it should be given for life, otherwise relapse may occur.

Tropical sprue may settle on folic acid or antibiotics.

The surgical conditions may be cured by reconstruction operations allowing a more normal passage or mixing of food. Malabsorption related to 'blind-loops' may improve on a broad spectrum antibiotic such as tetracycline.

In lactase deficiency milk and milk products must be avoided. Chronic pancreatitis may occasionally be helped by pancreatin (which contains the enzymes) sprinkled on food. Giardia lamblia infection responds to metronidazole (Flagyl) or mepacrine.

B. GENERAL. *Diet*. Diet should be high protein and low fat. Note that milk is the basis of many high protein diets and is undesirable if there is lactase deficiency. Medium chain triglycerides are better absorbed (via the portal system) than ordinary fats and can be given as the beverage Portagen which also contains protein and carbohydrate.

Supplements. Iron is given as ferrous sulphate 200 mg thrice daily or as injections of iron-dextran (Imferon) or iron-sorbitol complex (Jectofer) if there is no response to oral treatment. Folic acid 10 mg daily and hydroxocabalamin (vitamin B_{12}, Neo-cytamen) 1,000 μg injection 2-monthly, may also be required depending on the type of anaemia.

Vitamin B complex by mouth, vitamins K and D by mouth or injection, plus calcium lactate given as the effervescent preparation Sandocal, and potassium supplements may all be necessary.

Malabsorption syndrome is one of the few conditions requiring such 'polypharmacy' when there is not a reversible cause such as coeliac syndrome. Steroids such as prednisone sometimes cause improvement in malabsorption syndrome when all else has failed.

Summary and prognosis

Malabsorption syndrome has steatorrhoea, fatty stools, as its hallmark but steatorrhoea may not be gross and malabsorption should be suspected in patients with weight-loss and evidence of malnutrition or anaemia. Elaborate tests may be necessary to define the cause of malabsorption. Surgical operations on the stomach and intestine, and the coeliac syndrome of gluten-induced enteropathy are the important and treatable causes. Coeliac syndrome responds to a gluten-free diet, which must be continued for life, and the prognosis is good.

Where there is no definite or correctable cause, treatment is based on a low-fat high protein diet, with multiple mineral and vitamin supplements. Milk is the basis of many high protein diets but it will worsen symptoms if there is intestinal lactase deficiency. There is an increased risk of neoplastic change in the small bowel in malabsorption syndrome (neoplasm normally being most unusual). This apart, although the suggested measures in treatment benefit many patients and prevent severe recurrences of steatorrhoea. often the course is a downhill one over months or years.

Carcinoid tumour

Tumours of the small intestine are extremely rare, but it is worth noting the Carcinoid Syndrome—a 'carcinoid' tumour of the small intestine which metastasises to the liver, with the production of large quantities of an amine called serotonin. This is normally concerned in the regulation of vascular tone and in the function of the nervous system. In carcinoid syndrome there is diarrhoea, facial flushing and rashes, and effects on the pulmonary circulation. Diagnosis is confirmed by a raised degradation product of serotonin, 5 HIAA, in the urine. Treatment is unsatisfactory but includes serotonin antagonists such as methysergide (Deseril, used also in migraine), and surgery.

The large intestine (caecum, colon and rectum)

The large intestine is so called because it is of larger diameter than the small intestine but of course it is shorter—starting at the caecum (from which protrudes the appendix) in the right iliac fossa then the ascending, transverse and descending colon, the pelvic or sigmoid colon, rectum and anal sphincter. The external muscular layer is collected into three longitudinal bands which are shorter than the rest of the colon, causing puckering or 'haustration'. The function of the colon is the absorption of water and minerals, converting the intestinal contents to semi-solid faeces, about 150 G daily. The rectum is normally empty, entering faeces causing stimulation and defaecation of the pelvic and descending colon contents. The colon normally contains Esch. coli and large numbers of other bacteria which may cause serious disease in tissues outside the colon. Some bacteria synthesise vitamin B complex and vitamin K, but it is uncertain to what extent absorption occurs in man.

Constipation

Constipation is the infrequent and difficult passage of hard faeces. Most people have a bowel action daily, a normal "habit-time" being after breakfast as the result of the gastro-colic reflex stimulus. There is, however, considerable variation some people normally having a motion only three or four times per week. Many have been brought up to believe that constipation is a fact of life, and urged by the "inner cleanliness" type of advertisement take purgatives regularly— there is usually no need for this.

Causes

Failure to answer the call to stool—this may be due to inadequate time at breakfast, lack of w.c. facilities, forced use of the unpleasant bedpan, or physical weakness in the elderly. Fluid becomes absorbed from the stools in the rectum, resulting in hard motions or faecal impaction.

Abuse of purgatives—after powerful purgation, the whole colon may empty, take a day or two to refill so that further purgation is taken to attempt to produce a motion. The bowel may become dependent on such stimulation, and true constipation follow its withdrawal.

Dietary—a large part of the faeces is in fact of non-dietary origin; however, inadequate bulk in the diet and lack of fluids may cause constipation.

General illness especially febrile illness and bedrest with lack of exercise a possible factor. Depressive states and myxoedema (hypothyroidism) are also causes.

Disorders of the colon

Carcinoma: change in bowel habit, i.e. constipation in someone previously regular should raise suspicions.

Adhesions after operation.

Anal fissure making defaecation painful.

Hirschprung's disease in children, due to lack of nerve cells at the pelvi-rectal junction (analagous to achalasia of the cardia).

Symptoms and effects

The only symptoms of constipation are vague loss of appetite and abdominal discomfort, due to distension and not to 'toxic absorption'. Other symptoms ascribed to constipation are due to anxiety or other causes.

Constipation is, however, important in the elderly for it may result in faecal impaction in the rectum, as noted, and spurious diarrhoea, a little watery faeces being squeezed past the obstruction; impaction may also cause both faecal and urinary incontinence.

A heavy loaded colon may press on pelvic veins, worsening varicose veins in the leg, and possibly contributing to venous thrombosis. Urinary tract infections may be commoner if there is constipation, the mode of infection being uncertain. Straining at stool worsens haemorrhoids and is undesirable in those with cardiac and respiratory disease.

Management

Faecal impaction may require digital removal, a painful and unpleasant procedure before which the patient may be sedated with diazepam. *Enemas* such as the disposable phosphate type, or olive oil, or gentle soap and water, may next be required to clear the rectum and lower bowel of hard faeces. *Suppositories* of glycerine, bisacodyl (Dulcolax) or beogex (which has an effervescent action) may be effective in less severe blockage and are used periodically in the elderly or bedridden patient. It is often wisest to allow old people simply to continue to use a purgative they have been in the habit of taking, to avoid their becoming constipated after admission to hospital.

Retraining of a normal bowel habit is otherwise the objective. This may be achieved by adjustments in the tempo of life, allowing time for proper bowel movement around breakfast time. It may help to *increase the bulk of the diet* and the fluid intake, and foods such as All-Bran may be acceptable. Methylcellulose and proprietary preparations such as Isogel and Normacol act by absorbing water and the increased bulk of the colonic contents allows easy passage of a soft stool. Liquid paraffin acts as a lubricant, but prolonged use prevents the absorbtion of fat-soluble vitamins.

Purgatives (also called laxatives and aperients) are drugs taken by mouth to stimulate defaecation. A senna preparation (Senokot), bisacodyl, dioctyl sodium sulphosuccinate (contained in Dulcodos and Normax with other drugs) and Dorbanex act on the colon, Lactulose (Dulphalac) is a synthetic sugar which is not absorbed but renders the bowel contents more acid, producing a softer stool.

Purgatives should only be used temporarily until bowel regularity is regained—like any drugs, there must be a clear indication for their use, and they should be stopped when the indication no longer exists —this is usually possible except in the elderly. Gross over-use may be complicated by dehydration and potassium deficiency, itself a cause of muscle weakness and constipation.

Purgatives must never be given to patients suffering from acute abdominal conditions such as appendicitis or obstruction for perforation of the bowel and peritonitis may result.

Diarrhoea

Diarrhoea means the passage of frequent or loose stools. After defaecation in some cases there may be a residual feeling of unsatisfactory evacuation or 'tenesmus'.

Causes

A. ACUTE

1. *Gastro-intestinal infections* (see page 25)
   (a) Food poisoning, as part of a gastro-enteritis. Diarrhoea after 'dietary indiscretion' may have such an infective cause, or be due an irritant such as alcohol.
   (b) Typhoid and paratyphoid—pea-soup stools, but constipation in earlier stage.
   (c) Dysentery—stools contain blood and mucus, and often watery.
   (d) Cholera—profuse 'rice-water' stools with little faecal matter.
2. *Melaena* from bleeding peptic ulcer, aspirin ingestion, or oesophageal varices—stools loose, black and tarry.
3. *Excessive use of broad spectrum antibiotics* such as tetracycline, which cause upset in the normal bowel bacterial flora.

B. RECURRENT OR CHRONIC

1. *Small intestine*
   (a) Malabsorption syndrome—steatorrhoea (fatty stools).
   (b) Crohn's disease—stools loose and may contain blood, or steatorrhoea.
2. *Large intestine*—see below
   (a) Irritable colon syndrome.
   (b) Diverticular disease.
   (c) Ulcerative colitis.
   (d) Carcinoma.

3. *General causes*
   Anxiety and 'nerves'.
   Thyrotoxicosis (hyperthyroidism).
   Diabetes—nocturnal diarrhoea.
   Pellagra (a vitamin B factor, nicotinamide, deficiency).

Further investigations

The stool must always be inspected, and sent for bacteriological investigation if there is any suspicion of an infective cause. Occult blood tests and faecal fat estimation may also be required, sigmoidoscopy, barium enema or barium meal and follow through.

Effects of diarrhoea

Severe diarrhoea is debilitating (and may be fatal in infants). Large amounts of fluid, sodium and potassium may be lost leading to hypovolaemia, hypokalaemia, and collapse. Nutrients are lost in the steatorrhoea of malabsorption and blood in melaena.

Management

Treatment is that of the cause.

Mild attacks of food poisoning and dysentery should not be treated with antibiotics, for these may alter the bowel flora and allow superimposed infection with a resistant organism, such as a staphylococcus. Antibiotics may also prolong the carrier stage, and induced resistance to gram-negative organisms may become transferred to previously sensitive organisms, rendering them resistant. Antibiotics are of course specifically indicated for the treatment of typhoid.

For transient diarrhoea, time is the best cure but adsorbent powders such as kaolin or chalk may be given in mixture form, often combined with a small dose of opium. Codeine phosphate 60 mg twice daily for a few days may also be useful.

Severe cases of diarrhoea will in addition require supportive therapy with fluids and electrolytes intravenously as well as by mouth, and such cases, especially in children, should be managed in hospital.

Irritable colon syndrome (spastic colon)

This is an ill-defined disorder presenting as frequency of bowel movement, or urgency after meals—suggested causes include overactive gastrocolic reflex, intestinal hurry from lactase deficiency (when removing milk from the diet may help) and disturbance of motility of the large bowel, and anxiety. The motility disturbance of the colon merges into the condition of diverticular disease, and treatment is similar.

Diverticular disease of the colon

Diverticulosis is the presence of colonic diverticula—little out-pouchings of mucous membrane through the muscular wall, where blood vessels enter, of the pelvic and descending colon, but the whole colon may be involved. The cause is a disturbance of motility, often with muscle thickening, related possibly to the anxiety and tension of Western civilization, with *lack* of bulk in the diet, for the disorder is rare in under-developed countries. Diverticula are seen commonly in barium enemas of the bowel in the elderly, and may cause no symptoms.

Diverticular disease may result from the motility disturbance, or the diverticula. *Symptoms and signs* include abdominal discomfort colicky pain at the left lower abdomen, altered bowel habit and episodes of constipation or large bowel obstruction, with distension and later vomiting.

Diverticulitis is acute inflammation of the diverticulum with its complications. *Symptoms and signs* are acute pain in the left iliac fossa, tenderness, fever and malaise. A mass may become palpable from peridiverticular abscess, and there may be perforation with peritonitis, or fistula formation.

Further investigation may include barium enema. It may be difficult or impossible to differentiate the symptoms or findings from those of carcinoma.

Treatment of diverticular disease

The diet must be of adequate bulk (*not* a low-residue diet as previously recommended) to allow regular bowel actions—Isogel may be a helpful addition. Episodes of mild constipation can be treated with lactulose or a mild purgative such as Senokot, but strong purgatives and enemas are dangerous.

Anticholinergics such as propantheline (Probanthine) or the bowel antispasmodic mebeverine (Colofac) may relieve colicky pains; codeine phosphate 30 mg may help diarrhoea, but some authorities claim it worsens spasm, and morphine is dangerous.

Diverticulitis is treated with bed rest, a fluid diet initially and pethidine 100 mg to relieve pain. A broad spectrum antibiotic such as tetracycline is given orally or intravenously. Severe rectal bleeding

Where there is no definite or correctable cause, treatment is based on a low-fat high protein diet, with multiple mineral and vitamin supplements. Milk is the basis of many high protein diets but it will worsen symptoms if there is intestinal lactase deficiency. There is an increased risk of neoplastic change in the small bowel in malabsorption syndrome (neoplasm normally being most unusual). This apart, although the suggested measures in treatment benefit many patients and prevent severe recurrences of steatorrhoea. often the course is a downhill one over months or years.

Carcinoid tumour

Tumours of the small intestine are extremely rare, but it is worth noting the Carcinoid Syndrome—a 'carcinoid' tumour of the small intestine which metastasises to the liver, with the production of large quantities of an amine called serotonin. This is normally concerned in the regulation of vascular tone and in the function of the nervous system. In carcinoid syndrome there is diarrhoea, facial flushing and rashes, and effects on the pulmonary circulation. Diagnosis is confirmed by a raised degradation product of serotonin, 5 HIAA, in the urine. Treatment is unsatisfactory but includes serotonin antagonists such as methysergide (Deseril, used also in migraine), and surgery.

The large intestine (caecum, colon and rectum)

The large intestine is so called because it is of larger diameter than the small intestine but of course it is shorter—starting at the caecum (from which protrudes the appendix) in the right iliac fossa then the ascending, transverse and descending colon, the pelvic or sigmoid colon, rectum and anal sphincter. The external muscular layer is collected into three longitudinal bands which are shorter than the rest of the colon, causing puckering or 'haustration'. The function of the colon is the absorption of water and minerals, converting the intestinal contents to semi-solid faeces, about 150 G daily. The rectum is normally empty, entering faeces causing stimulation and defaecation of the pelvic and descending colon contents. The colon normally contains Esch. coli and large numbers of other bacteria which may cause serious disease in tissues outside the colon. Some bacteria synthesise vitamin B complex and vitamin K, but it is uncertain to what extent absorption occurs in man.

including skin sepsis and abscesses, erythema nodosum, arthritis (which may involve spinal joints, spondylitis), iritis, liver inflammation and cirrhosis, and a tendency to venous thrombosis.

Ulcerative colitis should be distinguished from Crohn's disease which sometimes affects the colon but spares the rectum, and ischaemic colitis in the elderly causing transient bloody diarrhoea.

Further investigations

Stool bacteriology—to exclude infections.

Sigmoidoscopy—this is an examination with a tube inserted through the rectum, and it must be done gently to avoid perforating inflamed mucosa. The mucosa is red, granular and bleeds easily and there may be mucus or a muco-purulent exudate.

Barium enema shows an irregular or ulcerated mucosal pattern, loss of haustrations, and in late stages a tube-like colon. Straight x-ray may show toxic dilatation in acute cases.

Blood examination may show anaemia, raised white cell count and E.S.R., and fluid and electrolyte depletion, especially a low potassium, from prolonged diarrhoea.

Treatment

A confident approach to the patient.

The patient may have been embarrassed or even disgusted by her symptoms. Kindness and understanding relieve her distress and an attitude of reassurance is a most important contribution to therapy.

Rest in bed is indicated in severe cases, but there should be easy access to the toilet, commode or bedpan. It may be preferable to nurse the patient in a side room until symptoms improve. Diazepam (Valium) 10 mg thrice daily may relieve anxiety.

Diet. This must be adequate in fluids, and in nutritive value. It is more important to allow an acceptable light diet with adequate protein than to insist on a low-residue regime, which is of dubious value though husky foods and fruit pips should be avoided in the acute stages. Indeed, some increse in bulk or a preparation such as Isogel may allow a formed stool later. Intolerance to milk may only be discovered by trial and error but is probably not common. Potassium supplements and vitamins may be indicated. Oral iron is irritant and should be avoided in the acute stages.

Specific drug therapy

Steroids are most useful in inducing remission, and are therefore indicated in the acute stages.

Rectal steroids. Hydrocortisone 100 mg dissolved in 120 ml warm water or saline is given by rectal drip, using an intravenous giving set, with the patient lying flat. If given slowly over 15–30 minutes retention for a few hours is possible, with good effect. The procedure is initially carried out night and morning. Prednisolone phosphate retention enemas (e.g. Predsol) are an alternative, but the hydrocortisone rectal drip is usually better retained in the acute stages. Prednisolone suppositories can be used later.

Oral steriods. Prednisone or prednisolone, 10–15 mg 6-hourly is also given, the dose being reduced within a week or ten days, when improvement has occurred.

Sulphasalazine (Salazopyrin) is a sulphonamide preparation taken up by the large bowel. It may be beneficial in mild attacks but is most useful in long treatment to prevent relapses. It is started in dosage of 1·0 G 4-times daily as the steroids are being tailed off, and continued in a dose of 0·5 G 3 or 4 times daily for a year. Sulphasalazine may cause gastric irritation and an enteric-coated tablet is available.

Propantheline and codeine may be used to attempt to relieve the diarrhoea, but are seldom effective.

Ulcerative colitis is not an infective process, and oral antibiotics should not be given, for they may worsen diarrhoea. Injectable antibiotics may, however, be required for complications such as abscesses.

Intravenous therapy—fluids, potassium and steroids, and *blood transfusion* may be required in fulminating cases.

The majority of attacks of ulcerative colitis settle if the above medical measures are applied promptly and efficiently, and recurrences may be prevented by sulphasalazine.

Surgical treatment

Surgical treatment should be considered in acute fulminating ulcerative colitis which is not responding to medical measures, in patients with many debilitating recurrences, and in longstanding cases with total involvement of the colon and risk of carcinoma. It is usually possible to improve the patient's general state sufficiently to permit operation, with measures such as intravenous therapy and blood transfusion, and if the indications are clear, many surgeons believe that operation should not be delayed too long. The operation is total colectomy (removal of the large bowel) and ileostomy (exteriorization of the ileum, its contents being discharged through the skin-opening). This sounds a drastic procedure, but the results are often gratifying, the patient's general condition and nutrition improving markedly after removal of the diseased large bowel. Patients adapt well to ileostomy, and with the convenience of adhesive, plastic disposable bags, can lead normal lives with full activity.

Carcinoma of the rectum and colon

Carcinoma of the large bowel is common, causing some 15,000 deaths annually in Britain, and therefore being second only to carcinoma of the bronchus in terms of mortality from cancer. The disease is most frequent in the middle-aged and elderly, but can occur in young people.

Symptoms and signs

Cancer of the rectum is commonest, symptoms include bleeding (often mistakenly ascribed to piles) and change of bowel habit, often with diarrhoea and passage of slime. The cancer may be palpable with the finger on rectal examination.

Cancer of the pelvic colon presents similarly.

In the descending and transverse colon, the change of bowel habit is likely to present as constipation rather than diarrhoea, and there may be stricture and obstruction with abdominal distension and later vomiting.

Growths in the caecum and ascending colon may be silent, the complaint being of vague deterioration in health, weight loss, and weakness from anaemia due to occult bleeding.

A mass may become palpable in colonic cancer in later stages. Sometimes the growth presents as metastases in the liver with jaundice, or as ascites.

Further investigations include stool tests for occult blood, sigmoidoscopy and barium enema. Blood examination may show anaemia and raised E.S.R. Laparotomy (surgical exploration of the abdomen) may be indicated in suspicious cases even when barium enema is negative.

Treatment and prognosis

Surgical resection of the affected segment of bowel is indicated where possible, and the prognosis may be good if the growth has been entirely removed. In elderly patients too weak for major surgery, colostomy is a palliative measure; the carcinoma may grow or spread only slowly, the patient succumbing to another condition.

The acute abdomen

Management of conditions such as bleeding peptic ulcer, pyloric stenosis and ulcerative colitis requires co-operation between medical and surgical disciplines. There is much to be said for admitting patients with such disorders to a unit combining these disciplines and supported by x-ray, clinical pathology and blood transfusion facilities.

When confronted with a patient with abdominal pain and vomiting the decision as to whether the condition is a 'surgical' one requiring operation may not be possible without careful observation and charting of pulse and temperature. Diabetic ketosis may present with abdominal pain and vomiting, operation is lethal in this situation, and the urine must be routinely tested for sugar and ketones to exclude it. Analgesics to relieve pain may obfuscate diagnosis of the acute abdomen, and should only be given when the course of management has been decided. In doubtful cases, it may be necessary to proceed to laparotomy. The following are some acute surgical conditions to be borne in mind.

Acute appendicitis is commonest in children and young adults, but may occur in the elderly. There is central abdominal discomfort followed by pain, tenderness and muscle guarding at the right iliac fossa, slight vomiting and raised pulse and temperature, but pyrexia may not be marked. Treatment is appendicectomy. Mesenteric adenitis is an inflammation of abdominal lymph glands in children and may have similar symptoms but these settle spontaneously.

Perforated peptic ulcer causes severe upper abdominal pain, tenderness and rigidity and has been considered above. *Acute cholecystitis, biliary colic*, and *acute pancreatitis* cause abdominal pain, and *renal colic* causes pain in loin or iliac fossa—these conditions are described in later chapters.

Ruptured ectopic pregnancy is a 'gynaecological' emergency; pregnancy has occurred in the ovarian tube instead of the uterus, the tube ruptures in the early weeks causing severe lower abdominal pain and usually vaginal bleeding. There is a history of a missed period. *Salpingitis*, inflammation of the ovarian tubes, is another cause of pain.

Intussusception is an invagination of one length of intestine into another; it occurs in infants, and in adults in association with a lesion such as a polyp or carcinoma. There is pain, vomiting, bloody diarrhoea and palpable mass. In infants barium enema investigation may cause spontaneous cure but generally operation is necessary.

Intestinal obstruction has many possible causes—herniae caught at the inguinal and femoral canals, adhesions from previous operations, carcinoma, mesenteric arterial thrombosis causing ischaemia and stasis, or volvulus (sudden twisting) of the bowel in the elderly. Symptoms include pain and vomiting, but if the large bowel is involved vomiting may not be marked and there is constipation. The abdomen becomes distended and 'fluid levels' are seen on x-ray. Treatment is surgical relief of the obstruction except in early mesenteric thrombosis where conservative management includes suction by nasogastric tube and intravenous fluid replacement.

Paralytic ileus is an atony of the small intestine post-operatively or complicating intestinal obstruction or peritonitis. Secretions continue to be poured into the intestine, which is unable to pass its contents onwards or to absorb them. The patient becomes increasingly dehydrated, with hypotension and collapse. Nasogastric suction and intravenous fluids and antibiotics are required until the causative condition is relieved or intestinal motility is re-established.

Peritonitis may complicate any of these conditions and is considered below.

Disorders of the peritoneum

The peritoneal membrane of the abdomen is similar to the pleural membrane of the thorax. The visceral layer of peritoneum covers the intestines and is not sensitive to pain, the parietal layer lines the abdominal wall and is pain-sensitive. The peritoneal cavity is the potential space between the two layers. A large fold of peritoneum called the greater omentum is spread like an apron over the intestines, separating them from the anterior wall of the abdomen.

PERITONITIS

Peritonitis is inflammation of the peritoneum. Just as pleurisy is usually a consequence of disease of the lungs, so peritonitis results from spread of inflammation from abdominal or pelvic organs. It is usually a 'surgical' condition complicating the disorders discussed above.

Symptoms and signs are pain, tenderness and muscle guarding, which may remain localized by the 'policeman' action of the greater omentum, with subsequent healing or abscess formation, or the peritonitis may become generalized with rapid pulse, pyrexia and toxaemia from infection. Gram-negative septicaemia causes circulatory failure and collapse. Paralytic ileus (described above) may worsen an already desperate situation.

Treatment is with antibiotics (ampicillin, carbenicillin and/or kanamycin may be required), nasogastric suction, intravenous fluids and surgery if appropriate. Hydrocortisone in massive dosage may afford circulatory support in collapsed cases.

Pneumococcal and tuberculous peritonitis are now rare—the latter occurred in children from infection with bovine (milk-borne) type tubercle bacilli. These conditions respond to penicillin and anti-tuberculous drugs (streptomycin, isoniazid and P.A.S.) respectively.

Infection may be introduced by careless paracentesis, patients with cirrhosis of the liver and ascites being especially at risk.

ASCITES
Ascites is the presence of fluid in the peritoneal cavity.

Causes

Congestive cardiac failure—here ascites is part of the generalized oedema from fluid retention.

Nephrotic syndrome (renal disease with albuminuria and oedema).

Cirrhosis of the liver—ascites is here due to low plasma albumin and raised portal venous pressure, causing fluid exudation into the peritoneal cavity.

Malignant ascites—from peritoneal metastases in carcinoma of stomach, large intestine or ovary.

Symptoms and signs

There is abdominal distension, but this is not marked in early stages. Here there is dullness to percussion over the flanks, the dullness shifting when the patient is asked to roll to one side. With increasing ascites the umbilicus becomes everted and the abdomen tense and uncomfortable.

Diagnostic tap may be required in suspected malignant ascites, a specimen of fluid being sent for cytology for malignant cells. The fluid may be blood-stained and often accumulates rapidly in such cases.

Treatment

Treatment is that of the cause. Diuretics such as frusemide, bendrofluazide and spironolactone are effective in relieving the ascites associated with cardiac failure or nephrotic syndrome, and are usually effective in cirrhosis; here it is important to give potassium supplements. Paracentesis may be required in a few cases of cirrhosis, but should generally be avoided as the procedure depletes the body of protein, and it may also precipitate hepatic coma.

Diuretics are of little value in malignant ascites and paracentesis may be required to afford the patient relief of discomfort. Cytotoxic drugs of the nitrogen-mustard group may be instilled into the peritoneal cavity in an attempt to prevent recurrence of malignant effusions. However, the prognosis in such cases is usually poor, treatment being largely palliative, with proper use of opiates to prevent pain and alleviate suffering.

Intestinal worms

Threadworms, roundworms and tapeworms have been considered on page 33.

7

Disorders of the liver, biliary tract and pancreas

Anatomy of the liver and biliary tract

The *liver*, the largest organ in the body, is wedge-shaped, and occupies the uppermost right part of the abdomen immediately below the diaphragm, sheltered by the ribs. The *portal vein* carries to it the food products absorbed in the intestine, and it receives arterial blood from the hepatic artery. The hepatic veins are behind the liver and discharge their blood into the inferior vena cava just below the diaphragm.

The hepatic duct carries *bile* from the liver and joins the cystic duct from the gall bladder to form the *common bile duct*. This usually unites with the main pancreatic duct just before opening into the second part of the duodenum. The *gall bladder* is a pear-shaped bag on the under-surface of the liver opposite the anterior end of the ninth costal cartilage. It stores and concentrates the bile.

Most of the liver cells are specialized *hepatic cells*, but the liver also contains cells of the *reticulo-endothelial system*. The reticulo-endo-thelial system includes cells in the spleen, liver, lymph nodes and bone marrow. It has a scavenger function for worn out cells and foreign material, and a function in the immunity mechanism, producing the immune globulins or antibodies. Thus the liver may become involved in blood diseases such as leukaemia and Hodgkin's disease.

Functions of the liver

1. *Metabolism and storage*

Carbohydrates are metabolized, and glucose stored as glycogen.

Proteins are synthesized from amino-acids. Thus the liver makes plasma-albumin and prothrombin, which is necessary for blood coagulation; vitamin K is required for its synthesis. In protein breakdown, ammonia is formed and is converted by the liver to urea which is excreted by the kidneys in the urine.

Fats are catabolized to fatty acids which provide a reserve source of energy when glucose metabolism is upset as in diabetic ketosis.

Vitamins A, D and B_{12} are stored in the liver.

2. *Detoxification*

The liver renders harmless the body's waste products. It also destroys toxic substances and drugs, or conjugates them chemically to prevent their further action and allowing their excretion in the urine or, in some cases, into the bile.

3. *Bile secretion*

The liver produces the bile salts, which by their 'detergent' action, cause the emulsification of dietary fats into small globules for digestion by pancreatic lipase in the intestine. Bile salts are necessary for the absorption of the fat-soluble vitamins A, D and K. Bile also contains bile pigment, bilirubin, which has no digestive function, but gives bile its colour.

Bilirubin metabolism. The red blood cells become worn out in 120 days, when they are taken up by cells of the reticulo-endothelial system. The haemoglobin is broken down, globin joins the protein pool; iron is detached from the haem and retained for further use; the remainder of the haem molecule goes to form bilirubin. At this stage bilirubin is insoluble in water. It is carried by the bloodstream to the liver where it is taken up by the hepatic cells, rendered water-soluble by conjugation and excreted as bile pigment, passing to the intestine, and becoming responsible for the brown colour of normal faeces. In the colon part of the bilirubin is converted by bacterial action to a colourless derivative called stercobilinogen or urobilinogen some of which is absorbed into the portal circulation to reach the liver. A healthy liver re-excretes urobilinogen into the biliary tract, but a small amount is passed through into the general circulation to be excreted by the kidneys in the urine. It should be clearly understood that *bilirubin* does not normally appear in the urine, but a tiny amount of colourless *urobilinogen* is present.

Jaundice

Jaundice is a yellow discoloration of the tissues due to excess bilirubin in the blood. Jaundice is often first noticed in the skin of the abdomen, or in the sclera (white part) of the eyes, but an observant nurse may note it in the plasma when reading an E.S.R.

Types

1. *Pre-hepatic—excessive production of bilirubin*

This is Haemolytic Jaundice or Haemolytic Anaemia, from abnormal red-cell destruction, considered further in Diseases of the Blood, Chapter 9. It is also known as Acholuric Jaundice, and it is worth remembering this term—'a' means 'without' and 'chol' means bile, i.e. there is *no bile* in the urine. This is because bilirubin is not water-soluble when just formed from red-cells. Because of the large amount of bilirubin reaching the colon in haemolytic jaundice, much urobilinogen is formed and reabsorbed, overwhelming the excretory capacity of the liver, so that an excess of urobilinogen appears in the urine. As noted, urobilinogen is colourless, and though an orange hue may develop in the urine on standing, urobilinogen can only be detected by special test—see below.

2. *Hepatic*

This is due to disordered function of the liver cells. It is caused by infections, such as hepatitis, poisons such as carbon tetrachloride (used in dry-cleaning and as a fire extinguisher) and benzene (a solvent), drugs (see below) and by some rare familial diseases. Depending on the degree of swelling and obstruction to bile outflow, the stools may be normal in colour or pale. Reabsorption of bilirubin rendered water-soluble by passage through the liver causes bile to appear in the urine. In the early stages of liver cell dysfunction, the capacity of the liver to re-excrete urobilinogen is one of the first functions to be impaired. Urobilinogen is at this stage detectable in the urine. In later stages with complete obstruction to the outflow of bile, no bile reaches the colon, so that urobilinogen cannot be formed.

3. *Post-hepatic or Obstructive Jaundice*

This is due to blockage of the bile duct by a *stone* from the gall bladder, or by *carcinoma of the head of the pancreas*. The jaundice is deep and the skin often itchy (possibly an effect of bile salts). The stools are pale and clay coloured, the urine dark brown from the presence of bile pigment, bilirubin. As bilirubin has not been able to reach the colon, urobilinogen cannot be formed and is absent from the urine in obstructive jaundice.

Effect

The bilirubin in the tissues is not in itself harmful in adults. In haemolytic disease of the newborn (which is due to Rhesus factor antibodies and is now preventable) the excess bilirubin is toxic to the infant brain.

In obstructive jaundice fat digestion is impaired and vitamin K cannot be absorbed. Prothrombin manufacture may also be impaired by hepatic jaundice. Failure of blood coagulation and bruising tendency results.

Summary of findings in jaundice

Type	Causes	Degree	Stool Colour	Urine Bilirubin (Bile Pigment)	Urine Urobilinogen
Pre-hepatic	Haemolytic Anaemia	Mild	Normal (or dark)	Absent	Excess
Hepatic	Virus hepatitis Drugs (also carcinoma, and rare familial)	Variable	Normal or Pale	Present	Increased then absent
Post-hepatic ('Obstructive')	Stone in Bile-duct Carcinoma of head of pancreas	Deep (+itch)	Pale	Present	Absent

Management

Jaundice is a sign, not a disease. The cause of the jaundice must therefore be sought from a consideration of the history, physical examination and findings in the stools, urine and blood-serial tests may be required. The importance of drugs as a cause of jaundice cannot be overstressed.

While the diet is traditionally a low-fat one, there is no evidence that fats are harmful, but jaundiced patients usually do not desire fatty foods. Vitamin K 10 mg daily by intramuscular injection should be given in prolonged jaundice. Cholestyramine, a resin which absorbs bile salts, may relieve pruritus in partial obstructive jaundice.

Surgery is indicated for relief of biliary obstruction due to a gallstone, and a palliative operation may be possible in carcinoma of the head of the pancreas. Patients with hepatic jaundice fare badly if operated on—proper evaluation should prevent this.

Urine tests

Bilirubin (Bile pigment) gives a brown colour to the urine, and on shaking in a test-tube, the froth is yellowish.

Ictotest tablets or *Bili-Labstix* reagent strips confirm presence of bilirubin.

Urobilinogen is colourless. Ehrlich's aldehyde reagent added to the urine causes a pink colour if excess urobilinogen is present. *Urobilistix* reagent strips may be used.

Further investigations in diseases of the liver and biliary tract

Liver function tests

These are carried out on a blood specimen obtained by venepuncture. They include serum bilirubin, proteins and enzymes. Techniques for proteins include paper strip electrophoresis and immuno-electrophoresis. Certain enzymes such as S.G.P.T. are raised in liver cell dysfunction—it will be recalled that similar tests are helpful in myocardial infarction. The serum alkaline phosphatase is raised in obstructive jaundice.

Liver biopsy

Using local anaesthetic, a special needle is inserted between the right lower ribs in the mid-axillary line, and passed into the liver from which a small specimen is withdrawn for microscopical examination. This investigation is contra-indicated if the patient has a bleeding tendency or is severely jaundiced.

Cholecystography—x-ray examination of the gall bladder

If a substance which is excreted by the liver into the bile also contains iodine, it will become radio-opaque when concentrated by a normal gall bladder, allowing demonstration of the latter on x-ray. The patient is given tablets of such an iodine compound (e.g. Telepaque or Solubiloptin) in the evening, no food overnight, and x-ray in the

morning should show the gall bladder shadow. Further films after
a fatty meal containing egg yolk will show contraction of a normal
gall bladder.

The biliary tract may also be visualized radiologically by intravenous biligrafin. Such investigations are, however, unsatisfactory
in a jaundiced patient.

Portal venography

This is carried out in special centres. A radio-opaque substance is
injected into the spleen and absorbed into the splenic vein, a tributary
of the portal vein, allowing x-ray demonstration of the portal venous
system.

Liver scanning is also possible using radio-active isotopes.

Diet and the liver

In underdeveloped countries protein malnutrition in infants causes
kwashiorkor, a condition characterized by oedema, diarrhoea and
liver swelling. It is possible that an extremely protein-deficient
diet in adults predisposes to liver damage with fatty infiltration and
fibrosis or even massive necrosis. Amino-acid supplements prevent
this in the experimental situation, but in practice it is better to ensure
an adequate normal diet.

The liver may be exposed to naturally occurring toxins in foods,
especially in the tropics where concoctions such as 'bush teas' are
taken. Again, fungal contamination of ground nuts produces a liver
poison called aflatoxin. Parasitic infestation further lowers resistance
and the virus or antigen associated with hepatitis may be more
persistent in the blood. Liver disease is therefore common in the
tropics.

In temperate climates alcohol is an important liver toxin, both by
a direct action on liver cells and indirectly from the effects of the
dietary deficiencies incurred by the alcoholic who neglects or cannot
afford a proper diet.

Drugs and the liver

Drug detoxification

If liver function is impaired drugs normally destroyed by the liver
may reach toxic concentrations in the bloodstream. Morphine and
barbiturates (excluding phenobarbitone which is excreted unchanged
in the urine) are such drugs and they must not be given to patients
suffering from disorders of the liver.

Enzyme stimulation (*Induction*)

It has recently been noted that certain drugs, e.g. phenobarbitone, may stimulate the detoxicating function of the liver, a process called enzyme induction. If another drug is given simultaneously it will be destroyed more quickly and have less clinical effect. Thus if a patient is receiving phenobarbitone as a sedative and is put on anticoagulants, these will have a lesser effect on blood clotting, and a higher dose will be ordered; if the phenobarbitone is subsequently stopped and the same dose of anticoagulants continued, bleeding may result.

It is important to be aware of such possible interactions when several potent drugs are being used.

Jaundice due to drugs

The mechanisms of drug-induced jaundice are complex. Substances such as carbon tetrachloride (used in dry-cleaning and in fire extinguishers), chloroform, and benzene are directly toxic, causing liver-cell necrosis, and very high concentrations of tetracycline and paracetamol may have a similar effect. The anaesthetic halothane if used repeatedly, and the mono-amine-oxidase inhibitors, used in treatment of depressive illness, may cause a hepatitis-like jaundice. Chlorpromazine (Largactil) and its derivatives, oral contraceptives and sex-hormones may cause a less severe sensitivity (cholestatic) jaundice, which clears when the drug is stopped.

In any patient with obscure jaundice, the possibility of a drug cause must be borne in mind.

Drug-induced bleeding

Anticoagulants such as warfarin and phenindione act by competing with vitamin K in the liver, lowering the production of prothrombin and other clotting factors. Large doses of aspirin have a similar action and may cause bleeding. (Another cause of drug-induced bleeding is platelet destruction from toxic effects on the bone marrow.)

Virus hepatitis—infectious hepatitis and serum hepatitis

Cause and mode of infection

Infectious hepatitis is caused by a virus present in the patient's stools and transmitted by faecal contamination of food or water. Cases may occur sporadically or in epidemics where hygiene is poor, and have followed the eating of shellfish from sewage-polluted waters. The incubation period is about 30 days. Jaundice is the hallmark of the infection but may be mild, and many cases go undiagnosed. The faeces are infective from about two weeks before to two weeks after the onset of jaundice. Infectious hepatitis is commonest in children and young adults.

Serum hepatitis is caused by a virus, possibly the same virus, in blood or blood products. Infection is spread usually by blood transfusion or by injection from contaminated syringes and needles. The incubation period is up to 120 days. Adults are mainly affected, the illness frequently being more severe than infectious hepatitis.

The blood of patients with serum hepatitis (and some with infectious hepatitis in the early stages) contains an antigen related to the presence of the virus. This antigen is called the hepatitis-associated antigen (or Australia antigen as it was first found in the serum of an aborigine) and may persist for many years, possibly due to deficiency of the immunity mechanism. The person's blood therefore remains infective although he is symptom-free. Outbreaks of serum hepatitis have occurred in renal dialysis units where much blood is used, but the screening of blood donors for the presence of the antigen may eliminate this risk.

Drug addicts who give themselves intravenous injections are at risk from contaminated syringes.

The virus is destroyed by autoclaving or dry heat sterilization but a better preventive measure is the use of disposable equipment where possible, and the avoidance of blood transfusion unless there is a clear indication for its use.

Gamma-globulin prophylaxis

Injections of this immune globulin may prevent the development of infectious hepatitis after exposure in epidemics. This measure is indicated in pregnant women. Gamma-globulin prophylaxis is of less value in serum hepatitis.

Symptoms and signs

Loss of appetite, malaise and generalized aches, fever, nausea and vomiting occur for a few days before jaundice becomes manifest. There may be abdominal discomfort with liver swelling and tenderness. The condition usually settles in a week or ten days.

Fulminating cases develop deep jaundice and high fever and may go into hepatic failure and coma, considered below.

Though liver cell function returns to normal over some weeks in most patients, mental depression is often marked. A very few cases have persistent liver dysfunction and may develop active chronic hepatitis or cirrhosis.

The stools become pale during hepatitis; the urine may contain excess urobilinogen in the earliest stages, but with liver cell swelling and obstruction to bile outflow this disappears and the urine becomes dark due to the presence of bilirubin, which clears as the jaundice lessens. The liver function tests in the blood are also abnormal.

Treatment

Mild cases of infectious hepatitis may be managed at home. As the stools are infective from before the onset of jaundice, other members of the household may have had contact with the infection and it is too late for isolation measures. Patients admitted to hospital should have modified barrier nursing, with access to their own toilet; alternatively, stools must be carefully disposed of, and proper hand-washing is essential to prevent the spread of infection.

Bed rest is indicated in the acute and febrile stages, and was formerly recommended until the jaundice cleared, but young patients who feel well may be allowed up despite the presence of jaundice. Patients tire easily, however, and proper rest is important for some weeks, then gradual resumption of normal activities.

Diet is traditionally a low-fat one but there is no benefit in the rigid exclusion of fats. Patients generally prefer a light diet, high in carbohydrate such as glucose drinks. With recovery, appetite is often voracious, and normal diet, with adequate protein is resumed. Vitamin supplements are not necessary. Alcohol should be avoided for at least six months.

Drugs are seldom needed, and sedatives are best avoided. Steroids lower the serum bilirubin in hepato-cellular jaundice, and this 'steroid whitewash' has been used in differential diagnosis from obstructive jaundice. Steroids do not, however, generally affect the underlying liver cell damage but may be tried in fulminating cases with risk of hepatic failure, considered below.

Other infections of the liver

GLANDULAR FEVER (INFECTIOUS MONONUCLEOSIS). Jaundice from liver involvement may occur in gladular fever.

WEIL'S DISEASE (LEPTOSPIROSIS). This is an infection of the liver and kidneys with an organism from the groups known as leptospira or the spirochaetes (syphilis is caused by a different spirochaete). The organism infects rats, is excreted in rat urine, and human infection occurs by eating contaminated food, or through abrasions in the skin. Workers in rat-infested mines, sewers, canals and in occupations such as fish-gutting are at risk. Symptoms include fever, jaundice and haematuria (blood in the urine). Penicillin may be effective if given early. Severe cases with renal failure require dialysis.

A similar but milder infection may be contracted from dogs (canicola fever).

TROPICAL DISEASES. The malaria parasite invades the liver, but usually it is the red-cell destruction that is clinically significant. Amoebiasis may cause swelling and liver abscess. Yellow fever is a virus infection (transmitted by mosquitoes) of liver, kidneys and heart. Schistosomiasis, a parasitic infection transmitted by water snails, is common in Egypt. Liver fluke infestation may follow ingestion of water-cress contaminated by sheep. A hydatid cyst, is due to the larval or cyst stage of infection by a tapeworm of dogs, and occurs where man has close contact with dogs, as in sheep-rearing countries.

Acute liver abscesses

Suppuration in the pelvis, e.g. appendicitis with abscess formation, may spread via the portal system of veins, portal pylephlebitis, to cause infection and abscesses in the liver.

Cholangitis, infection of the bile duct related to gall-stones or carcinoma, may also spread upwards to involve the liver; there is pain, high fever and jaundice.

These conditions are now uncommon, due to prompt management of the causative infections. Antibacterial drugs are indicated, and surgical drainage may be required.

Active chronic hepatitis

This occurs in young women and may follow virus hepatitis, but usually arises without such a history. There is persistent or recurrent jaundice over months or years. Other organs are involved including the joints and lungs, and the disorder may be a disturbance of immunity, the hepatitis-associated antigen playing a part. Corticosteroids or immuno-suppressive drugs may improve symptoms, but the prognosis is often poor, cases tending to go on to liver cell failure.

Cirrhosis of the liver

Cirrhosis is diffuse fibrosis of the liver with areas of nodular regeneration. The word cirrhosis is derived from a Greek word meaning tawny, the colour that the liver may acquire in this condition.

Types

There are two main types, portal cirrhosis and biliary cirrhosis.

Portal cirrhosis is the commoner type and is a disease of middle-aged men. The patient is not usually jaundiced (except terminally), the brunt of the trouble affecting the portal venous system, though the liver cells are also involved.

The term 'cirrhosis' used alone implies portal cirrhosis, described in detail below.

Biliary cirrhosis is associated with obstruction to bile outflow, cholestasis, which may be primary from intrahepatic disease or secondary from extrahepatic biliary obstruction, and the patients are jaundiced.

Primary biliary cirrhosis occurs in middle-aged women. The cause is unknown; like active chronic hepatitis, it may be a disturbance of immunity to hepatitis-associated antigen and certain antibodies are detectable in the blood. There is jaundice with dark urine and pale stools, and severe pruritus (which may be alleviated by cholestyramine). Treatment is unsatisfactory, and though steroids may be of temporary benefit, the course is a downhill one with liver cell failure and death in a few years.

Secondary biliary cirrhosis occurs if bile-duct obstruction from stone, stricture, or carcinoma goes unrelieved for months or years Improvement may follow surgical relief of the obstruction.

Portal cirrhosis

Causes

1. *Alcoholism*—the commonest cause in many countries although not in Britain.
2. *Dietary deficiencies* and effects of toxins and parasites especially in the tropics.
3. Following *virus hepatitis* but this usually resolves completely.
4. Right sided heart failure and constrictive pericarditis if untreated.
5. Rare diseases with liver fibrosis—haemochromatosis (bronzed

6—EM

diabetes) from iron deposition in pancreas and liver, and hepato-lenticular degeneration (Wilson's disease) from copper deposits in the liver and basal ganglia of the brain.

In many patients the cause is unknown.

Symptoms and signs

Cirrhosis is a chronic disease of insidious onset in middle-age, the type related to alcoholism being commoner in men than in women. Complaints include vague ill-health, anorexia and mild fever. The disease is suspected by the finding of an enlarged liver (especially in alcoholic cirrhosis, but in other cases the organ is shrunken from fibrosis) and enlarged spleen.

The clinical features are due to the two main effects of cirrhosis *portal hypertension* and *liver cell dysfunction.*

Portal hypertension. The liver fibrosis causes obstruction to the portal vein and back pressure on its tributaries. Distension occurs where veins of the portal system anastomose with the systemic veins, causing varicose veins at the lower end of the oesophagus, dilated vessels in the abdominal wall near the umbilicus and splenic enlargement. *Haematemesis* occurs from ruptured oesophageal varices, though bleeding may occur from peptic ulcer or gastric erosions commonly associated with alcoholism; anaemia is common. Splenic enlargement may inhibit the release of cells from the bone marrow (which remains active) resulting in deficiency of platelets causing bleeding, and of white cells with increased susceptibility to infections.

Liver cell dysfunction is associated with the appearance of vascular spiders on the face, neck and arms. These are little red spots consisting of a dilated arteriole from which tiny vessels radiate. The skin of the palms of the hands is pink, contrasting with the muddy colour of the skin as a whole in cirrhosis. These and circulatory disturbances may relate to disturbed hormone balance. Failure of prothrombin production is another cause of bleeding tendency.

Ascites is common, from the combined effects of portal hypertension and reduced serum albumin in the blood. Albumin normally maintains the osmotic pressure, the 'holding force' by which fluid is retained in the circulation. The leakage of fluid from the bloodstream to form ascites lowers the blood volume, and compensatory mechanisms to retain fluid in the body come into operation; these include secretion of the adrenal cortical hormone aldosterone which causes salt and water retention which further increases the ascites and causes *oedema*. Aldosterone also causes potassium loss with muscle weakness as a result.

Failure of detoxication by the liver cells results in ordinary doses of drugs having toxic effects. Protein breakdown products from the intestine are not detoxicated, and may also by-pass the liver via the anastomotic veins into the general circulation. Such patients may have a sweetish, slightly faecal smell in the breath, fetor hepaticus.

Jaundice is a *late* sign, heralding liver cell failure. Fetor hepaticus may become marked and build-up of these toxic nitrogenous substances causes depression of brain function or portal-systemic encephalopathy and coma, considered below.

Further investigations

The urine contains excess urobilinogen. Liver function tests in the blood are abnormal, and the electrolytes, especially potassium, must be checked. Liver biopsy may elucidate the type of cirrhosis. Barium swallow demonstrates oesophageal varices. Portal venography may be helpful.

Treatment

Bed rest reduces the demands on the liver and is indicated in active cases until tests show improvement in liver function. *Alcohol* is forbidden.

Sedatives should be avoided if possible, and morphine may precipitate hepatic coma.

Diet. Patients should be encouraged to take an adequate mixed diet, which should be palatable and attractively served. Fat need not be restricted. There is no advantage in giving protein supplements. In hepatic failure with impending coma, protein must be withdrawn, but otherwise a normal 80 G daily intake is reasonable.

It may be worth ensuring adequate vitamins by adding 100 mg ascorbic acid (vitamin C), and vitamin B factors (10 mg thiamine, (B_1), 2 mg riboflavine (B_2) and 15 mg nicotinic acid daily). Vitamin K_1 10 mg intramuscularly is given if there is bleeding tendency or impaired prothrombin activity in the blood.

Salt restriction is sometimes indicated in severe oedema.

Diuretics. Ascites and oedema respond to oral diuretics such as bendrofluazide, 10 mg daily, or the more powerful frusemide (Lasix) 40–160 mg daily but potassium chloride supplements are essential. Spironolactone (Aldactone-A) 25 mg four times daily is a most effective additional diuretic, acting by antagonizing the salt-retaining effect of aldosterone on the renal tubules. A new diuretic, Amiloride may prove useful.

Abdominal paracentesis should generally be avoided, and is only rarely indicated, to relieve discomfort if these measures fail. It depletes the body of protein. The procedure may itself precipitate hepatic coma.

Management of haematemesis from oesophageal varices. Blood transfusion is given. Vasopressin 20 units in 100 ml 5 per cent dextrose is given intravenously in ten minutes. This lowers the portal venous pressure by constricting the arterial channels supplying the gut. It also causes intestinal spasm and discomfort and constriction of the coronary arteries which may be dangerous in myocardial ischaemia.

The Sengstaken tube is a triple-lumen tube which is passed through the mouth into the stomach. A distensible bag causes compression on the veins at the lower oesophagus, thus diminishing bleeding. It may be used in severe cases, but its use is not without danger.

Emergency surgery is indicated if blood-loss cannot be controlled, and in acute cases should be limited to a minimal procedure such as ligation of the bleeding varices.

The treatment of hepatic coma is described below.

Prognosis and follow-up

The prognosis is good in patients in the early stages of alcoholic cirrhosis if they stop drinking, and abstention must be absolute. In such cases, the liver has considerable powers of recovery, and its size and function may return to normal.

Patients with portal hypertension and recurrent haematemeses or gastro-intestinal haemorrhages should be considered for surgical treatment by portal—systemic shunting operations, which lower the venous pressure. These are indicated in the few cases who retain good liver-cell function, but long-term results are uncertain.

In most patients with cirrhosis the changes in the liver are irreversible. Good management includes advice on the avoidance of alcohol and drugs which may be toxic to the liver, the maintenance of adequate nutrition, the treatment of ascites and oedema with diuretics, and the early recognition of liver cell failure. The course nevertheless tends to be a downhill one over a few years, rapidly recurring ascites and the development of jaundice being unfavourable signs. There is also an increased risk of primary liver carcinoma in cirrhosis of the liver.

Liver cell failure and hepatic coma

Hepato-cellular dysfunction has been described above, and may proceed to *hepatic failure* with jaundice, bleeding tendency and the ill-effects of increased circulating nitrogenous substances absorbed from protein breakdown in the intestine.

Causes

1. *Acute liver poisoning and necrosis* ('acute yellow atrophy of the liver') from chemicals such as carbon tetrachloride, benzene, and chloroform, and toxins.

2. *Fulminating virus hepatitis.*

3. *Cirrhosis of the liver.* Precipitating factors here include alcohol intake, intercurrent infections, gastro-intestinal haemorrhage causing excessive protein load, and potassium deficiency.

Symptoms and signs

These are those of the causative condition, of which the commonest is cirrhosis, increasing jaundice, fever and effects of the nitrogenous toxins. These cause marked fetor hepaticus, and the condition of *portal-systemic encephalopathy*, from effects on the brain. There is a flapping tremor of the outstretched hands, lethargy and variable mental confusion, inability to make simple figures with match-sticks being a useful sign. If untreated, the condition proceeds to hepatic coma and death.

The electro-encephalogram (E.E.G.) shows typical changes in the brain waves.

Treatment

All dietary protein is stopped, and to prevent endogenous protein breakdown, a high calorie diet is given. At least 1600 calories should be supplied daily in the form of glucose drinks or as 20 per cent glucose by nasogastric tube, or intravenously. Potassium chloride supplements are indicated.

The bowel is cleared by enema or purgative. Neomycin 1 G 6-hourly is given to sterilize the bowel and prevent protein breakdown by bacterial action. Lactulose (Duphalac) 10–30 ml 4 times daily may help by altering the bacterial flora, and loosening the stools.

Vitamin K_1 10 mg by intramuscular injection daily may improve the bleeding tendency. Sedatives, especially morphine must be avoided.

The condition is often a terminal one in cirrhosis, but where there is a recoverable cause such as acute virus hepatitis and if the above measures are not producing benefit in a few days, other methods may be tried. These include exchange blood transfusion, perfusion of the patient's blood through an isolated pig liver, and liver transplantation, which is still in the experimental stages in liver disease.

Carcinoma of the Liver

PRIMARY LIVER CANCER. This is rare in Britain. It may follow cirrhosis and should be suspected if a patient with cirrhosis shows sudden deterioration with increased size of the liver. There are geographical differences in the incidence of primary liver cancer. It is common in the Bantus of South Africa, and in China and the Far East. Environmental and food factors may be more important than genetic factors, for toxins such as the aflatoxin may be carcinogenic. Surgical removal of the tumour is rarely possible, so the prognosis is poor.

SECONDARY CARCINOMA. The liver is a very common site of metastatic growths, spread by the portal or systemic veins from primary carcinomas in the abdomen, such as stomach and large intestine, or in the chest, such as carcinoma of lung or breast.

Symptoms and signs

There may be evidence of the primary growth, but the secondary carcinoma in the liver may present first. There is malaise, lassitude, weight loss and abdominal swelling, partly from the liver, which may be huge and nodular, partly from ascites from peritoneal metastases. Jaundice may be mild or severe when major bile ducts are invaded.

The urine may contain bilirubin and/or urobilinogen. Ascitic fluid is often blood-stained and contains malignant cells.

Treatment and prognosis

Treatment can only be palliative, for, when the liver is thus involved, the prognosis is hopeless, often only measured in weeks. Tapping of ascites may afford symptomatic relief. Otherwise, management includes tranquillizing drugs such as chlorpromazine and the proper use of opiates (which are contra-indicated in recoverable liver diseases) to prevent pain and alleviate suffering.

Gall-stones and the biliary tract

Gall-stones are formed when some of the constituents of the bile are deposited from solution. As bile is concentrated in the gall-bladder, stones are most frequently formed here.

There are three types:

1. Pigment stones—composed of bilirubin, rare, but occur in haemolytic anaemia.

2. Cholesterol stones—which may be single or multiple.

3. Mixed stones—containing bilirubin, cholesterol and calcium. are commonest. It is their calcium content that renders some stones opaque to x-ray, others may be seen as 'negative shadows' on cholecystogram.

Gall-stones occur at all ages but are very common in middle-aged women who are obese and have borne many children—women fair, fat, fertile and forty. Hormonal effects on bile composition or gall-bladder motility, and infection may be causative factors.

Effects of gall-stones: may be symptomless, especially in the elderly.

associated with cholecystitis.

cause bile-duct obstruction with colic, jaundice and cholangitis from infection of the stagnant bile.

may rarely cause an intestinal obstruction (gall-stone ileus).

ACUTE CHOLECYSTITIS

This is acute inflammation of the gall-bladder, usually associated with a gall-stone obstructing the neck of the gall-bladder or the cystic duct, and there is super-added infection often with Esch. coli.

Symptoms and signs

Acute attacks occur against a background of previous biliary tract disease, and are commonest in obese, middle-aged women; they may be precipitated by a fatty or heavy meal.

There is epigastric discomfort soon followed by severe pain and tenderness at the right upper quadrant over the gall-bladder as the peritoneum becomes involved; pain may be referred to the right scapula or tip of the shoulder. There is anorexia, malaise and fever and occasionally vomiting, but jaundice suggests bile-duct obstruction. The inflamed gall-bladder is not usually palpable.

The white cell count is raised. Straight x-ray may show opaque stones.

Differential diagnosis includes abdominal conditions such as perforated peptic ulcer and acute pancreatitis, and conditions in the thorax such as diaphragmatic pleurisy (from lung infection or infarction) and myocardial infarction.

Treatment: Bed rest till fever settles.

Relief of pain: Pethidine 50–100 mg by injection (morphine may worsen biliary spasm).

Diet: Adequate fluids, low-fat.

Antibacterial drugs: Ampicillin 500 mg 6-hourly by mouth or rifamide 150 mg 8-hourly intramuscularly—these antibiotics are concentrated in the bile.

Acute cholecystitis usually settles with these conservative measures. However, some surgeons prefer to treat cholecystitis by immediate cholecystectomy. Surgical drainage may be required for cases with increasing gall-bladder distention and risk of rupture.

Once the acute attack has subsided cholecystography is carried out (the gall-bladder does not concentrate the opaque medium in the acute stages). The patient is instructed on diet and weight reduction, and elective cholecystectomy is advised some two or three months after the acute attack.

CHRONIC CHOLECYSTITIS

This presents as recurrent attacks of acute cholecystitis, or as dyspepsia and upper abdominal discomfort often provoked by fatty foods or a heavy meal. It is, however, important to consider other causes of pain such as peptic ulcer, with which cholecystitis may be associated. Flatulence may be attributed to cholecystitis, but may simply be due to air swallowing, or may be associated with hiatus hernia and oesophagitis. Again, 'bilious attacks' may indicate migraine, or a depressive state.

Thus the diagnosis of chronic cholecystitis must be confirmed by cholecystography, which shows gall-stones and a poorly functioning gall-bladder.

Treatment is weight-reduction followed by cholecystectomy. Carcinoma of the gall-bladder is rare, but may follow chronic cholecystitis.

BILE DUCT OBSTRUCTION

This is caused by a gall-stone passing into the common bile duct, resulting in *biliary colic, jaundice* and *cholangitis*.

Biliary colic is severe intermittent colicky pain or a more prolonged pain building up over an hour or two, felt in the epigastrium or right upper quadrant of the abdomen, and accompanied by vomiting.

Jaundice may be mild or deep and is obstructive in type with pale stools and dark urine, but the obstruction is rarely complete so that the stool colour may vary from day to day.

Cholangitis is inflammation of the bile duct from infection of the stagnant bile often with a Gram-negative organism such as Esch. coli. This causes fever, often of an intermittent type, accompanied by pain and jaundice. Severe cholangitis may spread to cause liver abscesses and septicaemia, with swinging pyrexia or severe toxaemia.

Further investigations include blood culture, cholecystography or cholangiography.

Differential diagnosis includes virus hepatitis, and carcinoma of the head of the pancreas—here the jaundice is deep and persistent.

Treatment

Bed rest in the acute stages or till fever settles.

Relief of pain—pethidine 100 mg may be preferable to morphine which causes spasm of the sphincter at the lower end of the bile duct, but atropine 0·5 mg or propantheline 15 mg may prevent this.

Appropriate antibacterial drug (e.g. ampicillin, and await blood culture results).

Vitamin K_1 10 mg daily intramuscularly.

Surgery is indicated if these measures fail, and may be necessary for diagnostic as well as therapeutic reasons if jaundice persists for six weeks.

Follow-up—the stone may pass uneventfully into the duodenum and intestine (rarely a stone causes obstruction here), or may remain in the bile duct after acute symptoms settle. There is risk of recurrence of attacks, biliary cirrhosis, and acute pancreatitis, so elective surgery is indicated for removal of calculi and exploration of the biliary tract.

The pancreas

The pancreas is an elongated gland that lies across the upper part of the posterior wall of the abdomen, its head in the loop of the duodenum, its body and tail extending to the left behind the stomach. It consists of two types of cells:

1. The *acinar* or *gland cells*, similar to cells in the salivary glands, which secrete the pancreatic juice containing enzymes which act on protein fat and carbohydrate. These enzymes are activated on meeting the duodenal juices. The main duct of the pancreas usually unites with the bile duct to form what is called the ampulla just before entering the second part of the duodenum. The sphincter of Oddi surrounds the ampulla and prevents reflux of duodenal contents into the pancreatic duct.

2. The *islet cells*, or islets of Langerhans, which secrete the hormone insulin into the bloodstream. Insulin is especially concerned with glucose metabolism, and deficiency of its action results in diabetes mellitus.

Acute pancreatitis

Cause

Acute pancreatitis is usually associated with disease of the biliary tract or gallstones, or with alcoholism. Reflux of duodenal contents into the pancreatic duct activates the enzymes resulting in self-digestion of the pancreas and necrosis of surrounding fat—a very acute inflammatory process.

Symptoms and signs

The condition is commonest in middle-aged men and may be precipitated by a heavy meal or high alcohol intake. There is sudden agonizing upper abdominal pain, nausea and vomiting. The abdomen is tender and rigid. There is pallor, rapid pulse and often hypotension and collapse, a picture commonly referred to as shock, here due to lowered blood volume from outpouring of fluid into the intestine.

Differential diagnosis includes perforated peptic ulcer, biliary colic and surgical conditions described above, and sometimes the picture simulates myocardial infarction. The diagnosis of acute pancreatis is confirmed by a very high serum amylase, one of the enzymes that leaks into the bloodstream; the serum amylase may however, be, slightly raised in other acute abdominal conditions.

Treatment

This should be conservative if the diagnosis is clear. Bed rest is indicated.

Relief of pain—pethidine 100 mg intramuscularly; morphine causes spasm of the sphincter of Oddi and is best avoided.

Nasogastric suction—to remove stagnant gastric and intestinal contents; removal of these secretions also helps by preventing further pancreatic stimulation.

Antisecretory drugs—atropine 0·6 mg or propantheline 15–30 mg intramuscularly are anti-cholingergic drugs which inhibit the effect of vagal stimuli on the pancreas.

Aprotinin (Trasylol) given intravenously antagonizes pancreatic enzymes but opinions are divided on its value.

Intravenous fluids—saline, dextrose, plasma or blood are needed for hypovolaemia. Calcium may be required to combat hypocalcaemia from the combination of calcium with breakdown products of fat.

Follow-up

Disease of the biliary tract such as gallstones, and alcoholism should receive attention, to prevent recurrent attacks—relapsing acute pancreatitis; this is associated with deposits of calcium, seen on x-ray, in the pancreas.

Chronic pancreatitis

In chronic pancreatitis there is a gradual destruction of the pancreatic cells with replacement fibrosis and permanent impairment of function.

The cause is often unknown, but alcoholism and dietary deficiencies in underdeveloped countries may be responsible. Many authorities now state that chronic pancreatitis is a rare sequel to acute pancreatitis or biliary tract disease but a gallstone pressing on the pancreatic duct could cause obstruction, and gradual pancreatic fibrosis. Carcinoma of the pancreas may also be associated with chronic pancreatitis and it may be difficult to distinguish the two conditions.

Symptoms and signs

Middle-aged men are mainly affected. There are bouts of upper abdominal pain, persistent and demoralizing often precipitated by a heavy meal or alcohol. Pain may be worse lying flat and antacids do not help. There may be slight jaundice, and fever.

Sometimes there is no pain, the condition presenting as *pancreatic insufficiency*. This has two effects:

1. *Malabsorption syndrome* from lack of digestive enzymes. There is weight loss and steatorrhoea—loose, pale, offensive, fatty

stools. Unlike the malabsorption of intestinal cause, anaemia is rare.

2. *Diabetes* in the late stages, from destruction of the insulin-secreting islet-cells. There is polyuria and thirst.

Further investigations

Straight x-ray may show pancreatic calcification.

The serum amylase may be slightly raised.

Stools show a high fat content (normally less than 6 G per 24-hours).

Glucose tolerance test may show a high diabetic curve instead of the flat curve of intestinal causes of malabsorption, and xylose absorption is normal.

Pancreatic secretion tests—a tube is passed into the duodenum, and the pancreas stimulated with injection of secretin-pancreozymin, or by placing bile salts in the duodenum. The pancreatic juice obtained by aspiration is tested for volume, and bicarbonate and enzyme content. Such tests are difficult in practice.

Radio-isotope scanning of the pancreas is sometimes helpful.

Treatment

Analgesics may be necessary for pain.

The diet should be low in fat and rich in protein.

Pancreatin and proprietary pancreatic enzyme preparations may be sprinkled on food or mixed with meals but are not always helpful.

Insulin injections are required for diabetes; its control is not usually difficult.

Prognosis

This is variable—the condition may remain static for years, or the course may be a downhill one and here carcinoma should be suspected.

Fibrocystic disease of the pancreas (muscoviscidosis)

This is a disease of recessive inheritance. The pancreas is one of the secreting glands involved, its ducts being blocked with viscid mucus (mucosviscidosis) followed by fibrosis and cyst formation. An affected baby may have intestinal obstruction from thick meconium filling the intestine. In infancy and childhood, there is steatorrhoea. The sweat glands are also affected, excessive salt in the sweat confirming the diagnosis and distinguishing mucoviscidosis from coeliac disease. Bronchial gland involvement causes bronchiectasis and cyst formation, with recurrent lung infections.

The pancreatic steatorrhoea is treated with a low fat, high protein diet and enzyme supplements. Lung infections require antibacterial drugs.

Carcinoma of the pancreas

This occurs in the middle-aged and elderly.

Symptoms and signs

The onset is insidious, and the condition often difficult to diagnose. There may be upper abdominal pain similar to that in chronic pancreatitis, anorexia and weight loss—this is usually the cachexia of malignant disease, but may be partly due to steatorrhoea from associated pancreatic insufficiency. Similarly the condition may present as diabetes in middle-age, and despite control of the diabetes, the patient deteriorates.

Obstructive jaundice may be the first sign in carcinoma of the head of the pancreas. The jaundice is deep with itchy skin, pale stools and dark urine containing bilirubin but no urobilinogen.

Metastases are frequently the first clinical indication—thus, there is ascites from peritoneal deposits, or liver swelling and jaundice. Involvement of the inferior vena cava causes venous obstruction and oedema.

Sometimes recurrent phlebitis is associated with carcinoma of the pancreas.

Further investigations

Barium meal may show distortion of the loop of the duodenum. The E.S.R. may be raised, as in any malignant disease.

Radio-isotope scanning of the pancreas may be helpful.

Treatment

Palliative surgery may relieve the biliary obstruction in carcinoma of the head of the pancreas. It is, however, rarely possible to remove a pancreatic growth, and the risks of auto-digestion and fistula formation render operations hazardous.

Treatment is therefore generally conservative, with the proper use of analgesics and opiates to prevent pain and alleviate suffering, and the course is a downhill one, with death in months or weeks.

Haemochromatosis (bronzed diabetes)

Haemochromatosis is an inborn error of metabolism, sometimes familial. There is excessive iron absorption and deposition in the pancreas and liver, the resulting fibrosis causing diabetes and cirrhosis. Deposits in the skin and increased melanin production cause the slaty-blue or bronze pigmentation characteristic of the disorder. It occurs mainly in men, for women utilize the iron to make up for the blood-loss of menstruation, but is not a common disease—cases may be discovered at a diabetic clinic.

Diagnosis is confirmed by tests including high serum iron.

Treatment is by repeated venesection to deplete the body's iron stores and prevent further fibrosis. Insulin injections are required for the diabetes, control being usually quite easily achieved on doses of about 40 units daily.

It is important to investigate the patient's sons and male relatives, for if serum iron studies reveal the trait, venesection may prevent the development of the condition.

Islet cell tumour (insulinoma)

This is a tumour of the islet cells of the pancreas resulting in excessive insulin secretion and attacks of *hypoglycaemia*, low blood sugar. This provokes the outpouring of adrenaline in an attempt to raise the blood sugar. Thus the attacks are characterized by weakness, tremor, sweating and collapse. They may occur after a long period without food. Alternatively attacks may follow a high carbohydrate meal as this stimulus causes over-production of insulin. In some patients hypoglycaemia may be induced by the amino-acid leucine contained in certain protein foods. The administration of sugar rapidly corrects the symptoms.

Diagnosis may be confirmed by fasting the patient to provoke an attack, but glucose must be available, orally or by intravenous injection, for its correction. Other investigations include glucose tolerance test, and the response to tolbutamide and to glucagon, with serum insulin assays.

Insulinoma is rare, but diagnosis is important for the tumour is not usually malignant, and surgical removal results in complete cure.

Diabetes mellitus is described on page 264.

8

Disorders of the kidney and urinary tract

Anatomy

The *kidneys* are a pair of organs which lie behind the peritoneum on the posterior abdominal wall and diaphragm. Examined from the back, they are deep to the muscles of the loin and to the twelfth rib. Each renal artery arises from the aorta. A blood supply equal to one fifth of the cardiac output reaches the kidneys, indicating the importance of their work. The urine each forms is passed into the renal pelvis, the funnel shaped expansion of the upper end of the ureter. The *ureters* pass down along the line of the transverse processes of the vertebrae to reach the *bladder*, the muscular bag in which urine accumulates. Urine is voided along the *urethra*, which runs from the lower end of the bladder to the exterior, having a short course in the female but a longer course through the prostate gland and penis in the male.

Functions of the kidneys

The kidneys have two main functions, 1. an *excretory* function and 2. a *regulatory* function.

1. *Excretory function*

The obvious function is to make urine, an aqueous solution containing the soluble waste products of metabolism, such as urea from proteins. Drugs and their metabolites are also excreted.

2. *Regulatory function*

The kidneys maintain the body fluids at a constant composition despite wide fluctuations in fluid intake and metabolic demands.

(a) *Salt and water regulation.* The *tonicity* or *osmolality* of the plasma depends on the concentration of electrolytes such as sodium, potassium and chloride dissolved in it, that is, the number of such ions in solution. In states of dehydration when the tonicity of the plasma is tending to rise, the posterior pituitary gland releases its anti-diuretic hormone. This acts on the renal collecting tubule causing water retention and a return to normality.

The *total body water* is controlled by 'volume receptors', some of which are in the kidney related to the small arteries. The substance renin is released. This forms angiotensin in the plasma. One action of angiotensin is on the adrenal cortex, causing release of aldosterone. Aldosterone in turn affects the renal tubule, causing sodium retention and with it water retention. (The diuretics bendrofluazide and fruse-mide act by causing sodium and therefore water loss at the renal tubule. Spironolactone acts by competing with aldosterone, with the same effect.)

(b) *Blood pressure regulation.* The blood pressure depends partly on the amount of sodium and water retained, and partly on a second action of the renin—angiotensin mechanism: angiotensin has a constrictor effect on small blood vessels, raising the blood pressure.

(c) *Acid-base balance.* Tissue respiration results in the production of carbon dioxide which goes to form carbonic acid. This is duly excreted as carbon dioxide by the lungs. Exercise, and protein and fat breakdown are metabolic processes which are also acid-forming, that is they cause the production of hydrogen-ions. These are excreted by the kidney, which also controls the 'buffer' system of chemicals, such as bicarbonate, which bind hydrogen-ions harmlessly in the bloodstream.

Thus the kidney keeps constant the acid-base balance of the blood. This can be expressed as the pH. Neutral point is pH7. Acids have a pH of *less than* 7, alkalis have a pH *greater than* 7. The pH of plasma is maintained at 7·4, just on the alkaline side of neutral. Urine is generally acid and the pH can drop to 4 in acidotic states such as diabetic ketosis (keto-acidosis).

Acid base balance can be controlled only if the kidney is provided with a sufficient circulation to do its work. If water and sodium are lacking, acidosis results.

In renal failure (and some rare diseases of the renal tubule) the control mechanism fails and again there is acidosis.

(d) *Calcium and phosphorus balance.* Parathyroid hormone acts on the renal tubule causing phosphate excretion. In renal failure phosphate builds up in the blood and calcium is lowered. This may cause tetany, but the calcium and bone changes are complex.

(e) *Red cell production.* The kidney produces the hormone erythropoietin which stimulates the bone marrow. Lack of erythropoietin may be partly responsible for the anaemia of chronic renal disease.

The structure of the kidney and formation of urine

Each kidney contains a million units of *'nephrons'*. Each nephron is a long, fine tube with a cup-shaped, upper blind end. This contains the capillary tuft or *glomerulus* through which the fluid constituents of the blood are filtered into the nephron, the red cells and plasma proteins being retained in the capillaries. The glomerular filtrate passes into the proximal tubule of the nephron where much of the water and electrolytes, and all the glucose, are reabsorbed into the bloodstream. The nephron now leaves the outer region of the kidney or cortex, descending and rising again in a loop in the inner, medullary region. Near the top of the loop is the distal tubule, which opens into collecting tubules again descending in the medulla. Electrolyte exchange and hydrogen-ion excretion occur along the course of the nephron, and the final concentration of the filtrate to form urine takes place in the collecting tubule, under the influence of antidiuretic hormone. The collecting tubules pass downwards through the renal papillae to empty into the cup-shaped 'calyces' of the renal or ureteric pelvis.

Important concepts in clinical practice

From the blood reaching the kidneys 125 ml of glomerular filtrate is formed every minute—this is the glomerular filtration rate. This in 24 hours amounts to 180 litres, yet only 1·5 litres of urine are produced. The work of healthy *glomeruli* is to produce a protein-free filtrate. The work of the *tubules* is to produce a concentrated urine.

In pure glomerular disease, such as the nephrotic syndrome, there is a leakage of protein, mainly albumin, into the glomerular filtrate, resulting in albuminuria.

Isolated tubular disease is rare.

Chronic renal disease results in *destruction of nephrons* and ultimately there are only a few intact nephrons left to do all the work. There may be little or no albuminuria, but the important aspect is that the *concentrating power* of the kidneys is impaired. The residual nephrons can excrete the body's waste products only by passing large quantities of dilute urine of fixed, low specific gravity. Further destruction of nephrons, or their complete non-function as in acute renal failure, causes retention of waste products with serious clinical effect unless treatment, possibly including dialysis, is carried out.

Examination of the urine

Appearance

Colour. The normal yellow or amber colour is due to urochrome. Dark urine may simply be concentrated urine or due to the presence of bile (bilirubin). Blood in the urine, haematuria, causes a dark, smoky urine. Haemoglobinuria is port wine in colour and is rare. denoting intravascular haemolysis. In the rare disease porphyria, the urine darkens on standing. Ingestion of beetroot and the drug phenindione can cause a pink colour, and the dye methylene blue in some patent medicines turns the urine green.

Deposits. Urates form a brown or pink deposit when urine cools on standing. Phosphates are white and appear in neutral or alkaline urine. A cloud of mucus may be seen. These are normal findings and should be distinguished from pus in the urine, pyuria (which may be creamy and offensive) and from haematuria, but microscopic examination may be necessary.

Volume and specific gravity

The volume varies from 500–3,000 litres per 24-hours, average 1,500 litres, and depends on the fluid intake and water vapour losses through the skin. *Polyuria* is an increased output of urine, *oliguria* a diminished output, and *anuria* complete suppression of urine. The urine volume must be carefully charted—weighing the patient daily gives a further check of output.

The specific gravity is measured by a hydrometer (urinometer) and in health varies between 1,002 and 1,032. It indicates the amount of dissolved substances, largely urea. Healthy kidneys can produce a concentrated urine or a dilute urine, adapting to variation in fluid intake and metabolic demand. In compensated chronic renal failure, the kidneys cannot produce a concentrated (or very dilute) urine, and can only get rid of the body's waste products by passing large quantities of pale urine with specific gravity fixed around 1,010. Other causes of polyuria include compulsive water drinking and diabetes insipidus (lack of posterior pituitary antidiuretic hormone) where the specific gravity may be 1,000–1,002, and diabetes mellitus. Here much sugar is dissolved in the urine, and although it looks pale, it is of high specific gravity (may be over 1,032), an exception to the usual association of pale urine with low specific gravity.

Reaction (*Acidity*)

This is tested by litmus, or preferably pH indicator paper strip Urine is normally slightly acid, pH 6. The pH may drop to 4 if metabolism is increased, or in states of acidosis. Ingestion of alkalis and fruits (fruits are really alkali-forming), renders the urine alkaline, pH above 7. Drug excretion is affected by the urinary pH. In aspirin poisoning it is important to render the urine alkaline to pH 8, for this speeds the excretion of salicylate formed from aspirin.

Presence of sugar

Glucose is present in the urine in diabetes mellitus, and in patients with a low renal threshold for glucose reabsorption. Other sugars are rare, but lactose may be found in the urine of nursing mothers. The Clinistix strip test detects only glucose. The Clinitest tablet test is not so specific, being affected by glucose and other sugars and substances such as salicylate, but it gives a better guide to the *amount* of sugar in the urine.

Acetone—really Keto-acids

Ketonuria occurs in severe vomiting, starvation, and diabetic ketosis and coma. It is detected by Ketostix strip test or Acetest tablet. These are very sensitive tests and if they are positive, it is desirable to carry out the less sensitive ferric chloride test in addition, which if positive will denote a serious degree of ketosis. A positive ferric chloride test (that is, purple coloration on adding the solution to the urine) also occurs in aspirin (salicylate) poisoning. Boiling a further sample of the urine destroys keto-acids but not salicylate, allowing differentiation on retesting with the cooled specimen.

Protein

Glomerular damage is the commonest cause of proteinuria. Proteinuria is persistent and often heavy in the nephrotic syndrome. It occurs in acute nephritis, hypertensive kidney disease and in chronic renal failure but is much less marked in these conditions. In urinary tract infections, pus in the urine may cause slight proteinuria but this is *not* a reliable index of such infection.

Proteinuria may occur in high fever, cardiac failure and poisoning with a heavy metal such as gold (used in treatment of rheumatoid arthritis). In toxaemia of pregnancy there is hypertension, oedema and proteinuria.

Strenuous exercise may cause proteinuria, and in some people it follows prolonged standing, but is absent in a specimen tested after a period of recumbency.

In all these conditions, the protein present is albumin, which has a small molecule so that it escapes through leaky glomeruli. In the blood disease myelomatosis, an abnormal protein is present in the bloodstream and this appears as Bence Jones protein in the urine.

Tests: Albustix strip test is sensitive, and should be carried out on a fresh specimen. False positives occur with soap or cetrimide contamination of containers.

The boiling test is carried out on urine slightly acidified with acetic acid to dissolve phosphates. Albumin appears as a cloud or white curd at boiling point. Bence Jones' protein appears at about 70°C but redissolves before boiling point is reached.

The amount of albumin can be gauged roughly by these tests and by Esbach's albuminometer, but an accurate estimation demands laboratory examination of a 24-hour specimen of urine. Up to 5 G albuminuria may not cause symptoms, but heavy albuminuria of 10 G or more per 24-hours is a serious loss to the body—see Nephrotic Syndrome.

Bilirubin and Urobilinogen

These may be found in the urine in diseases of the liver and biliary tract. Urobilinogen may be found in haemolytic anaemia and is detected by Ehrlich's aldehyde reagent (turns the urine pink) or Urobilistix strip test.

Blood—Haematuria

Blood in the urine is called *haematuria*. If arising from the kidneys the blood will be intimately mixed with the urine. If from the prostate or urethra blood may only be present at the start of micturition. Painless haematuria most commonly arises in the bladder or prostate, but a renal lesion may be responsible.

Causes

1. *Systemic*   blood disorders such as purpura; anticoagulant overdosage.

2. *Renal*   acute glomerulonephritis.
                acute pyelonephritis is not a common cause, but
                urinary tract tuberculosis is a rare possibility.
                renal infarction from arterial thrombosis or embolism;
                in subacute bacterial endocarditis there may be mul-
                tiple small emboli.
                hypernephroma (carcinoma)—this is painless, there
                may be a palpable mass, secondary spread to the
                lungs and obscure pyrexia.
                polycystic disease of the kidneys.
                trauma.
3. *Ureteric*   stones—usually associated 'renal colic'.
4. *Bladder*   papilloma and carcinoma (industrial hazard with dye-
                stuffs and benzidine).
                schistosomiasis, a parasitic infection common in East
                Africa.
                haemorrhagic cystitis, a toxic effect of the drug
                cyclophosphamide.
5. *Prostate*   carcinoma and
6. *Urethra*   caruncle, and trauma.

A large amount of blood is obvious, lesser quantities give the urine
a smoky appearance, or the amount may be so small that microscopical examination is necessary to detect the red cells. If the cause
is not clear, investigations such as cystoscopy and x-rays may be
necessary to locate the site of bleeding and allow early and appropriate treatment.

Combined strip tests of the urine

Paper or plastic strips are available, such as *Bili-labstix* which
combines test areas for pH, protein, glucose, ketones, bilirubin and
blood.

Microscopical examination in the side-room

This allows the detection of red cells, pus cells (pyuria) and casts.
Casts are formed in the renal tubules, and the presence of cellular
casts indicates active renal disease.

Specimens for bacteriology

Mid-Stream Urine (M.S.U.). A catch specimen in midstream is
taken into a sterile wide-mouthed container (preliminary cleansing
of the labia in the female with sterile water may be advisable).
Catheterization should be avoided, as it carries risk of infection.

The specimen should reach the laboratory within one hour. If this is impracticable, then a procedure such as Uricult or Oxoid Dip Slide should be used. The special slide, which is coated with culture-medium, is dipped into the freshly voided urine, replaced in its container and sent or posted to the laboratory. Coliform organisms may grow at room temperature allowing diagnosis even before incubation is carried out. The number of colonies of organisms grown, the Colony Count, is a better index of urinary tract infection than the amount of pus cells present, a colony count of over 100,000 per ml urine being significant.

Cytology. An early morning specimen is examined for malignant cells in patients with suspected carcinoma of the urinary tract, especially bladder carcinoma.

Further investigations in renal disease

Urine concentration test

The patient is given no fluids after 6 p.m.; the bladder is emptied at 10 p.m. The following morning, the urine specific gravity should be 1,022 or higher. While theoretically a test of tubular function, the concentrating power of the kidney becomes impaired in disease such as chronic renal failure, the specific gravity being fixed at 1,010.

The specific gravity parallels the urea concentration, a healthy kidney being able to produce a urinary area of at least 2 G per 100 ml.

Dilution tests are not helpful in clinical practice.

Blood urea

The normal blood urea is 20–40 mg per 100 ml. The level is raised in renal failure and may reach 300 mg per 100 ml in neglected cases; the rate of rise is more important than the absolute level. A raised blood urea is quite late evidence of renal disease, as more than half the total nephrons must be destroyed before a rise occurs.

The waste products urea, creatinine and uric acid are all raised in renal failure but they are not in themselves toxic, other unknown metabolites being responsible for the symptoms of 'uraemia'—the syndrome associated with a high blood urea.

Other routine blood tests include the serum electrolytes sodium, potassium and chloride, acid-base measurements such as pH and bicarbonate, and estimation of calcium and phosphorus.

Clearance tests

The amount of a substance cleared from the plasma by the glomerular filter can be estimated by measuring its plasma concentration, and its urine concentration over a set time. This 'clearance' is a guide to the glomerular filtration rate. A substance can be injected intravenously for this test, or alternatively one of the substances already present in the plasma can be utilized, for example urea or creatinine. Thus the *creatinine clearance test* (estimated on a 6 or 24 hour urine collection) is used clinically as a measure of the glomerular filtration rate and is normally 120 ml per minute. The test becomes impaired before there is any rise in blood urea, and is a guide to therapy in renal failure.

Radiography

Plain x-ray may show the kidneys, and any opaque stones. In intravenous pyelography (I.V.P.) an iodine-containing, radio-opaque substance is injected into a forearm vein. It is excreted by the kidneys, demonstrating their size and function, and showing also the renal pelvis, ureters and bladder.

Cystoscopy is the examination of the bladder through an instrument passed by the urethra under general anaesthetic. Catheters can be passed into the ureters and a radio-opaque medium allows 'retrograde pyelography'. Modern I.V.P. technique has, however, curtailed the need for this investigation, which carries risk of introducing infection.

Isotope renogram

Radioactive hippuran is excreted by the kidneys, and counters placed over the renal tract measure its function and detect obstruction such as a stone in a ureter.

Renal biopsy

A tiny specimen of kidney tissue is obtained by a special needle inserted through the lumbar region using local anaesthesia. The biopsy is examined by ordinary and electron microscopy. Renal biopsy is proving of value in the understanding of renal disease and may be necessary to ensure proper treatment. The procedure is contra-indicated in bleeding diseases and severe uraemia, and carries a risk of causing a renal haematoma.

Arteriography

A radio-opaque medium is injected into the aorta near the renal arteries by direct puncture through the lumbar region, or through a catheter inserted from below via the femoral artery. This demonstrates the renal arteries and circulation.

Urinary tract stones (calculi)

In bygone times, bladder stone was common, but in developed countries today, a stone is more likely to originate at the kidney.

Types

The calcium oxalate stone is commonest, occurs mainly in men, and may be associated with excessive calcium in the urine (hypercalciuria) or in the blood (hypercalcaemia). Mixed phosphate stones are often associated with urinary tract infection and sometimes form a 'staghorn calculus' in the renal pelvis. Rarer types include uric acid stones, occurring in gout, leukaemia or with excessively acid urine, and cystine stones in the rare recessive condition cystinuria.

Symptoms and signs

Renal colic is really *ureteric* colic from the passage of a stone, which tends to become impacted at the lower end of the ureter. There is pain at the loin, radiating to the groin, building up to maximum severity over about half an hour, then declining only to recur or disappear if the stone is passed into the bladder. Haematuria may occur. The stone may eventually pass out through the urethra.

Complications include stasis and infection. Obstruction may have a back-pressure effect on the kidney, causing *hydronephrosis*, a dilatation of the renal pelvis, which if infected becomes a pus-containing *pyonephrosis*. (Other obstructions may cause these conditions.) Renal function becomes impaired.

Further investigations

Most urinary stones (except uric acid stones) are radio-opaque and visible on plain x-ray, but I.V.P. is usually helpful. 24-hour urine calcium, and serum calcium and phosphorus tests may be indicated.

Treatment

1. Relief of pain—pethidine 100 mg by intramuscular injection may be required in renal colic.

2. Copious fluids.

3. Surgical removal of the stone—this may be possible during a cystoscopy, or open operation may be necessary.

4. Prevention of recurrence—this includes search for a metabolic cause such as hyperparathyroidism in hypercalcaemia. Hypercalciuria can be treated with bendrofluazide which, as well as being a

diuretic, lowers the urinary calcium, or with sodium cellulose phosphate, which lowers intestinal calcium absorption.

Urinary tract infection

Cause

Urinary tract infection occurs from bacterial invasion, and the organisms can be cultured from the urine, a colony count of 100,000 per ml being significant, as explained above. Symptoms such as painful or frequent micturition may be due to inflammation of urethral glands without proven infection, precipitated by stimuli including exposure to cold, bubble baths, and sexual activity ('honeymoon cystitis'). However, a true *cystitis* (inflammation of the bladder) from bacterial infection is very common in women, the short urethra in the female allowing entry of bacteria such as Esch. coli (the bowel organism), the commonest cause of urinary tract infection.

Infection ascends the ureters and reaches the renal pelvis, inflammation of which is called pyelitis, but the renal substance tends to be invaded and the term *pyelonephritis* is now preferred. However, pyelonephritis may also be caused by infection reaching the kidney by the bloodstream.

Predisposing factors

Urinary stasis in pregnancy, from lack of tone of the ureters, and pressure from the gravid uterus.

neurological disease affecting the bladder, such as multiple sclerosis and paraplegia.

prolonged recumbency, often with inadequate fluid intake in geriatric patients.

Obstruction from stone, or carcinoma of bladder or prostate.

Deformity abnormality at ureteric orifice in children, allowing reflux of urine from bladder; scarring of the developing kidney following pyelonephritis in childhood; diverticulum of the bladder.

Catheterization especially if sterile precautions are haphazard— organisms other than the usual Esch. coli may also be introduced here.

Analgesic abuse phenacetin preparations may damage the renal papillae and infection follows.

In men, urinary tract infection is nearly always associated with some such abnormality.

ACUTE PYELONEPHRITIS

Symptoms and signs

Women are mainly affected. Frequency, pain or burning on micturition is largely due to associated cystitis, and there may be tenderness over the bladder. There is pain and tenderness at one or both loins, rigors and fever which may be the only presenting sign. Vomiting is common in children. Rarely, in debilitated patients a septicaemia with severe toxaemia and hypotension may follow.

Further investigations

The urine may be cloudy and nearly always contains pus cells, but the diagnosis can only be established bacteriologically. As explained above, a mid-stream urine bacterial colony count of 100,000 per ml is significant. The sensitivity of the organisms to antibacterial drugs is ascertained.

Intravenous pyelography is indicated later.

Treatment

1. *Bed rest* in febrile stage.
2. *Copious fluids.*
3. *Antibacterial drugs.* Pending bacteriology report, a sulphonamide or the combined sulphamethoxazole-trimethoprim drug Septrin or Bactrim, 2 tablets twice daily is given. If clinical improvement occurs, the drug chosen should be continued. Infections in hospital may be resistant, and depending on the bacteriology report, nalidixic acid (Negram), nitrofurantoin (Furadantin), ampicillin or cephalexin may be used. Gentamicin, carbenicillin or kanamycin by injection may be required for resistant organisms or in septicaemic states.

Follow-up

Usually a 10–14 day course of the appropriate antibacterial drug is sufficient in adults, a further urine sample being checked bacteriologically four weeks later. Longer courses and more detailed radiological investigations may be necessary in children.

CHRONIC PYELONEPHRITIS

This may present as recurrent attacks of acute pyelonephritis and loin aches, or there may be symptomless bacteriuria. Antibacterial drugs may be given at the first sign of recurrent infection, or long-term trimethoprim-sulphamethoxazole used in prophylaxis. It is important to seek and if possible eliminate any predisposing factor.

Renal function may become impaired as a result of chronic pyelonephritis but there is now doubt as to the significance of uncomplicated attacks of pyelonephritis in adults, most cases of renal scarring probably having occurred in childhood. It is in children that proper management of urinary tract infection is therefore so vital.

Further scarring, possibly from repeated infection and contraction of the kidneys may present as renal failure in adult life, or result in hypertension.

TUBERCULOSIS OF THE URINARY TRACT

This was a complication of pulmonary tuberculosis and may still be seen in patients whose drug therapy was non-existent or inadequate, from a lurking focus of infection. The kidneys and bladder are involved, symptoms are those of pyelonephritis as above, and there may be haematuria. Thus it is important to consider the possibility of tuberculosis if the more common organisms are not found, especially if there is lung scarring or a previous history. The urine should be examined for the acid-fast tubercle bacilli, and culture or guinea pig inoculation may be necessary. Cystoscopy and pyelography may be diagnostic. Treatment is usually with streptomycin, isoniazid and P.A.S.

The kidneys and hypertension

Renal disease as a cause of Hypertension

Renal damage, or impairment of blood supply to the glomeruli, is frequently associated with a raised blood pressure. This may be temporary in acute nephritis, or permanent in chronic bilateral renal disease (chronic glomerulonephritis and chronic pyelonephritis).

Unilateral renal disease may also cause hypertension and if the other kidney is normal there need be no outward evidence of renal dysfunction. The causes are scarring from childhood pyelonephritis, and renal artery stenosis (due to arteriosclerosis, and rendering the kidney ischaemic); the poor blood supply to the glomerular region causes release of renin and formation of angiotensin with rise of blood pressure, the kidney here acting as an endocrine organ. I.V.P. and arteriography, and blood hormone tests aid the diagnosis. Provided the other kidney is functioning normally a diseased kidney can be removed, or its artery reconstructed, curing the hypertension. Results of surgical treatment of renal artery stenosis have, however, proved disappointing and the present trend is towards the use of hypotensive drugs in treatment.

Effects of hypertension on the kidneys

Not only may kidney disease cause hypertension, but hypertension from any cause may in turn damage the kidneys. In mild cases of essential hypertension, although the renal arterioles are affected, renal function is not usually seriously impaired, though there may be slight proteinuria. Treatment with hypotensive drugs delays the progress of renal disease but gradual destruction of nephrons over a period of years is associated with polyuria, renal shrinkage and ultimately chronic renal failure.

In malignant or *accelerated hypertension* it is uncertain how far the kidneys are responsible for initiating or maintaining the very high diastolic pressure, which is associated with arteriolar necrosis (and papilloedema). The renal vasculature is itself severely damaged and renal failure is rapid, with haematuria and casts, or proteinuria, and often salt and water retention. Hypotensive drugs may lower the blood pressure and break the vicious circle, but where the patient presents with a high blood urea the underlying renal damage may be irreversible. The management is that of chronic renal failure, but the prognosis is poor in these cases.

Polycystic disease of the kidneys

This is due to a congenital defect, but patients present in adult life. The condition is relatively rare. Both kidneys become converted into big cystic masses, easily palpable in the abdomen. Signs include haematuria, hypertension, or renal failure. Conservative management may be possible for many years, and some cases may be suitable for renal transplantation.

Drugs and the kidneys

Drugs causing renal damage

Analgesic (pain-relieving) drugs containing *phenacetin* taken over a period of years, have caused renal papillary necrosis (predisposing to pyelonephritis) and chronic renal failure—this is called *analgesic nephropathy*. Phenacetin has therefore been withdrawn from these preparations, being replaced by paracetamol in 'tab. codeine co.'. Phenacetin actually forms paracetamol in the body, but paracetamol does not appear to be toxic. Aspirin increases the urinary cell count, but does not cause lasting damage.

The antibiotics streptomycin and kanamycin in large doses damage the kidneys. Tetracycline increases protein breakdown and should not be used in renal failure.

Troxidone (used in petit mal epilepsy), heavy metals such as gold, (used in rheumatoid arthritis) and mercury can cause the nephrotic syndrome (see below). Excess vitamin D causes renal calcium deposition (nephrocalcinosis).

Drugs affecting renal mechanisms

Probenecid increases uric acid excretion, and is used in gout (aspirin may antagonize this action). Probenecid also blocks the excretion of penicillin and is used where high blood levels of penicillin are required, as in subacute bacterial endocarditis.

Increasing the renal excretion of drugs

The promotion of a diuresis by intravenous fluids is used in the treatment of poisoning with aspirin or phenobarbitone—the excretion of these drugs is further enhanced if the urine is made alkaline using intravenous bicarbonate. Pethidine excretion is increased if the urine is acid.

Impaired excretion of drugs in renal failure

Commonly used drugs such as morphine and chlorpromazine (Largactil) may build up to toxic levels when excretion is impaired, causing cerebral and respiratory depression. Tissue levels of antibiotics are similarly raised, and in the case of streptomycin this may result in disturbance of balance and deafness from damage to the inner ear. Thus reduction of dosage, or the use of alternative drugs may be required in renal failure.

The classification of renal disease. 'Nephritis'

The old term for kidney disorders was Bright's Disease. This was later replaced by the word *'nephritis'* which means bilateral inflammation of the kidneys, cause unspecified, though acute nephritis was known often to be a reaction in the kidneys to preceding streptococcal throat infection. Septic infection of the urinary tract was not included in the term nephritis, but we have seen above that the kidney substance may be involved by such infection for which the separate term pyelonephritis is used.

Attempts were then made to classify nephritis by clinical and post mortem appearances—hence the terms acute (Type 1) glomerulonephritis, subacute (Type 2) nephritis and chronic nephritis. However, this classification is proving unsatisfactory for renal biopsy (during life) has shown that different clinical presentations can have the same microscopical appearances (and vice versa), and it is the histology of the kidney which determines prognosis and guides treatment. Indeed, just as the diagnosis and management of leukaemia depends on the examination of the blood film, so the management of 'nephritis' may depend on the biopsy appearances. As in leukaemia, we remain ignorant of the cause of many kidney diseases.

There are two fairly clear cut clinical syndromes—acute glomerulonephritis, and the nephrotic syndrome (which is often due to 'subacute nephritis'). These are described below, followed by a description of *acute renal failure*, which may complicate both. The term chronic nephritis is not very helpful clinically, for while it may follow acute or subacute nephritis, the patient may present without such a history suffering from *chronic renal failure* (uraemia). The kidneys are small and scarred and it may be quite impossible to know what the cause of the destruction has been, possibilities including chronic glomerulonephritis (which may have followed acute or subacute glomerulonephritis), chronic pyelonephritis, or the effects of hypertension.

The availability of renal dialysis and transplantation has transformed attitudes towards management of these conditions, which are increasingly the province of specialized renal units. In the long term, an understanding of the nature of renal disease may lead to its prevention. Meantime, we must be aware of current concepts.

Acute glomerulonephritis (Type 1 nephritis).

This is commonest in schoolchildren but may occur in adults.

Causes

The commonest cause is an antecedent throat infection with certain strains of haemolytic streptococci. It is an allergic response in both kidneys about ten days after such infection. It thus resembles serum sickness, antigen-antibody complexes being formed and producing an inflammatory, cellular reaction at the capillaries of the renal glomeruli—hence *glomerulo*nephritis.

Other diseases involving small blood vessels may be causative—anaphylactoid (Henoch-Schonlein) and other purpuras, systemic lupus erythematosus, and polyarteritis nodosa. These immune disorders are important in adult cases and the picture may be less benign than that of post-streptococcal nephritis.

Symptoms and signs

There is *oedema*, especially of the face, giving a pale, puffy appearance, but peripheral oedema may not otherwise be marked. The urine is initially diminished in amount, and there is haematuria giving a smoky appearance.

The onset is usually abrupt (but there may be history of sore throat), with malaise, shivering, fever and aches at the loins. The blood pressure is slightly raised.

Usually the illness is short, diuresis occurring in a few days and followed by disappearance of oedema and haematuria.

Complications. 1. Rarely, hypertension is severe and associated with headache, vomiting and convulsions (hypertensive encephalopathy) or with left ventricular failure and pulmonary oedema.

2. Persistent oliguria or anuria with rising blood urea and acute renal failure—see below.

Investigations

Urine contains red cells and casts, is of high specific gravity, and may contain protein, but heavy proteinuria suggests underlying chronic renal pathology.

Throat swab and anti-streptolysin O (A.S.O.) titre may confirm antecedent streptococcal infection. The E.S.R. is raised. Blood urea and electrolytes are checked.

Important nursing observations include pulse and temperature chart, blood pressure, daily urine volumes and daily weighing of the patient.

Treatment

1. *Bed rest*—indicated in febrile stage or until obvious haematuria clears.

2. *Penicillin*—½ mega unit intramuscularly twice daily for a few

days to clear any residual streptococci from the throat; long term oral penicillin (penicillin V 250 mg twice daily) may prevent recurrent throat infection.

3. *Diet*. The object is to maintain fluid balance and give adequate calories until there is spontaneous recovery of renal function, which usually occurs in a few days.

Fluid—in the oliguric stage, restrict to 400 ml daily plus an amount equal to the volume of urine passed during the previous 24 hours. Salt is restricted if there is oedema or hypertension—usually it suffices not to add salt at meals, and to avoid obviously salty foods such as bacon and kippers.

A high calorie intake comprising carbohydrates and fat prevents endogenous protein breakdown, but protein restriction is only indicated if the blood urea is rising, when the management becomes that of acute renal failure.

4. Treatment of *hypertensive complications* includes pentolinium 2 mg injections to lower the blood pressure, frusemide (Lasix) 80 mg orally for pulmonary oedema, and diazepam (Valium) 10 mg slowly intravenously if there is marked restlessness or convulsions.

Follow-up

Most children, possibly 100 per cent of those whose acute nephritis follows streptococcal throat infection, recover completely—continued oral penicillin may diminish reinfection of the throat but has no effect on any existing renal damage.

The occurrence of severe hypertension, persistent proteinuria or rising blood urea (a state of affairs which may occur in adult acute nephritis) makes the prognosis much less satisfactory, such cases merging into nephrotic syndrome or renal failure.

Nephrotic syndrome

This is a clinical picture characterized by:

1. Oedema of insidious onset, resulting from
2. Heavy proteinuria (5 G or more/24 hours), with a reduced serum albumin level.

The nephrotic syndrome is commonest in young children but can occur at any age, usually without preceding history.

Causes

1. *Subacute glomerulonephritis (Type 2 Nephritis).*

This is responsible for about 75 per cent of the cases. The cause is unknown, most cases presenting from the start with this type of renal disease, but cases may follow an episode of acute glomerulonephritis. It is probably a disorder of immunity with glomerular damage classified as minimal change, membrane thickening, and cellular proliferation—the more marked these changes, the worse the prognosis.

2. *Renal vein thrombosis.*

3. *Systemic disease affecting the kidneys*—amyloid disease (complicates chronic infection or rheumatoid arthritis or occurs alone), systemic lupus erythematosus, diabetes and in Nigerian children especially, malaria.

4. *Poisons and drugs*—carbon tetrachloride, troxidone (used in petit mal) and gold (used in rheumatoid arthritis).

In all these disorders the renal glomeruli have become abnormally porous, leaking out albumin (and other plasma proteins in severe cases) into the urine. The plasma albumin level therefore falls. Albumin in the plasma maintains the osmotic force which attracts water into the circulation. The fall in the plasma albumin results in water passing from the circulation into the tissues, causing oedema. The tendency for the circulating blood volume to fall causes excess aldosterone secretion, with salt and water retention, worsening the tissue oedema.

Symptoms and signs

The first complaint is often ankle swelling, then oedema spreads to the legs, body and face which is pale and puffy. There may be ascites, and pleural effusion. There need be no urinary symptoms, perhaps some frothing at micturition due to the albumin in the urine, but renal function is preserved for months or years, and the blood pressure need not be raised. Due to the protein loss, which includes some antibodies, resistance is lowered and patients are prone to infection, such as respiratory tract infections.

The course is variable, and proteinuria may diminish as diseased nephrons are destroyed but total renal function deteriorates, the patient passing into renal failure.

Investigations

Urine contains 5 G or more albumin per 24 hours, but initially is of normal specific gravity. The plasma albumin is low, and for unknown reasons the cholesterol high. Blood urea and electrolytes are initially normal. The L.E. latex test is positive in cases due to systemic lupus erythematosus.

Renal biopsy may be necessary, for knowledge of the underlying renal lesion is required for correct management.

Nursing observations include blood pressure, urine volume and daily weighing of the patient.

Treatment

1. *Bed rest*—helps to mobilize gross oedema, but is unnecessary in mild cases.

2. *Diet.* Normal fluids are given, but moderate salt restriction (1–3 G daily) is advised while oedema persists—no added salt, avoidance of foods such as bacon and kippers. A *high protein* intake (at least 100 G daily) is encouraged provided the blood urea is normal.

3. *Diuretics.* Frusemide (Lasix) 80–480 mg daily will usually initiate a diuresis, and potassium supplements (slow-K or Sando-K) are added. Spironolactone (Aldactone-A), which antagonizes the effect of aldosterone on the renal tubules, is often used in combination with frusemide. An intravenous infusion of albumin may promote a diuresis, but its effect on the plasma albumin is usually short-lived.

4. *Corticosteroids.* In children and in adults with 'minimal change' lesion, prednisone 10–15 mg four times daily is given for 2–6 weeks and if proteinuria improves, it can be continued long-term on smaller dosage. Patients with more severe glomerular changes do not benefit from steroids and side-effects such as protein breakdown cause a rise in the blood urea, while their salt-retaining action worsens oedema and may cause hypertension. Steroids are also contra-indicated in diabetes and possibly in amyloid disease.

Immunosuppressive (cytotoxic) drugs such as cyclophosphamide may prevent relapse in a proportion of cases responding to steroids.

It is now seldom necessary to resort to mechanical methods for removing oedema, such as Southey's tubes inserted under the skin, or paracentesis for ascites.

Antibacterial drugs are not given routinely but may be necessary for treatment of the infections to which the patient is prone.

Prognosis

Remission or cure is possible in minimal lesion cases, which includes most children but in adults with nephrotic syndrome the prognosis is generally more serious, only about 10 per cent cases recovering completely. Many have a slowly progressive course over years, but can be reasonably maintained on the treatment described. Others, especially if there is accompanying hypertension, deteriorate within a year or two, with muscle wasting, fatigue, infections and progression to chronic glomerulonephritis with destruction of nephrons, rising blood urea and renal failure.

Acute renal failure

Causes

1. *Pre-renal*—lack of blood supply to the kidneys.
   (*a*) haemorrhage—injury, haematemesis (so-called 'haemorrhagic shock');
   (*b*) fluid loss from vomiting, diarrhoea or severe burns;
   (*c*) prolonged hypotension from cardiac failure, or Gram-negative septicaemia (so-called 'septic shock').

2. *Renal*
   (*a*) some cases of acute nephritis;
   (*b*) renal cortical necrosis in pregnancy, and the renal damage that may complicate operations in jaundiced patients;
   (*c*) mis-matched blood transfusion, and following crush injuries causing sludging of blood and nephron damage;
   (*d*) tubular blockage or damage by sulphonamide drugs, or poisons such as carbon tetrachloride.

3. *Post-renal*. Obstruction in the ureters, bladder or prostate, such as stones, carcinoma, or fibrosis following x-irradiation or the drug methysergide (used in migraine).

Symptoms and signs

There is diminished output of urine: complete anuria suggests a post-renal, obstructive cause. About half the cases presenting in hospital are in fact 'acute on chronic'—in such cases there will be a history suggestive of renal disease such as polyuria, or anaemia, and the event may have been precipitated by an infection or lowered fluid intake.

Where there is no such history, and no evidence of pre-renal circulatory inadequacy, suppression of urine has little clinical effect for about ten days, when symptoms from retained waste products— *acute uraemia*—begin to occur—drowsiness, twitching and vomiting.

Where there has been much tissue destruction or severe infection, the 'hyperkatabolic' cases, uraemia is of rapid onset, but it is malpractice to await gross signs such as convulsions, coma or the appearance of deposits of 'urea frost' on the skin.

Investigations

Except in pre-renal cases, the urine is of low specific gravity and urea content, and may contain red cells, casts and protein. Straight x-ray may be helpful, for small kidneys suggest a chronic cause. I.V.P., radio-isotope renogram and cystoscopy are helpful if a post-renal cause is suspected. Blood urea, electrolytes, especially potassium, and acid-base balance are checked. Catheterization of the bladder may be necessary to see if any urine is being formed.

Important observations are urine volume and daily weighing of the patient.

Treatment

Prompt treatment of circulatory inadequacy is important in the prevention of the pre-renal causes, measures include adequate blood transfusion and fluid replacement in such conditions. If there is doubt as to whether blood volume is adequate, it may be justified to give blood or saline intravenously, monitoring the central venous pressure with an indwelling cannula in the superior vena cava, until normality is attained. Mannitol 200 ml of 10 per cent solution intravenously may, by its osmotic effect and possibly direct action on the kidney, initiate a diuresis in very early cases, but it is dangerous to repeat mannitol unless a urine flow is established.

Established acute renal failure—there are two important principles:

I. To maintain the body's fluid and metabolic requirements as near normal as possible until spontaneous recovery occurs: this is *Conservative Treatment*.

II. If the patient deteriorates, and the blood urea is rising, *dialysis* is indicated early rather than late. Dialysis may also be required to bring a neglected patient into suitable conditions for surgical measures for correction of post-renal obstruction.

I. Conservative treatment

1. *Fluids* are restricted to 400–500 ml daily plus a volume equal to the previous 24-hour urine output.

2. *Diet*. Protein breakdown products are responsible for the symptoms of uraemia and therefore dietary protein should be

restricted, but it is equally important to give adequate calories in the diet otherwise there will be excessive endogenous protein katabolism. Dietary protein should be restricted to 18–20 G daily provided it can be given as protein of high biological value, as in the modified Giordano-Giovanetti diet—1 egg, 6½ oz milk, plus low protein (0·5 per cent) bread and salt-free butter or margarine, with the amino-acid methionine 500 mg daily. However, an easier regime is to give about 20 G egg-protein, and supply 1,700 calories daily with 4 bottles (each 180 ml) of Hycal, a liquid dextrose concentrate, or use Caloreen if Hycal proves unpalatable.

3. *Antibacterial drugs* may be required for infection, but tetracycline should be avoided.

4. *Potassium-exchanging-resin* such as Calcium resonium 15 G orally or rectally (or intravenous calcium gluconate in emergency), lowers high blood potassium levels, which may provoke cardiac arrhythmias.

The emotional needs and the comfort of the patient must not be neglected during such a tedious regime and it is unwise to pursue it unless spontaneous diuresis occurs within a few days, when careful fluid and electrolyte balance is also necessary. New methods such as heparin injections in certain types of renal failure are being tried in special centres.

II. Dialysis

Peritoneal dialysis can be carried out in a general hospital if biochemical facilities are adequate. *Haemodialysis* is carried out in special units. These are considered below.

Chronic renal failure—uraemia

Chronic renal failure is a disorder of gradual onset, the end result of many chronic diseases of the kidneys. Biochemical evidence of deteriorating renal function, such as a rising blood urea precedes the clinical picture, for symptoms do not appear until 75 per cent of the renal function has been destroyed.

Causes

1. Chronic glomerulonephritis.
2. Chronic pyelonephritis.
3. Hypertensive kidney disease.
4. Chronic urinary tract obstruction (stones, enlarged prostate).

Less common causes are amyloid disease, systemic lupus erythe-matosus, gout, diabetes and polycystic disease of the kidneys.

The kidneys are small and scarred, so it may be impossible to establish the cause, but the effect is the same. Most of the nephrons have been destroyed, the remaining ones are working hard, but there is a lack of sufficient numbers to excrete the body's waste products and to control fluid, electrolyte and acid-base balance.

Uraemia literally means a high blood urea, which is the hall-mark of renal failure. The term uraemia may be used to describe the clinical picture. Urea is itself non-toxic (except possibly to the gut from breakdown to form ammonia). The raised urea proves that renal failure exists, but it is unknown toxic end products of protein metabolism, plus the systemic effects of the disordered renal function that cause the symptoms.

Symptoms and signs

Chronic renal failure occurs in middle-age, men being more commonly affected (from the effects of hypertension). Presenting features include malaise, lack of energy, anaemia, raised blood pressure and polyuria—the important symptom of rising at night to pass urine may, however, only be elicited on questioning. The urinary and blood findings may lead to the diagnosis in a symptom-less patient. Any system may gradually become affected:

cardiovascular system: hypertension, pulmonary oedema, arrhyth-mias from high potassium, terminal pericarditis.

respiratory: deep, sighing breathing of acidosis (blowing off CO_2).

alimentary: anorexia, nausea, vomiting, hiccups, dry tongue and stomatitis, later diarrhoea which may be bloody.

haemopoietic: anaemia and bleeding tendency.

nervous system: twitching, convulsions, coma; peripheral neuro-pathy.

skin: muddy, yellow pigmentation, pruritus, purpura.

skeletal: bones may be decalcified (osteomalacia), calcium deposited in tissues, or tetany may occur from a low blood calcium.

Patients may tolerate mild symptoms for many years. Deteriora-tion may be provoked by infection or inadequate fluid intake.

Investigations

The urine is of large volume, fixed specific gravity around 1,010 and poor urea content (less than 1 G/100 ml). Proteinuria may be present but is not gross. A mid-stream specimen should be cultured, so that any infection can be recognized and treated. Frequent weighing of the patient is a guide to fluid balance.

Straight x-ray shows small kidneys. I.V.P. may be performed, but the kidneys may be unable to concentrate the medium adequately for visualization.

The *blood urea* (normal 20–40 mg/100 ml) is raised; a level of 100–200 mg/100 ml may be tolerated for years, and a sudden rise is more significant than the absolute level. The blood creatinine (another protein metabolite) is raised and its level is independent of protein in the diet. The creatinine clearance test is a guide to the glomerular filtration rate, roughly parallels residual renal function, and may drop to 10 per cent of normal or even less in the terminal stage. The serum sodium, potassium and degree of acidosis (low pH or bicarbonate) are measured.

Treatment

Any *obstruction* of the urinary tract should be relieved, and *infection*, whether renal or systemic, is treated with appropriate antibacterial drugs; tetracycline should be avoided as it increases protein breakdown.

Hypertension should be treated, using methyldopa (Aldomet) 250–500 mg 3-times daily, or more powerful hypotensives such as guanethidine or bethanidine, provided they do not cause a rise in the blood urea. Hypertension may be due to salt and water retention, and dietary restriction, frusemide and even dialysis may be required to remove this excessive fluid.

Fluid and electrolyte balance. Provided the urine output remains high, *fluid* intake should be liberal, but it may be dangerous to 'push' fluids unless the patient's weight and serum sodium levels are watched. While normal *salt* intake is often permissible some patients retain salt excessively leading to hypertension and oedema, others lose salt, leading to hypotension. Suitable dietary adjustments are necessary. For *raised serum potassium*, the potassium-exchanging resin Calcium resonium is given orally (15 G) or by retention enema. *Acidosis* is rarely severe enough in itself to warrant intravenous bicarbonate therapy.

Diet. The aim is to cut the load of toxic protein breakdown products that the kidneys are required to excrete. This is achieved by *trimming the dietary protein* to the essential basic requirement, and at the same time *giving adequate calories* to suppress the unnecessary katabolism of bodily protein for energy purposes.

Dietary restrictions are tedious and a symptom-free patient can often be adequately maintained on any palatable diet which avoids excessive meat or fish.

The special low-protein high-calorie diets relieve the gastrointestinal symptoms of uraemia such as vomiting and diarrhoea. These diets are also indicated when renal function falls to about 10 per cent of normal, when a 40 G protein (of high biological value) plus at least 2,000 Calories (from carbohydrate and fat) intake may be prescribed. When renal function falls even lower, conservative treatment may still be successful using the modified Giordano-Giovannetti diet, described under Acute Renal Failure, and containing only 18 G protein; iron and vitamin supplements are necessary. Such low-protein diets may cause a raised serum potassium and acidosis. Their proper use may, however, prevent the need for dialysis, which has to be considered when this stage of renal failure has been reached.

Anaemia is usually present in renal failure, a haemoglobin of 40–50 per cent being common, but patients adapt to this. Drugs are not usually of value. Blood transfusion produces only a transient rise and should be avoided as it introduces antigens which may complicate subsequent transplantation, and may transmit serum hepatitis.

Calcium gluconate may be required for tetany, and vitamin D for renal bone disease, which is often resistant to the usual therapeutic doses (0·5–1·0 mg/day for osteomalacia).

Where these conservative measures fail, the patient should be considered for an intermittent dialysis—renal transplantation programme. If age or complicating conditions preclude this, then it is important that the patient's life be as free from discomfort as possible. In the terminal stages of uraemia nursing care in hospital includes especially attention to the mouth, and medical measures include chlorpromazine (Largactil) to allay distress and vomiting, and diazepam (Valium) as a sedative.

Renal dialysis

Dialysis really means a process of separating substances in solution, but used medically the term has come to mean the *removal of the waste products of metabolism* in renal failure. Urea and protein breakdown products will diffuse from an area of high concentration in the tissues or blood on one side of a membrane into a solution of low concentration on the other side. The electrolyte content of the solution is isotonic (isosmotic) with the blood, but can be adjusted to cause the removal of excess potassium or water from the body. The acid-base upset is also corrected.

Methods

Peritoneal Dialysis. The principle is to run a volume of solution into the peritoneal cavity, allow time for excess urea and waste metabolites to diffuse into it, drain the fluid off and then repeat the cycle.

The bladder is emptied. Then, using local anaesthesia, a catheter (mounted on a stylet) is inserted through the anterior abdominal wall below the umbilicus into the peritoneal cavity. One (or two) litre of warmed sterile peritoneal dialysing solution (such as 1·36 per cent Dialaflex Dianeal or Difusor) is run in, left for 20 minutes then drained off via a two-way tap into a plastic drainage bag and the volume measured. As soon as drainage is complete the process is repeated with fresh solution, it being possible to make two exchanges each hour over a 36–48 hour period. Careful checking of drainage volume and of the patient's serum electrolytes (especially potassium) is necessary. Hypertonic (6·36 per cent) solution can be used if it is desired to remove water from a patient with fluid retention. Skilled and kind nursing, attention to pressure areas and mouth care are important, but fluids in the diet may be more liberal during the process, as excess water can be removed.

Techniques of peritoneal dialysis vary, but if 2 litre instead of 1 litre volumes are used, the patient tends to have some discomfort from the induced ascites, and increased risk of pneumonia following poor chest expansion. Other complications of dialysis include peritonitis, and protein losses in the dialysing fluid.

Haemodialysis using some type of Artificial Kidney. This is a much more efficient method but can only be carried out in special centres. It involves cannulation of an artery and a large vein in the arm or leg. As the process may need to be repeated, a 'shunt' of plastic tubing may be inserted between artery and vein, uncoupled for dialysis and replaced between dialyses. An alternative technique to cannulation is the creation of a subcutaneous arterio-venous fistula, the arterial and venous supply being 'needled' for dialysis.

The arterial supply is fed through plastic tubes to a pump which assists it on its way to the kidney machine. There are two main types, the Kolff disposable coil kidney, and the Kiil kidney. In the Kolff machine the blood flows through a 'sausage skin' tube of cellophane (which retains the red cells and proteins in the plasma) coiled round a supporting bobbin place in a bath of dialysing fluid. In the Kiil kidney the blood flows over layers of cellophane or cuprophane membrane. In each case, the outer surface of the membrane is bathed by dialysing fluid, warmed and isotonic with plasma, but it need not be sterile as it does not come into contact with the patient's blood. The excess urea, toxic metabolites and potassium pass into the dialysing fluid, and the purified blood flows onwards into the patient's vein. The process takes 6–12 hours.

Indications

Acute renal failure. Dialysis 'buys time' until spontaneous recovery occurs. It should be used before uraemia complications occur. If they already exist, dialysis will cause improvement, allowing investigation, and surgical relief of urinary obstruction if present. Dialysis is essential in hyperkatabolic cases, and its use permits the dietary supplementation necessary for tissue repair.

Poisoning. Dialysis hastens the excretion of certain poisons, and its use is occasionally necessary in very severe aspirin or barbiturate poisoning.

Chronic renal failure. Dialysis is indicated to tide the patient over an acute crisis—infection, trauma, or operation (all of which increase protein katabolism), and for fluid retention and hypertension. It should also be considered in long-term therapy in association with a renal transplantation programme. Intermittent haemodialysis three times weekly (often carried out overnight) can be given for months or years. Complications include clotting and infection at the cannulation site, anaemia and calcium upset. Following repeated blood transfusions and failure of immunity, patients may become carriers of the hepatitis-associated (Australian) antigen, and outbreaks of hepatitis have affected patients and staff in dialysis units. This may be prevented by detection of carriers and special isolation centres. Patients who have understanding relatives can now be treated with intermittent haemodialysis using machines installed in their own homes.

Renal transplantation

This involves the replacement of the patient's kidneys by a donor kidney, with restoration of renal function. Some 3,000 persons whose lives might be saved die annually in Britain from renal disease, and dialysis-transplantation facilities are being expanded to provide treatment. A transplant from an identical twin has 90 per cent success rate. Using a kidney from other living blood relatives, the success rate is no higher than that of a cadaver transplant. Current procedure therefore involves the use of the kidneys from persons who had given their consent to such organ donation before death. The British register of such volunteers, with their tissue type (red and white cell antigens) is at Bristol, and there is a Eurotransplant scheme. Patients on a dialysis programme are also typed, and when a suitable kidney becomes available, transplantation is carried out within a few hours. Rejection reactions can be prevented by immunological methods, or suppressed with steroids and cytotoxic drugs such as azathioprine, but improved tissue typing is lowering their incidence.

If renal transplantation fails, nothing is lost, for the patient can be maintained by haemodialysis until a further opportunity presents. The technique is steadily becoming more successful and 50 per cent of transplanted kidneys are still functioning after two years. The actual survival rate of patients on the programme, is of course, considerably higher.

Renal dialysis and transplantation have not only improved and prolonged life, they have also contributed to the understanding of renal diseases, and raised the hope of their prevention in the future.

9

Diseases of the blood and lymph glands

Physiology of the blood

Blood consists of red cells, white cells and platelets suspended in the plasma.

Red cells (erythrocytes, R.B.C.'s) are formed in the bone marrow and contain haemoglobin, the red pigment which carries oxygen to the tissues and removes carbon dioxide. The normal haemoglobin is 100 per cent, 15 G/100 ml., the red cell count 5,000,000/cu mm. Other indices include packed cell volume (P.C.V., normal 45 per cent), mean cell volume (M.C.V.) and mean corpuscular haemoglobin concentration (M.C.H.C.). The red cell has a life of 120 days, when it is taken up and destroyed by cells of the reticulo-endothelial system in the lymph glands, spleen and liver. The iron content of the 'haem' is re-utilized for blood formation, the remainder goes to form bilirubin (which becomes bile pigment), and the globin part of haemoglobin joins the body's protein pool.

White cells (leucocytes) are of three types:

1. Polymorphonuclear ('many-shaped nuclei') leucocytes (*polymorphs*, granulocytes) formed in the bone marrow, concerned in the inflammatory reaction, and in the destruction of bacteria in infections forming pus cells. The polymorphs are subdivided into neutrophils, basophils and eosinophils by the staining properties of their granules with dyes.

2. *Lymphocytes*, formed in the lymph glands and probably of two groups, one related to immune globulin (antibody) production, the other dependent on the thymus gland and concerned with tissue or 'cellular' immunity.

3. *Monocytes*, fewer in number but, like the polymorphs, phagocytic in function (engulfing foreign matter).

The total white cell count (W.B.C.) is 4,000–9,000 mm^3. An increase is called a leucocytosis and may occur in any inflammation. In bacterial infection the polymorphs are especially raised. In virus infection the total white count may not be raised, the increase being confined to the lymphocyte series, lymphocytosis.

Platelets (thrombocytes) are much smaller, are produced in the bone marrow and are concerned in blood clotting.

Plasma contains water and electrolytes (such as sodium, potassium, chloride and bicarbonate) concerned in normal tonicity and acid base balance and the plasma proteins, albumin, globulins, fibrinogen and prothrombin. Albumin (formed in the liver) helps to maintain the osmotic pressure, keeping fluid in the circulation. The globulins include the immune globulins, some of which are antibodies. They are formed partly by lymphocytes and partly by 'plasma cells', a bad term as these cells are normally confined to the bone marrow and lymph glands and do *not* enter the plasma. Fibrinogen and prothrombin are concerned in blood clotting by the formation of fibrin. Blood also contains a 'fibrinolytic' mechanism to prevent excessive deposition of fibrin.

Blood groups

A person is of group A, B, AB or O, the blood group antigen(s) being carried in the red cells. Group O people lack such an antigen, and their blood can be transfused into others without causing a reaction. Group AB people, who are rare, can be given blood of any of these groups, for their cells already contain both antigens. Now let us consider a person of blood group A. His serum contains antibodies, called agglutinins, to cells of group B or AB. If he is wrongly transfused with such blood, the cells will agglutinate (clump) and then haemolyse (break up) causing a severe reaction.

Eighty-five per cent of persons carry the Rhesus (Rh) factor in their red cells; the factor has three components, c, D, and e, D being the important one; these persons are Rh (D) positive. A developing foetus may be Rh positive from paternal inheritance although its mother is Rh negative. At childbirth, when the placenta is separating from the uterus, some of the baby's red cells may pass into the maternal circulation, causing the formation of antibodies. In a subsequent pregnancy these can pass across the placenta and destroy an Rh positive baby's red cells causing haemolytic disease of the newborn. This sequence of events can now be prevented by giving a susceptible mother anti-D immunoglobulin immediately after childbirth to prevent her own production of this antibody.

These are the important blood groups. Before transfusion, the recipients group must be ascertained, then some of his serum must be cross-matched against the donor cells to ensure compatibility. Apart from incompatibility, hazards to the recipient include infection (such as serum hepatitis, but screening for the antigen is now possible), calcium depletion (from the citrate in massive transfusions) and non-specific fever—but the most important hazard is human error; names and bottles must be carefully checked.

Blood groups have been found to have some disease associations— thus peptic ulcer is commoner in those of blood group O, itself the commonest group.

Investigations in blood diseases

Minimum investigations are haemoglobin, white cell count, and erythrocyte sedimentation rate (E.S.R.). Cell counts are done by microscopy, or electronically. R.B.C.s and their indices are worked out. It is usually necessary also to stain and microscopically examine a blood film.

For an E.S.R., venous blood is added to anticoagulant, such as citrate solution (0·5 ml to 2 ml blood) in the Westergren method, drawn into a capillary tube and stood for an hour. The red cells tend to sink, leaving clear plasma above. The normal E.S.R. is up to 10 mm in males, and 15 mm in females. The rate of fall depends on the plasma proteins, and is high in inflammation and infection, neoplasms, leukaemia, myeloma and auto-immune diseases—due to the raised globulins in the latter. It is lowered in congestive cardiac failure. The plasma proteins may also be measured chemically, and by a method called electrophoresis, on a paper strip or immunologically.

Special tests such as serum iron, vitamin B_{12} and folic acid levels in the blood may also be required.

Sternal marrow puncture, using a special hollow needle (local anaesthesia) and biopsy of enlarged glands may be indicated.

In the *urine*, urobilinogen will be increased (positive Urobilistix) in haemolytic anaemia. The *stools* will give a positive test for blood (guaiac, Hemoccult) if there is gastrointestinal bleeding.

Anaemia

Definition
Anaemia is a reduction in the number of the red cells, or their haemoglobin content, or both.

Causes
There are three possible mechanisms:

1. BLOOD LOSS
2. DECREASED BLOOD FORMATION
3. INCREASED BLOOD DESTRUCTION

When confronted with an anaemic patient, consider which one of these is likely to be responsible.

Classification
Anaemias are best classified by these three causes, as follows:

1. ANAEMIA DUE TO BLOOD LOSS

The blood loss may be *acute* or *chronic*. Chronic blood loss is the most important cause of 'Iron-deficiency anaemia', which will be considered in this section.

2. ANAEMIAS DUE TO DECREASED BLOOD FORMATION

   (a) *Lack of building factors* such as iron, vitamin B_{12} and folic acid. This may occur from:

      (i) *inadequate dietary intake:* iron deficiency is common, dietary B_{12} lack very rare, folic acid lack is rare but may occur in the elderly on a diet poor in greens.
      (ii) *failure of absorption:* pernicious anaemia will be considered in this group.
      (iii) *increased demands:* anaemia of pregnancy.
      (iv) effect of *anticonvulsant drugs.*

   (b) *Lack of bone marrow*—from infiltration (leukaemia), or desstruction (aplastic anaemia).

   (c) *Disordered function* of the bone marrow.

3. INCREASED BLOOD DESTRUCTION—HAEMOLYTIC ANAEMIAS

   (a) Faults in the red cell.
   (b) Faults in the plasma.
   (c) Effects of drugs.

General symptoms and signs of anaemia

Any system may be affected. *Cardio-respiratory* symptoms are weakness, breathlessness, ankle oedema and sometimes angina. In the *nervous* system, effects include tiredness and faint feelings. Peripheral neuritis, leg pains and loss of reflexes, may complicate any form of anaemia (but is commonest in pernicious anaemia). In the *gastrointestinal* system, symptoms include loss of appetite, constipation or sometimes diarrhoea.

The characteristic sign is *pallor*—this may be noted classically in the conjuntivae, but pallor of the fingers and hands may be a better guide.

Confirmation of the diagnosis

The appearance of the patient can be deceptive, and to establish the existence of anaemia the haemoglobin must be checked. This will be reduced, but there is no fixed level below which symptoms appear. If blood loss has been acute, symptoms may be present with a haemoglobin of 75 per cent. If the anaemic process has on the other hand been slow, then the patient may not complain until very low levels of 40 per cent or less have been reached.

Anaemia is a *symptom*, not a diagnosis in itself, and search must be made for its cause.

Anaemia due to blood loss

Acute blood loss may be obvious in injuries and gastrointestinal bleeding such as haematemesis, but less obvious with closed fractures or intra-abdominal conditions such as ruptured spleen or retroperitoneal haemorrhage complicating anticoagulant treatment. Rapid loss causes pallor, clammy skin, apprehension, fast pulse and low blood pressure—the picture of haemorrhagic shock, requiring transfusion. The body compensates for such haemorrhage by haemodilution causing a temporary anaemia until the red cells have been replaced by the activity of the bone marrow, given sufficient iron.

CHRONIC BLOOD LOSS. IRON DEFICIENCY ANAEMIA

The normal dietary iron content is 10–15 mg daily, meat and coloured foods being rich sources, but milk containing little iron. Though only a proportion of this food iron can be absorbed, it is more than enough to compensate for the tiny daily iron losses in men, about 1–2 mg. Thus, men cannot get 'iron deficiency' anaemia from dietary inadequacy—there must be another cause, usually occult blood loss. In women due to menstrual blood loss, the need for iron is greater and the demand is increased by pregnancy and childbirth. The diets of many women do not meet these needs and 'iron deficiency' anaemia will ensue. (Traces of iron off old-fashioned cooking pots gave protection not afforded by modern methods of food preparation.)

Causes of iron deficiency anaemia

(i) *Blood loss:* heavy menstrual bleeding (menorrhagia).
   chronic aspirin ingestion (causes gastric erosions).
   peptic ulcer.
   carcinoma, especially of rectum, colon or stomach.
   bleeds from the nose (epistaxis), and from haemorrhoids.

(ii) *Increased demand*—foetal needs during pregnancy.

(iii) *Dietary inadequacy*—occurs only in women.

(iv) *Defective absorption*—coeliac disease; following gastrectomy or stomach operation.

Symptoms and signs

These are the general symptoms of anaemia. Rarely, iron deficiency anaemia presents as the Paterson Kelly (Plummer Vinson) syndrome of flat or spoon-shaped nails (koilonychia), smooth tongue and dysphagia from a pharyngeal web (seen on barium swallow).

Blood examination shows a low haemoglobin, and some decrease in the red cell count; the cells are pale (hypochromic) and small (microcytic)—iron deficiency gives the picture described as a hypochromic, microcytic anaemia.

Treatment

Blood loss must be sought and its cause corrected if possible.

Iron. This should be given by mouth as ferrous sulphate 200 mg 3 times daily. Though best absorbed on an empty stomach, iron is rather irritant and usually given with meals. Other preparations such as ferrous succinate (Ferromyn-S), or single-dose capsules of iron, may be used in the few patients who are upset by ferrous sulphate. Vitamin C (ascorbic acid) given with iron theoretically aids absorption, but is not necessary. Treatment should be continued for some weeks after the haemoglobin is normal, to replenish the body's iron stores.

Iron injections (Imferon, Jectofer) may cause pain and staining if given intramuscularly, and hypersensitivity reactions may follow the use of intravenous preparations. In most cases, such injections have no advantage over oral iron—failure to respond to the latter usually being due to failure to take the tablets. In the iron malabsorption of coeliac disease, injections may be required (and they also have a place in the anaemia associated with rheumatoid arthritis).

Blood transfusion may be necessary in severe and neglected cases, in the elderly and if an operation is required. However, blood is a precious commodity and its use is not justified in the average case simply to 'speed the therapy'. There are also risks of transfusion reactions and transmission of serum hepatitis.

2. Anaemias due to decreased blood formation

PERNICIOUS ANAEMIA

Cause

Pernicious anaemia has a familial tendency and is thought to be a disturbance of immunity arising in adult life. There is an auto-immune destruction of the parietal cells of the stomach, and antibodies are detectable in the circulation. The parietal cells produce hydrochloric acid and also *intrinsic factor*. Their destruction is followed by atrophy of the gastric mucosa, and lack of intrinsic factor. Intrinsic factor is essential for the absorption of vitamin B_{12} in the lower ileum. In pernicious anaemia, intrinsic factor is lacking and vitamin B_{12} cannot be absorbed.

Vitamin B_{12} is essential for normal bone marrow function, and in its absence red cell development is defective. Thus abnormal large cells called megaloblasts are formed (in great quantity)in the marrow. From these there is produced a diminished number of red cells which appear in the circulation and are called macrocytes—these are large, well-haemoglobinized cells, but fragile, tending to haemolyse easily.

Thus pernicious anaemia is due to malabsorption of vitamin B_{12} from lack of intrinsic factor following gastric mucosal atrophy, and is characterized by a megaloblastic bone marrow and a macrocytic anaemia plus an element of haemolysis.

Pernicious anaemia is only one manifestation of vitamin B_{12} deficiency. The vitamin is essential for the normal function of cells other than those in the bone marrow, such as cells in the nervous system. Thus vitamin B_{12} deficiency may affect cerebral function causing deterioration of intellect (dementia) before there is any gross anaemia. A late effect is a degeneration of the posterior and lateral columns of the spinal cord, called subacute combined degeneration.

Symptoms and signs

Pernicious anaemia occurs in the middle-aged and elderly and is commoner in women. The symptoms are those of any anaemia, but the onset is slow over years. During this period the patient may have managed in a limited way before presenting with pallor, low haemoglobin and often mild fever. The skin has a lemon yellow tint from the mild jaundice associated with haemolysis. The tongue is smooth (like the stomach, its mucosa is atrophic) and often red and sore. There is anorexia, constipation or diarrhoea. The spleen may be palpable. Peripheral neuritis presents as leg pains and loss of sensation, motor weakness and absent tendon reflexes (lower motor neurone lesion). If the patient has subacute combined degeneration (which is unique to pernicious anaemia) there is ataxia and loss of vibration sensation from posterior column degeneration, and upper motor neurone signs (spastic weakness, increased reflexes, extensor plantar responses) from the lateral column degeneration.

There is an increased incidence of other auto-immune disorders such as hypothyroidism (myxoedema) in patients with pernicious anaemia and in their relatives—white patches of depigmented skin (vitiligo) may occur with this trait.

Investigations

The diagnosis is confirmed by:

1. Low haemoglobin, and the typical macrocytic blood film.

2. Megaloblastic marrow on sternal puncture; this rather unpleasant test is often omitted nowadays as other tests suffice. (A few megaloblasts may spill over into the circulation and be found in a special 'buffy coat' peripheral blood preparation.)

3. Low serum vitamin B_{12}.

Treatment will restore these three tests to normal, and should generally be started as soon as the specimens have been taken off. The following tests are not affected by treatment:

4. Histamine- or pentagastrin-fast achlorhydria. The gastric contents (obtained by tube) are found to contain no hydrochloric acid, and none is secreted after an injection of histamine (0·04 mg/Kg body weight subcutaneously after a preliminary dose of an antihistamine drug, which suppresses the circulatory but not the gastric

secretory effects of histamine). Pentagastrin (Pentavlon) 0·006 mg/ Kg is an alternative gastric secretory stimulant which does not require antihistamine cover.

5. The Schilling (Dicopac) test, which shows poor absorption of vitamin B_{12} using a radioactive-labelled preparation and measuring its urinary excretion.

The response to specific therapy also confirms the diagnosis.

Treatment

This is by injections of vitamin B_{12}. It is given as hydroxocobalamin (Neo-cytamen) 1,000 micrograms intramuscularly daily or alternate days for 3 or 4 doses with a further injection at one or two weeks, then an injection every two months for life.

Iron therapy (ferrous sulphate by mouth) is not necessary as a routine, but is indicated if there is accompanying evidence of iron deficiency.

Blood transfusion should generally be avoided in pernicious anaemia, as it may precipitate heart failure.

Results

The patient usually feels better within a few days, as though given a new lease of life, and blood film shows a 'reticulocyte response'— reticulocytes are early but normal red cells rushed into circulation as the marrow function becomes normal. The haemoglobin level rises to 100 per cent over a few weeks. Although the anaemia is cured, the malabsorption of vitamin B_{12}, of course, persists, and injections of hydroxocobalamin must be continued for life, otherwise relapse will occur. The results of therapy are, however, most gratifying, the patient being able to resume a full and normal life.

ANAEMIAS OF MALABSORPTION

Iron deficiency anaemia, as we have seen, occurs most commonly from blood losses or physiological demand in the face of relative dietary inadequacy. Iron deficiency anaemia follows malabsorption of iron in chronic atrophic gastritis (when it may complicate pernicious anaemia) possibly due to lack of hydrochloric acid which aids but is not essential to, the absorption of food iron. Iron absorption occurs largely in the duodenum. Malabsorption may also follow gastrectomy, where a large part of the hydrochloric acid secreting area of the stomach is removed. The anaemia responds to oral medicinal iron. Iron malabsorption occurs in coeliac disease, and sometimes injections of iron are necessary here, but once the benefit of the gluten-free diet takes effect, continued iron therapy may not be required.

Vitamin B₁₂ malabsorption causes pernicious anaemia as described. Gastric surgery leads to lack of intrinsic factor, causing the same picture but it may be delayed for many years until the body's own stores of vitamin B_{12} in the liver are exhausted. Thus, patients after stomach or extensive intestinal operations should be screened annually for iron and B_{12} deficiency, to prevent subsequent anaemia. Vitamin B_{12} deficiency anaemia may also occur in coeliac disease and other malabsorption conditions, especially Crohn's disease which affects the terminal ileum where B_{12} is absorbed.

(Dietary B_{12} deficiency is extremely rare, occurring only in the strictest of vegetarians, the Vegans—the tiniest amount of animal protein supplies enough).

Folic acid deficiency can occur from dietary lack in the elderly (from inadequate fresh vegetables) and from increased demands in pregnancy, but is usually due to malabsorption from the small intestine in tropical sprue and adult coeliac disease, gut infiltrations and following operations.

The clinical picture is similar to that in pernicious anaemia, with megaloblastic bone marrow and macrocytic peripheral blood film, but normal gastric hydrochloric acid. Subacute combined degeneration does not occur. The serum folic acid level is low.

Treatment is with folic acid, the oral route being usually effective, dose 5–10 mg daily. If vitamin B_{12} deficiency is also present, this must be corrected first, otherwise subacute combined degeneration may be worsened.

ANAEMIA OF PREGNANCY
This is due to dietary iron deficiency relative to the demands of the foetus and placenta. In addition, folic acid requirement is increased in late pregnancy. Thus it is customary to give pregnant women supplements of iron and small (100 micrograms daily) doses of folic acid, using a combined once-a-day preparation.

Rare cases of true pernicious anaemia (B_{12} deficiency) have occurred in the puerperium.

ANAEMIA OF ANTICONVULSANT DRUGS
Long-term treatment with phenytoin (and rarely primidone and phenobarbitone) for epilepsy may be associated with a folic acid

deficiency anaemia. This responds to folic acid by mouth, and the anticonvulsant drugs can be continued.

ANAEMIA FROM BONE MARROW INFILTRATION OR DESTRUCTION

Anaemia in leukaemia, or in marrow infiltration by cancer metastases (such as from the breast or prostrate) is due to the red cell production line being replaced by these abnormal proliferating cells.

Marrow destruction can be caused by x-rays (or nuclear emissions), poisons such as benzene and lead, and drugs including gold, and chloramphenicol. These may first depress platelet production (causing thrombocytopenia), or white cells (causing agranulocytosis) only later affecting red cell production, destruction of which causes *aplastic anaemia*. This may, however, be primary and of unknown cause.

Treatment of aplastic anaemia is to withdraw the offending poison, if known, and to give blood transfusions until spontaneous marrow regeneration occurs. Anabolic steroids such as oxymetholone are occasionally helpful but often the condition is irreversible, the patient is liable to bleeding and infection (from lack of platelets and white cells) and the prognosis is poor.

ANAEMIAS DUE TO DISORDERED FUNCTIONAL ACTIVITY OF THE BONE MARROW

Bone marrow function may be depressed in chronic infections and toxaemia, carcinoma and in renal failure (possibly due to lack of erythropoietin). The resulting anaemia does not respond to the usual haematinics such as iron, vitamin B_{12} or folic acid. A similar anaemia in rheumatoid arthritis may respond to iron by injection, for unknown reasons.

In the rare 'sideroblastic anaemias' there is a defect of iron utilization; some cases respond to pyridoxine (a B-group vitamin). In some patients with enlargement of the spleen and 'hypersplenism' there is anaemia (and leucopenia) despite an active and apparently normal bone marrow; the release of the cells into the circulation appears to be impaired.

3. Increased blood destruction—the haemolytic anaemias

Haemolytic anaemia may be due to defects in the red cells, or to circulating factors in the plasma which cause their destruction, or to the effects of drugs.

FAULTS IN THE RED CELLS

I. Inherited

(i) *Hereditary Spherocytosis (Congenital Haemolytic Anaemia, Acholuric Jaundice)*. Here the red cells are wrongly shaped, assuming a spherical form instead of their biconcave disc appearance. These spherocytes are fragile and haemolyse easily. The spleen is enlarged. The condition occurs mainly in children, but is rare.

(ii) *The Haemoglobinopathies*. Here the haemoglobin molecule is defective.

Sickle-cell disease occurs in negro races and is common in tropical Africa and the West Indies. It should be remembered as a cause of anaemia (which may be mis-diagnosed as refractory iron-deficiency anaemia) in immigrants. In affected persons, states of anoxia (from high altitudes or following infections) disturb the abnormal haemoglobin molecule causing change in shape of the red cells. They become sickle-shaped, fragile and haemolyse easily causing episodes of haemolytic anaemia. Interestingly, the trait affords protection against severe forms of malaria.

Thalassaemia (Cooley's Anaemia) occurs in Mediterranean countries and is due to a foetal type of haemoglobin persisting into adult life, the affected red cells having a 'target' appearance.

(iii) *Enzyme deficiencies*, which increase the susceptibility of the red cells to haemolysis by substances ranging from broad beans to many drugs (see below).

II. Acquired

An example is malaria, where the red cell is invaded by the plasmodium parasite, causing its subsequent rupture.

FAULTS IN THE PLASMA

Severe infections and chronic diseases. In some cases of severe pneumonia and in carcinoma, leukaemia and renal failure there may be circulating toxins or 'haemolysins' which destroy the red cells.

In *auto-immune diseases* such as systemic lupus erythematosus and rheumatoid arthritis these haemolysins may be identifiable as antibodies, immune globulins.

In certain vascular diseases and nephritis, excessive deposition of fibrin in small vessels may trap the red cells leading to their fragmentation (microangiopathic haemolytic anaemia).

Incompatible blood transfusion. Here the fault is in transfusing cells of the wrong group and, as already explained, the agglutinins in the plasma of the recipient cause clumping followed by haemolysis of the transfused cells, causing a severe reaction. Regarding the Rhesus factor, antibodies in a previously sensitized mother, reaching the baby's circulation, will cause haemolysis of the foetal red cells if the baby is Rh positive. This state of affairs, haemolytic disease of the newborn, can be prevented by giving a susceptible mother anti-D immunoglobulin as explained before, and by making sure that an Rh negative woman of child-bearing age receives only Rh negative blood should a transfusion be required.

EFFECTS OF DRUGS

Very many drugs are capable of causing haemolytic anaemia, especially in persons whose cells are predisposed from enzyme deficiencies, or who are already suffering from auto-immune diseases. Antimalarials and sulphonamides are common culprits, but chloramphenicol, nitrofurantoin, phenacetin and methyldopa may be responsible.

Symptoms and signs of haemolytic anaemia

Haemolytic anaemias classically cause 'acholuric jaundice'. The jaundice is often slight, and not deep as in obstructive jaundice. As explained in Jaundice (page 145) in haemolytic anaemia the urine shows no bile (bilirubin) but contains an excess of urobilinogen, detected by Ehrlich's aldehyde reagent (which turns the urine pink) or Urobilistix test. The spleen is enlarged and often palpable. In severe haemolytic reactions, as may occur with incompatible blood transfusions, there are rigors, fever, prostration and often severe backache. In very severe cases, haemoglobin is released into the blood stream and appears, with breakdown products, in the urine, causing a port-wine colour. There is danger of sludging of cells in the kidneys, causing acute renal failure. In sickle cell disease, such sludging occurs in peripheral vessels causing pain and leg ulceration.

Mild cases of haemolytic anaemia may only be detected using radio-isotopes (such as radioactive chromium) to 'tag' the red cells and confirm that their normal 120 day life span is decreased.

Further investigations include the Coombs' test which detects antibodies in the blood. It is positive in many 'auto-immune' haemolytic anaemias, and in that due to the drug methyldopa (Aldomet) used in hypertension.

Treatment

This will depend on the cause, which should be eliminated if possible. It is important to remember that almost any drug may be causative in a susceptible person, and often withdrawal of all drugs is indicated.

Corticosteroids such as prednisone (10–20 mg 6-hourly) may suppress, the haemolytic process, especially in patients with a positive Coombs' test.

Splenectomy is indicated in congenital spherocytosis and is sometimes required in intractable cases of other cause. There is no satisfactory therapy for the sickle-cell trait and anaemia, but avoidance or early treatment of states causing anoxia may prevent haemolytic crises.

The Haemorrhagic diseases

THE PHYSIOLOGY OF HAEMOSTASIS AND ITS DISTURBANCES

Platelet functions

The platelets can be regarded as plugging up potential holes which tend to occur in the capillary walls through wear and tear. Lack of platelets or deficiency of their 'stickiness' results in purpura and spontaneous bleeding. When a blood vessel wall is injured platelets collect at the site and liberate substances which aid vasoconstriction thus minimizing the haemorrhage until clotting occurs.

The clotting (coagulation) mechanism

This has two stages:

1. The conversion of prothrombin in the plasma to thrombin.

2. The action of thrombin on the soluble protein fibrinogen converting it to strands of fibrin, which forms a meshwork, trapping R.B.C.s and platelets in a clot which becomes firm by retraction.

Though platelets and calcium are involved in the first stage, only small quantities are required—even in severe deficiency of platelets, blood *clotting* can proceed. The many other factors needed in stage 1 include prothrombin, factor VII and antihaemophilic globulin (factor VIII). Deficiency of any of these factors results in a clotting defect, with a prolonged 'clotting time' (normally 3–5 minutes).

In stage 2 a deficiency of fibrinogen could prevent clotting. There is a rare primary congenital lack of fibrinogen, but an important clinical situation occurs when all the fibrinogen has been used up in the formation of fibrin for coagulation—defibrination syndrome, see below. The snake venom Arvin is being evaluated for its antifibrinogen action.

Excessive deposition of fibrin in small vessels may occur in certain vascular diseases, nephritis and malignant hypertension, causing microangiopathic haemolytic anaemia as described, and heparin is being tried in therapy.

Some of the clotting factors may be increased by the oestrogen component of the combined oestrogen-progestagen contraceptive 'pill', causing raised incidence of venous and cerebral thrombosis on those on such tablets. Lowering their oestrogen content may minimize this risk.

The Fibrinolytic system

The clotting of blood after injury is valuable, but the occurrence of intravascular clotting, thrombosis, is undesirable. The clotting mechanism is therefore balanced by the fibrinolytic mechanism which prevents intravascular thrombosis and breaks down (lyses) clots that do form, by digesting fibrin. Arteriosclerosis and conditions such as coronary thrombosis have long been thought to be due to excessive thrombosis—they may equally be due to inadequate fibrinolysis. The use of activators of the fibrinolytic system such as streptokinase in the treatment of thrombo-embolic disease and pulmonary infarction has been referred to earlier. The drug combination phenformin-ethyloestrenol, and the common onion may also stimulate fibrinolysis.

Overactivity of the fibrinolytic system again results in the defibrination syndrome and bleeding.

Classification of the Haemorrhagic Diseases

Abnormal bleeding may be due to:

1. *Damage or defect in the capillary wall.*
2. *Lack of platelets (thrombocytopenia).*

These result in spontaneous haemorrhages into the skin, mucous membranes and internal organs. The reddish purple spots in the skin (and mouth) are called *purpura,* and the spots do not fade on pressure—the red spots in the condition telangiectasia and the spider naevi of cirrhosis do fade, as they are vascular. Small purpuric spots are called petechiae, and large confluent areas are called ecchymoses which are bruise-like discolorations, occurring spontaneously. There may be bleeding from the nose (epistaxis), mouth and alimentary tract, and haematuria from renal involvement.

Senile purpura, seen at the wrists and hands in the elderly is due to loss of elasticity of the tissues and slight oozing of blood from shearing stresses; it is not of serious significance, and not due to capillary or platelet deficiency.

3. *Clotting* (*coagulation*) *defects*. Deficiency of one of the blooding clotting factors. The clinically important ones are prothrombin, and antihaemophilic globulin (factor VIII), deficiency of the latter causing haemophilia.

4. *Defibrination syndrome.*

1. HAEMORRHAGE DUE TO CAPILLARY DEFECT

Causes

(i) *Infections:* severe pneumonia, meningitis (meningococcal septicaemia), subacute bacterial endocarditis (may be embolic), haemorrhagic chicken pox and smallpox—toxaemia may be operative in these conditions.

(ii) *Vitamin C* (*ascorbic acid*) *deficiency—scurvy.* Occurs in elderly from lack of fruit, and fresh greens or potatoes; blotchy haemorrhages especially on legs and thickening of the skin around the hair follicles, bleeding from the gums.

(iii) *Allergic disorders*—severe urticaria. *Henoch-Schonlein* (*anaphylactoid*) *purpura* occurs especially in children; intestinal bleeding may cause pain, melaena and precipitate intussusception (herniation of one segment of intestine into another); there are pains and swellings of the joints. Acute nephritis and renal failure may occur. However, most cases of Henoch-Schonlein purpura are mild, settling in a few days—steroids may be tried but are not usually required in treatment.

(iv) *Drug sensitivity*—penicillin, sulphonamides, carbromal (a hypnotic)—causing a haemorrhagic or urticarial rash.

2. HAEMORRHAGE DUE TO LACK OF PLATELETS— THROMBOCYTOPENIC PURPURA

Causes

(i) *Poisons and drugs.* The platelets are often the first to be depressed by a poison or drug affecting the bone marrow and later causing aplastic anaemia—benzene, heavy metals and gold, chloramphenicol, phenylbutazone and sulphonamides. Quinine (present in tonic water) may cause platelet antibodies to be formed. Aspirin interferes with platelet stickiness but seldom causes thrombocytopenia.

(ii) *Aplastic anaemia*—often a complication of these poisons and drugs.

(iii) *Leukaemia and secondary carcinomatosis of the bones*—here the platelets are crowded out of the marrow; severe bleeding is common in acute leukaemia.

(iv) *Auto-immune diseases*, such as systemic lupus erythematosus.

(v) *Idiopathic chrombocytopenic purpura.*

The marrow is active here, but platelets are not properly released. There may be an auto-immune basis, for some patients later develop systemic lupus erythematosus.

Children may be affected, the condition in them often settling spontaneously. In young women there are recurrent episodes of purpura, spontaneous 'bruising', and they may have menorrhagia (heavy periods). In middle-age, symptoms can be more severe with haemorrhage from mucous membranes and alimentary tract, haematuria and anaemia. The nurse may be the first to notice purpura at the flexure of the elbow after taking the blood pressure: the tourniquet (Hess) test utilizes a short period of venous occlusion by the sphygmomanometer cuff in suspected cases. The spleen may be enlarged, but it is not necessarily palpable.

In thrombocytopenia, purpura is liable to occur when the platelet count (normal 150,000–350,000 per cu mm) falls below 40,000 per cu mm. Symptoms are severe when the level drops to 10,000 or below, and this is commonest where the thrombocytopenia is a complication of leukaemia or aplastic anaemia. At these low levels, haemorrhages may be seen in the retinae using the ophthalmoscope, and there is danger of intracranial haemorrhage, causing acute stroke or sudden death.

Treatment

A known cause should be eliminated, if possible.

Corticosteroids such as prednisone up to 80 mg daily may help, but if continued high dosage is required to maintain the benefit, side effects occur.

Blood transfusion may be needed for anaemia; fresh blood, collected in plastic containers as platelets stick to glass, supplies some platelets, but their life is short. Special *platelet infusions* may be tried in severe cases.

Splenectomy may be required if these measures fail, especially in severe idiopathic thrombocytopenic purpura. Here, the spleen may be a site of excessive platelet destruction. However, although its removal is followed by a rise in the platelet count, this is often only temporary. Nevertheless the symptoms may be improved although the platelet count is little greater than it was before splenectomy.

3. COAGULATION DEFECT—haemorrhage due to clotting-factor deficiencies

Prothrombin (and Factor VII) deficiency

These are formed in the liver by vitamin K, a fat-soluble vitamin contained in eggs and greens, but dietary deficiency is unknown, and normally some vitamin K is manufactured by bacteria in the intestine. Prothrombin deficiency is therefore due to:

(i) Failure of vitamin K absorption—obstructive jaundice, where there is a lack of bile salts, and, rarely, in malabsorption syndrome.

(ii) Liver dysfunction—cirrhosis, and in the newborn (haemorrhagic disease of the newborn, probably due to immaturity of the hepatic cells).

(iii) Effects of drugs—the anticoagulant drugs phenindione and warfarin compete with vitamin K in the liver, blocking the formation of prothrombin—this is the basis of their therapeutic effect. Large doses of aspirin have a similar action. The breakdown of these drugs is increased by barbiturates and if the latter are added and subsequently withdrawn, rebound bleeding may occur.

The dosage of these oral anticoagulants is controlled by estimations of the 'prothrombin time' or Thrombotest using venous and capillary blood (finger prick) respectively. (It should be noted that heparin has a different anticoagulant action, mainly an anti-thrombin action, reversible only with the substance protamine.)

Anticoagulant overdosage may present with haematuria, epistaxis or skin haemorrhages, and in all coagulation defects, the blood is slow to clot after injury.

Treatment. Vitamin K_1 (Aquamephyton injection, Konakion injection or tablet) 10 mg intramuscularly daily is indicated in obstructive jaundice and may improve the hypoprothrombinaemia of cirrhosis. For oral anticoagulant overdosage cases, the vitamin can be given by mouth—10 mg is rapidly effective.

Haemophilia

Haemophilia is due to deficiency of factor VIII, antihaemophilic globulin. It is a sex-linked genetic disorder. Thus it is transmitted by apparently normal females carrying the trait in one of their X chromosomes, and it affects only males. Queen Victoria carried the trait, but it no longer exists in the British Royal family.

Young boys are affected, but most now reach adult life. Patients bruise easily, and their blood does not clot well after injuries or dental extractions—there is a slow persistent ooze. Haemorrhage may occur into joints, causing pain and severe deformity if untreated. Cases of haemophilia should preferably be referred to special treatment centres; emergency treatment is with blood 'cryoprecipitate' which contains the antihaemophilic globulin, or, if not available, fresh blood can be used. Social management and genetic counselling are important.

Christmas disease is a similar but less severe inherited defect of coagulation.

4. DEFIBRINATION SYNDROME

This presents as continued severe bleeding and occurs in two important clinical situations—concealed accidental haemorrhage in pregnancy (retro-placental bleeding), and following operations on the prostate or lungs. In both these situations there has been much bleeding and its continuation is due either to massive intravascular coagulation using up all the body's fibrinogen, or to excessive action of the fibrinolytic system attempting to dissolve the clots.

The diagnosis is established by finding a lack of fibrinogen in the blood, and there is failure of clot retraction when blood is allowed to clot in a test tube.

Treatment:

Blood transfusion, preferably fresh blood to supply clotting factors.

Fibrinogen transfusion.

Heparin. Heparin is actually given in the *treatment* of this bleeding state—it acts by blocking the continued intravascular coagulation that is occurring.

Antifibrinolytic drugs such as aminocaproic acid (Epsikapron).

Polycythaemia

In polycythaemia there is an excess of circulating red cells, perhaps 7–8 million instead of the usual 5 million per cubic millimetre, with a raised haematocrit (packed cell volume, normal 45 per cent) and raised haemoglobin (over 120 per cent).

Polycythaemia may be *secondary* to the anoxia of living at high altitudes, chronic lung disease (such as chronic bronchitis and emphysema) or cyanotic congenital heart disease. It also occurs in some renal diseases, especially carcinoma of the kidney (hypernephroma) and Cushing's syndrome (over-activity of the adrenal cortex).

Polycythaemia vera, *primary* polycythaemia, occurs in middle-age, especially in men and is a disorder of the bone marrow of unknown cause. There is an excessive marrow production not only of red cells, but usually also of the white cells and platelets.

Symptoms and signs: There is a feeling of fullness in the head, giddiness and fatigue. Patients have a high coloured, plethoric appearance—a ruddy cyanosis. There is a tendency to venous and arterial thrombosis and strokes. Although the platelets are increased in number, their function is defective, causing a bleeding tendency too. Often there is pruritus. The spleen is enlarged in two thirds of the cases. There is a raised incidence of peptic ulcer, and of gout.

Treatment is directed to reducing the circulating red cell mass, and includes repeated venesections, removing 500 ml of blood at a time over weeks or months. This may be technically difficult, for the blood is of high viscosity and tends to clot in the needle. Radio-active phosphorus (^{32}P) is given intravenously—it is taken up by the bone marrow and depresses its activity. Repeat doses may be required over months or years. As ^{32}P carries a small risk of inducing leukaemia, some doctors prefer to use the cytotoxic drug busulphan. However, radio-active phosphorus is generally a very satisfactory treatment, and many patients do well for 10 years or more.

Myelo-fibrosis and myelo-sclerosis

This disorder, or group of disorders has some similarity to polycythaemia, but presents rather in middle-aged women. There is mild anaemia, raised white cell count and enlargement of the spleen. The bone marrow is replaced by fibrous tissue, or becomes bony and 'sclerosed', and a specimen is characteristically difficult to obtain at sternal puncture, so that open bone biopsy may be necessary to establish the diagnosis.

Treatment is by blood transfusions as necessary. It was formerly assumed that the spleen 'took over' blood manufacture but its enlargement is in fact part of the disease process. If the enlargement is gross, splenectomy may be indicated. Many patients survive for years, but myelofibrosis may terminate as leukaemia.

The leukaemias

Definition

Leukaemia is a neoplastic, malignant process affecting the white cells of the blood. Either the polymorph (here called the myeloid series), lymphocyte or monocyte series may be involved. There is an abnormal, progressive accumulation (hyperplasia) of cells in the haemopoietic tissues (bone marrow, lymph glands, spleen and liver) throughout the body and in chronic leukaemias increased circulating white blood cells.

Classification and cause

Until recently it was assumed that leukaemia (and cancer) cells were characterized by an abnormally rapid proliferation from an increased rate of division (mitosis), but this is not the case. In the leukaemias there is in fact no evidence that the cells divided more rapidly than others, but in acute leukaemia they fail to differentiate properly and build up in the bone marrow or lymph glands. In chronic leukaemia the accumulation may be due to a disturbance of the mechanism regulating the number that is normally produced.

The clinical presentation is as follows:

Acute Leukaemia—lymphatic (lymphoblastic), myeloid or the rare monocytic
or *Chronic Myeloid* (*polymorph*) *Leukaemia*
or *Chronic Lymphatic Leukaemia.*

The cause or causes are often obscure, but there is an increased incidence of leukaemia after exposure to x-rays or thermo-nuclear emissions as in the survivors of the atomic bomb explosions at Hiroshima and Nagasaki in 1945. A virus cause, an enzyme defect or a disorder of immunity are other suggestions. However, as chronic myeloid leukaemia is unique in its association with a specific chromosome abnormality, it may be wise to regard the leukaemias as separate entities.

Current concepts in therapy. Cytotoxic drugs

X-rays damage dividing cells, and as cells in the bone marrow and lining the alimentary tract have the highest rate of division, they are the first to be affected by excessive exposure. It was noted that exposure to mustard gas was followed by depression of the white cells (leucopenia) and this observation led to the development of *cytotoxic drugs* which, like x-rays, depressed actively dividing cells. Their initial use was based on the assumption, referred to above and now known to be untrue, that malignant cells divide more quickly than normal cells and could therefore be selectively destroyed. In fact cancer cells may accumulate because of decreased cell losses. The chemotherapy of leukaemia (and cancer) is based on the use of drugs that interfere with the metabolic processes of cells, different drugs acting at different stages of nucleo-protein production.

These drugs have been grouped into the *alkylating agents* (which includes nitrogen mustards such as mustine, chlorambucil, cyclophosphamide, and the drug busulphan), the *antimetabolites* (such as folic acid antagonists, 6-mercaptopurine, and cytosine arabinoside), *vegetable extracts* (vinblastine and vincristine) and the *antineoplastic antibiotics* (such as daunorubicin). Experience has shown that there is a certain selectivity in their clinical effects. Moreover if two or more drugs are known to be effective yet have different toxic effects, they can be given in combination at maximum dosage, summating their therapeutic actions but not their toxic effects.

Asparaginase (colaspase) is the only drug known to be truly selective in its action against malignant cells. Some malignant cells are unable to synthesize the amino-acid asparagine—for them it is an 'essential amino-acid'. Asparaginase destroys it, cutting off the supply and causing cell death. Normal cells can synthesize their own asparagine and are not affected. Asparaginase has been used in acute leukaemia but unfortunately resistance develops to it. However, it may pave the way for future selective drugs.

Corticosteroids such as prednisone inhibit proliferation of lymphoid cells and suppress immunity reactions. Thus steroids may have a beneficial effect in lymphatic leukaemia and similar states which may represent disturbances of immunity. The effect of steroids is a more discrete and selective one than that of the cytotoxic drugs described above which are also *immunosuppressives* as a result of their impairing the production of the cells that mediate the immune response.

Immunotherapy using injections of irradiated leukaemic cells and

B.C.G. vaccination, and fever therapy (malignant cells may be destroyed more easily than normal cells by high temperatures) are currently being evaluated in the treatment of leukaemia.

Acute leukaemia

Acute leukaemia occurs especially in children and the cause is unknown. There is an accumulation of early cells ('blast' cells) in the marrow and lymph nodes. These cells fail to differentiate properly into their appropriate series, and crowd out other white cells, red cells and the platelets. The most common type in children is acute lymphatic (lymphoblastic) leukaemia, but in adults acute myeloid leukaemia is equally common.

Symptoms and signs

There is a rapidly developing anaemia, and there are haemorrhages (from platelet-lack) from the gums and into the skin, bones and joints (causing severe pain in the latter) and internal organs, including the brain. There is fever, and great susceptibility to infections. There is enlargement of lymph glands and spleen, but this may not be gross. Investigations include blood film and bone marrow examination, and it is now important to distinguish the type of cell involved as the treatment and prognosis differ.

Treatment

Chemotherapy

Acute lymphatic leukaemia. There are two approaches. The first is to secure a remission using prednisone (or prednisolone) orally plus vincristine (injection weekly), dosage based on surface area. Maintenance therapy is then given using the drug 6-mercaptopurine orally. The other approach is to use combinations of cytotoxic drugs in high dosage to cause 'total kill' of the leukaemic cell population in the hope of producing a complete cure. Such patients are very prone to infections, and treatment can only be carried out in special centres in a 'germ-free' environment.

Acute myeloid leukaemia. A combination of cytosine arabinoside and daunorubicin is the most effective, but even so, results are disappointing.

General measures

Blood transfusions, platelet infusions and the treatment of

infections with appropriate antibacterial drugs are usually indicated. Nursing care of the mouth is essential.

Though the prognosis of acute myeloid leukaemia remains poor, measured in weeks or months, the outlook in acute lymphatic leukaemia, especially in children, is becoming more promising, some patients being maintained in remission for years, and a true 'cure' may be possible. It is therefore important to maintain an attitude of hope. The patient's relatives must be interviewed and therapy discussed—this will do much to assure the continued confidence of the patient in his attendants. When rapid deterioration and bleeding is occurring despite all therapy, then, of course, suffering must be allayed and comfort maintained by the proper use of drugs such as chlorpromazine (Largactil) and opiates.

Chronic myeloid (granulocytic) leukaemia

Here the bone marrow and lymph glands are taken over by an abnormal line of cells usually found to contain an abnormal chromosome called the Philadelphia chromosome. There is a progressive accumulation of granulocytes (polymorphs) with an excess in the peripheral blood.

Symptoms and signs

Chronic myeloid leukaemia occurs at any age but is commonest in young adults. There is gradually increasing tiredness and weakness due to anaemia. There is enlargement of lymph glands, liver and spleen, the latter often reaching a considerable size (larger than in other forms of leukaemia) and causing discomfort and dragging sensation in the abdomen. Purpura and haemorrhages may occur. There may be leukaemic deposits in the skin and pruritus. The disordered cell production causes a raised metabolism with weight loss, sweats, and raised blood uric acid causing gouty symptoms such as joint pains.

The diagnosis is confirmed by finding a raised white cell count, sometimes over 100,000 per cu mm (normal 4,000 to 9,000 per cu mm), in the peripheral blood, and by sternal marrow puncture.

Treatment

Chemotherapy. The object is to reduce the total mass of accumulated leucocytes. Busulphan (Myeleran) is the cytotoxic drug of choice, initially 4–6 mg by mouth daily, reducing to a maintenance dose of 1–2 mg daily to keep the white cell count between 10,000–20,000 per cu mm: daily and then monthly checks are required. Toxic effects include aplastic anaemia, brownish skin pigmentation and lung fibrosis. Drugs such as dibromannitol may be required if resistance to busulphan develops. Chemotherapy has proved more successful than x-ray therapy.

Steroids may be required for associated haemolytic anaemia.

Blood transfusion is required if the haemoglobin is falling despite chemotherapy.

Prognosis

The course is variable and though there is no cure, proper management allows a practically normal way of life for many patients, some surviving for up to 10 years. At some stage, the process becomes transformed to an acute leukaemic one, treatment of which is of little avail, the patient succumbing usually in a matter of weeks.

Chronic lymphatic leukaemia

Here the bone marrow is gradually infiltrated and eventually replaced by an accumulation of lymphocytes, also present in lymph nodes, spleen, liver and in the peripheral blood. In addition to progressive anaemia, the immunity function becomes defective and patients are prone to infection.

Symptoms and signs

Chronic lymphatic leukaemia is commonest in middle-aged and elderly men. Symptoms include tiredness, weakness, gland swellings and enlargement of the spleen, though this organ is not usually as big as in chronic myeloid leukaemia. Chronic lymphatic leukaemia may be remarkably benign in the elderly, being discovered sometimes at a blood count during investigation of pneumonia or other infection, or incidentally at a hospital attendance for another reason.

The diagnosis is confirmed by a total white cell count of up to 100,000 per cu mm, 90 per cent of the cells being lymphocytes.

Treatment

None may be necessary—treatment is only required if there is increasing anaemia or discomfort from gland swellings.

Chlorambucil (Leukeran) is the cytotoxic drug of choice, initially 4–12 mg by mouth then a maintenance dose of 1–5 mg daily to keep the white cell count at 10,000–20,000 per cu mm. Corticosteroids such as prednisone are preferable initially if marrow function is severely impaired, and are indicated for any associated haemolytic anaemia.

X-ray therapy is still occasionally used for local lymph node enlargements.

Blood transfusion is occasionally required. Appropriate anti-bacterial drugs should be given early if patients have evidence of an infection.

Prognosis

The average duration of life from diagnosis is 6 years, but many elderly patients may survive comfortably for 10 years or more.

Agranulocytosis

Agranulocytosis is an absence or greatly decreased number (leuco-penia) of white blood cells of the 'granular' series, the polymorphs, in the peripheral blood.

The cause is bone marrow depression, and the factors responsible are the same as in aplastic anaemia and thrombocytopenia, though some substances are more selective in destroying the white cells than the red cells or platelets.

Thus heavy metals such as gold, benzene and drugs containing the benzene ring (which includes the sulphonamides) may be responsible, but in practice the following drugs are the important causes:

phenylbutazone (Butazolidin) used in rheumatoid arthritis.
chloramphenicol, used in typhoid fever.
anti-thyroid drugs such as carbimazole and methylthiouracil.
the cytotoxic drugs—but careful dosage prevents this complication of their use.

Symptoms and signs

The patient is prone to infection, and the first symptom is often a sore throat. Thus if a patient has been prescribed a drug such as carbimazole with which there is a slight but known risk of agranulo-cytosis, he (or usually she, thyrotoxicosis being commoner in women) must be warned to stop the tablets if he develops a sore throat. This may precede any gross depression of the white cell count, and with carbimazole occurs as a sensitivity reaction in the first few weeks of treatment. The phenylbutazone marrow depression occurs over a longer period, and in the few instances where it is necessary to maintain this drug, periodic white cell counts are indicated.

In neglected cases the patient is febrile and toxic and may succumb to pneumonia or to septicaemia, his resistance to infection being zero if white cells are completely absent.

Treatment

The important aspect is preventive, using drugs such as the above only if there is a clear indication for them, and being aware of their side effects.

Where agranulocytosis exists, the offending drug must be stopped or all drugs stopped if the cause is unknown. Patients should ideally be nursed in a germ-free environment, but a side-ward may be the only compromise. It is probably justifiable to give penicillin, ampicillin and cloxacillin prophylactically; existing infections should be treated with the appropriate antibacterial drug. Steroids such as prednisone are often used to 'stimulate' the bone marrow though such an action is dubious, and they may promote the spread of existing infection.

In early cases, marrow recovery occurs within a week or two, but in severe cases, especially those following the misuse of chloramphenicol the marrow destruction may be irreversible and the patient succumbs.

The spleen and lymph nodes—the lympho-reticular system

Physiology

Along with the bone marrow the spleen and lymph nodes form an important part of the reticulo-endothelial or lympho-reticular system of cells. In the embryo, tissues are formed from one of three cell types —ectoderm which goes to form skin and cells of the nervous system, endoderm forming the gut, and mesoderm which forms the skeleton and framework or reticulum of certain organs including the spleen and lymph nodes. From the reticulum cells the bone marrow is formed, and while the red and white cells are therefore part of the reticulo-endothelial system, it is probably best to regard it separately as a defensive mechanism with two main functions—phagocytosis, and the immune response.

Phagocytosis is the ingestion of particulate matter or bacteria by living cells, phagocytes, derived from endothelial, lining, cells.

There are several types of cell with this action, including fixed and wandering tissue cells, and circulating white blood cells of the polymorph and monocyte series. Phagocytosis is an immediate response to invasion or infection, the offending organisms being engulfed.

The immune response can itself be sub-divided into two components—the formation of humoral (circulating) antibodies, and the production of cell-mediated immunity. The lymphocytes play the cardinal role in both mechanisms, which come into play when an antigen, which may be inhaled, ingested or injected, reaches a lymph node. Humoral antibodies are formed partly by lymphocytes but largely by 'plasma cells' which may be formed from lymphocytes. Thus the plasma cells are largely responsible for producing the immuno-globulins which include antibodies. They are especially important in the defence against bacteria, but also play a part in resistance to viruses. Derangement causes the immediate and serum-sickness allergic reactions described on page 14. Cellular immunity is mediated by a different group of lymphocytes which have a much longer life (months or years rather than days) and are produced by the thymus gland rather than by the lymph nodes. Cellular immunity is important in the defence against virus infection and in recognition of 'self' and tissue rejection reactions. Deranged cellular immunity is responsible for the 'delayed-hypersensitivity' type reaction. Disturbance of the immune response may cause auto-immune diseases.

The spleen and lymph glands are the important filters in the defence system against foreign matter or organisms. The spleen is the filter for the circulating blood. The lymph glands are the filter for organisms arriving from the mucous membranes and skin via the lymphatics.

THE SPLEEN

Anatomy and structure

The spleen is a red pulpy organ 12 cm long by 6 cm wide in the uppermost part of the left side of the abdomen below the diaphragm, lying along the line of the ninth, tenth and eleventh ribs. It consists of a spongy framework (reticulum) containing red blood cells, lymphoid tissue, and other cells of reticulo-endothelial function. It receives arterial blood from the aorta and its structure is unique in allowing close contact between circulating red cells and the lymphoid tissue. The splenic vein joins the mesenteric vein from the intestine to form the portal vein to the liver.

Functions

1. *Blood formation*—the spleen normally plays little part in red and white blood cell formation, but its haemopoietic function can be increased if there is undue demand or in marrow failure. The spleen has little reservoir function for red cells in man, but may store platelets.

2. *Blood destruction*—the reticulo-endothelial cells remove red cells from circulation at the end of their 120-day life span.

3. *Defence* against infection and participation in the immune response.

Causes of enlargement (splenomegaly)

1. *Infections*—any severe, acute infection especially if there is bacterial invasion of the bloodstream as in typhoid fever or septicaemia (septic spleen):

subacute bacterial endocarditis.

chronic infections, especially tropical parasitic infections such as malaria and kala-azar (trypanosomiasis).

2. *Blood diseases:*

polycythaemia; myelosclerosis.

the leukaemias.

haemolytic anaemia; idiopathic thrombocytopenic purpura.

3. *Diseases of lymphoid tissue*—Hodgkin's disease.

4. *Cirrhosis* of the liver—causes portal venous obstruction.

Effects of splenomegaly

The spleen has to enlarge to about three times normal size before it becomes palpable. Enlargement is greatest in the tropical diseases, myelosclerosis and chronic myeloid leukaemia, where the size of the organ may cause discomfort. The spleen has an influence on bone marrow function, possibly hormonal, and 'hypersplenism' prevents release of cells from the marrow, causing anaemia, leukopenia or thrombocytopenia.

Removal of the spleen (splenectomy) may be indicated following trauma (ruptured spleen), in congenital haemolytic anaemia, idiopathic thrombocytopenic purpura and myelosclerosis. Patients can live normally without the spleen, the other lympho-reticular structures taking over its function, but there is a slightly increased liability to infections, especially in children.

THE LYMPHATIC SYSTEM

Lymph is tissue fluid that enters the tiny lymphatic capillaries which join to drain it into the regional lymph nodes, where lymphocytes are added. The larger lymphatics terminate mainly in the thoracic duct, which enters the left subclavian vein at the root of the neck thus reaching the great veins near the heart. The lymphatic drainage of the small intestine is also an important route of fat absorption.

The lymphoid follicles in the lymph nodes produce the lymphocytes concerned in humoral antibody and plasma cell formation.

The thymus gland behind the sternum is a different type of lymphatic structure, especially important in foetal life and infancy, and relatively much smaller in adults. It produces many lymphocytes but most are quickly destroyed for unknown reasons; the remaining small percentage carry cellular immunity. The thymus gland also has an effect on the other lymphoid tissues, possibly hormonal.

Causes of lymph gland enlargement

1. *Infections:*
local, as from a septic focus or sore throat; tuberculosis (and sarcoidosis) generalized, as in *Glandular Fever.*

2. *Metastatic:*
from spread of tumour cells along the lymphatics, for example axillary gland involvement from carcinoma of the breast.

3. *Primary malignant conditions* of the haemopoietic system such as leukaemia, or of the lympho-reticular system—the reticuloses, such as Hodgkin's disease.

The reticuloses

The term 'the reticuloses' can be widely defined, but is generally restricted to a group of disorders of malignant nature involving the lympho-reticular system—that is organs such as the lymph nodes and spleen, but the equivalent cells in the bone marrow may also be involved. The cause or causes of the malignant reticuloses is unknown, but interest has been aroused by the finding of a rather similar tumour affecting the jaw and pharynx of children in tropical East Africa. This tumour was recently described by Burkitt and is called Burkitt's lymphoma. In some cases the cells contain a virus which may be transmitted by mosquitoes, and a similar virus may be found in glandular fever. There is, however, as yet no proof that diseases such as Hodgkin's disease have a virus cause.

HODGKIN'S DISEASE (LYMPHADENOMA, MALIGNANT LYMPHOMA)

Symptoms and signs

The disease is commonest in young adults. There are swellings of the lymph glands, often first in the neck, the glands being rubbery but not tender. Glands in the mediastinum (root of the lung) or abdomen may, however, be involved first, making diagnosis difficult— lymphatic blockage here may cause chylous ascites, or pressure on the veins cause leg oedema.

The disorder may remain local for months or years, or may present as generalized glandular enlargement with enlarged spleen and liver.

General symptoms include fever, weakness from anaemia, loss of weight and pruritus. The taking of even a small amount of alcohol often causes pain in the affected glands, a useful diagnostic sign. Patients are prone to infections.

Differential diagnosis includes glandular fever, leukaemia and malignant deposits from a primary tumour in another organ.

Investigations. Apart from anaemia and raised E.S.R., there are no specific findings in the peripheral blood. There may be infiltration of the bone marrow but the diagnosis of Hodgkin's disease is best confirmed by gland biopsy; lymphangiography defines its extent.

Treatment

Localized Hodgkin's disease is best treated with intensive radiotherapy. If there is a group of large accessible gland swellings these are sometimes surgically removed.

Generalized Hodgkin's disease. Chemotherapy with cytotoxic drugs is the treatment of choice. While cyclophosphamide or chlorambucil orally can be used alone, better results are achieved using a combination of the following four agents simultaneously—prednisone (or prednisolone) 40 mg daily, vinblastine (or vincristine) 10 mg intravenously weekly, mustine 10–40 mg into a fast-flowing drip (2 injections a week apart), and oral procarbazine 50–300 mg daily for two weeks. The course of treatment is repeated every four weeks, but close control of the blood count is necessary.

Cyclophosphamide and mustine may be given intrapleurally or intraperitoneally after aspiration of effusions to prevent their recurrence.

General management includes blood transfusion and prompt treatment of infections with appropriate antibacterial therapy and is similar to the management of the leukaemias. Pruritus may be helped by promethazine (Vallergan). Antiemetics such as prochlorperazine (Stemetil) may be useful for the nausea and vomiting induced by radio-therapy and some of the cytotoxic drugs (such as mustine).

Prognosis

The prognosis of Hodgkin's disease is variable, and true cure has been described in some localized types of the condition. Generalized disease is fatal in months or years, but complete remission has been achieved for up to two years with modern combined therapy, and the quality and quantity of life can be improved for five or even ten years.

LYMPHOSARCOMA AND RETICULUM CELL SARCOMA

These are malignant tumours of lymphoid tissue, involving lymphocytes and reticulum cells respectively. One of these cell types displaces all the others in lymph nodes, spleen, bone marrow or thymus gland. The process is much more rapid than in Hodgkin's disease and the cells spread into neighbouring tissues as well as spilling out via the lymphatics and bloodstream causing widespread dissemination of the growths. The conditions may terminate as acute leukaemias.

Symptoms and signs are similar to Hodgkin's disease, one group of nodes being first involved or the process presenting in several areas. Mediastinal and retroperitoneal lymph nodes are frequently involved, causing discomfort, pressure symptoms, and recurrent pleural or peritoneal effusions. Lesions may start in the tonsils, stomach or other part of the alimentary tract, or present in the skin. There is malaise, fever, sweating and weight loss. Anaemia occurs, sometimes haemolytic in type.

The diagnosis is confirmed by biopsy, which shows sheets of neoplastic cells of one cell type, different from the mixed cells in Hodgkin's disease tissue.

Treatment: Local excision and radiotherapy may help. Generalized disease can be treated with cytotoxic drugs such as cyclophosphamide (Endoxana) orally, its side effects include haemorrhagic cystitis and alopecia (loss of the hair); mustine is given by injection into an intravenous drip. Prednisone may be required for haemolytic anaemia. Antibacterial drugs are indicated for infections. Blood transfusion may be necessary.

The prognosis is poor, most patients surviving only a few months.

Myelomatosis (multiple myeloma)

This condition occurs in the middle-aged and elderly, is commoner in men, and is a malignant process usually arising in the bone marrow. Thus the marrow of flat bones such as the vertebrae and skull becomes infiltrated with plasma cells, here called myeloma cells. There are single or multiple osteolytic (bone-destructive) lesions in the bony skeleton. The myeloma cells produce abnormal immuno-globulins, a product of which may appear as Bence Jones protein in the urine. The cause is unknown.

Symptoms and signs

There is bone pain and backache, fever, weight loss, anaemia and sometimes a bleeding tendency from thrombocytopenia. Patients are prone to infection. The weakened bones may fracture causing root pains such as a bilateral 'sciatica' if the vertebrae are involved. The abnormal proteins may be deposited as amyloid tissue in nerves or organs including the tongue (amyloidosis involving spleen and liver used to be seen in patients with chronic suppurative processes such as osteomyelitis and bronchiectasis). Deposits of protein in the renal tubules may cause renal failure.

Investigations: The E.S.R. is raised—myelomatosis is a condition often associated with a very high E.S.R., 100 mm per hour or more; such a finding may lead to the diagnosis in a patient with few symptoms. The abnormal proteins can be characterized by the procedure called paper strip electrophoresis, or by immunological methods.

On heating the *urine*, Bence Jones protein is detectable as a cloud around 70°C, which disappears on boiling and reappears on cooling. When present, it is virtually diagnostic of myelomatosis.

X-rays show rarefaction or punched-out areas in the bones.

Treatment

Local bone pains can be helped by x-ray therapy. Cytotoxic drugs are used for generalized cases—melphalan 5–10 mg orally daily in courses, or cyclophosphamide 50–150 mg daily, with frequent checks of the white cell and platelet counts. Prednisone may be added. Blood transfusion may be required.

Some elderly patients have few symptoms, so that therapy with cytotoxic drugs may not always be justified. However, there is evidence that their use improves the quality and duration of life for months or even a year or two.

The Macroglobulinaemias

These are disturbances of immune globulin production from plasma cell dysfunction, without the discrete lesions of myelomatosis. There may be lymph gland swellings, bleeding tendency, liability to infection and to Raynaud's syndrome from cold temperatures precipitating the abnormal proteins in small blood vessels. Elderly men are affected, and treatment includes melphalan or cyclophosphamide, and plasmapheresis—removal of the abnormal proteins from the blood, but the outlook is poor.

Immunoglobulin deficiency

This occurs as hereditary hypogammaglobulinaemia in children, and various acquired types in adult life. Patients are prone to infection, and injections of immuno-globulin are available (for treatment) through the Medical Research Council.

10

Nutritional disorders

The Normal Diet

The normal diet contains, 2,500–3,000 Calories daily—the dietetic Calorie is in fact a kilocalorie, 1,000 times a chemical 'calorie'. Of the daily calorie intake 40–50 per cent is derived from carbohydrate, about 12 per cent from protein, and 42 per cent from fat in Western countries. It will be remembered that 1 G of carbohydrate or protein produces 4 calories, and 1 G of fat 9 calories. Thus an average diet contains 350–400 G carbohydrate, 70–90 G protein and 110–140 G fat. A mixed diet supplies adequate minerals (salt, potassium, calcium, magnesium, iron) trace elements such as iodine, and vitamins. The relative excess of carbohydrate, especially refined carbohydrate such as sugar, has been blamed for many of the ills of civilized society—especially diabetes and arteriosclerosis. Dental caries is related to a high sugar and sweet intake. Too much animal fat in the diet is associated with a raised cholesterol level and possibly a raised incidence of arteriosclerotic coronary disease. The substitution of certain vegetable oils for fats lowers the blood cholesterol, but it has yet to be shown that this prevents coronary disease. Much research is being carried out into the relationship between dietary habits in the West and the high incidence of arterial disease in the population.

Protein contains the amino-acids necessary for body building and tissue repair. Animal protein such as meat has been classed as 'first class' protein as it contains essential amino-acids that the body cannot make for itself, and vegetable protein such as peas and beans was thought to be 'second class' as it lacked these amino-acids. This division has less importance than was assumed, for mixing a small amount of animal protein with vegetable protein greatly enhances the nutritional value of the latter. Thus an adult diet, even if low in meat, generally contains a nutritionally adequate protein content, the minimum requirement being about 40 G daily. Protein is often regarded as a food of special virtue, but there is no evidence that high protein diets are of value in those in a normal state of health, a diet of adequate calories supplying sufficient protein. Moreover, protein can only be utilized for tissue repair if calorie intake is adequate.

Due to over-population, wars with their refugee problems and natural catastrophes such as earthquakes, typhoons and floods, much of the world's population suffers from *under-nutrition*, and in adults the important aspect is total *calorie-lack*. New varieties of rice with higher crop yields have improved calorie supplies, and new sources of protein are being sought. Inadequate calories in children results in stunting of growth. Inadequate protein despite adequate calories can occur in growing children, and causes *kwashiorkor*—oedema, fatty liver enlargement, pigmentary changes in skin and hair, apathy, proneness to infection and some retardation of development. Kwashiorkor occurs even when protein is available, where ignorance or prejudice prevents proper feeding of children.

In Western countries, the main nutritional disorder is not under-nutrition, but over-nutrition—too many calories, resulting in obesity. Dietary vitamin-lack is rare, but occurs in alcoholics and food fads, and sometimes in the elderly.

Obesity

Obesity is a condition of excessive deposition of fat—adipose tissue—in the body. The accumulation of fat is generalized in so-called simple obesity. The degree of obesity can be estimated from the subcutaneous fat by measurement of the skin-fold thickness using special calipers. Thus obesity exists if the skin-fold thickness over the triceps in the upper arm is greater than 23 mm in males or 30 mm in females.

In practice, obesity corresponds to being *overweight*, and it is sufficient to weigh the patient to confirm the condition, which is usually obvious. Ideal weight tables, based on life assurance statistics, give the weight for a given sex and height at which insured subjects live longest. Obesity is present if a person exceeds this ideal weight by 20 per cent or more—weight should not increase with age, and a middle-aged person weighing more than he (or more usually she) did in his twenties is probably too fat.

Incidence

In India obesity is a sign of affluence and success. In Britain, on the other hand, obesity is more common in the lower socio-economic groups, but occurs in all classes. It is predominantly a disorder of middle-age, almost half the population over forty being overweight. Obesity is commoner in women and at any time one out of five women are on some form of 'slimming diet', though fashion-consciousness rather than medical necessity may dictate the prevalence of such regimes.

Causes

1. *Genetic and environmental.* Obesity can start in childhood and there may be a genetic basis in some children who have inherited a greater number of adipose tissue cells than others. However, environment is largely responsible as children tend to follow the eating habits of their parents. Thus obesity often runs in families.

2. *Disturbed calorie balance.* In all cases of obesity, there must at some time have been an excess of calorie intake over metabolic requirement, so that fat has been laid down. Disturbance of the balance could be due to *excessive appetite*, or *deranged metabolism*.

Appetite is delicately controlled by an appetite centre in the hypothalamus—the small area of the brain below the cerebrum concerned also with emotion and sleep, connected with the autonomic nervous system, and with the pituitary gland below. The control of appetite may be upset in obesity, but the mechanism for this is generally obscure—endocrine and psychological factors are discussed below.

Deranged metabolism. Obese people often claim to eat no more than their thinner fellows. Again, some people eat a lot yet do not become fat. As the muscles of the obese are not more efficient in their use of calories than those of the thin, the explanation must lie in different energy expenditure—and this has been found to be the case. Thus thin people increase their metabolic rate in response to food consumption, channelling the glucose to be utilized in muscle activity. Fat people fail to do this, for in association with an increased insulin production characteristic of obesity, their glucose is directed towards the fat depots instead. It is uncertain how this abnormality has come about, but it has been shown that the obese are less active and take less exercise than thin people. Moreover excercise and weight-loss correct this metabolic abnormality of the obese.

Thus obesity may be due to inadequate exercise in a modern society where physical activity at work is no longer required by the use of machinery, and even the benefits of walking to work have been removed by buses, cars and trains. The gradual onset of obesity in middle-age is usually due to decreased energy expenditure with an unchanged calorie intake.

3. *Endocrine.* The obesity of Cushing's syndrome affects only the trunk, the arms and legs being thin, and the skin is thinned. This is a clinical picture which is distinct from the generalized obesity under consideration. The obese rarely have overt evidence of 'glandular disturbance', but as obesity often follows childbirth or the menopause, endocrine factors may play a part, possibly through effects on hypothalamic control.

4. *Stopping smoking* may be blamed for obesity—an increased sweet consumption is probably the real reason.

5. *Psychological.* There does not seem to be a particularly high incidence of psychiatric disturbance in obese people attending hospitals. A proportion may be of tense and anxious disposition and they gain solace from their worries by overeating. The obese are not a happier lot than their thinner fellows, but obesity is a state that is maintained, if not entered, voluntarily by the patient.

Effects

Cardiovascular. There is a raised incidence of hypertension and arteriosclerotic disease especially ischaemic heart disease—the mechanical burden on the heart and altered blood fats are responsible. Strokes and renal failure are commoner in the obese. Varicose veins, thrombo-embolism and pulmonary infarction are well known complications.

Respiratory. The layers of fat impede ventilation, with increased tendency to bronchitis and pneumonia, or chronic anoxia in extreme cases ('Pickwickian syndrome').

Joints and ligaments. Backache, arthritis especially of the knees and hips.

Metabolic. Greatly increased incidence of diabetes, the insulin produced being ultimately unable to cope with the demands of the great bulk of fatty tissue. Increased tendency to gall-stones and cholecystitis from cholesterol upset.

Accident-proneness. The increased bulk and relative slowness of the obese makes them liable to accidents at home, work, or in the street.

Surgical problems. Access at operations is difficult, wound healing is impaired with risk of incisional hernia, and post-operative pneumonia and pulmonary infarction are commoner in the obese.

Thus obesity is a grave medical and social problem. The obese have a shortened life-expectancy and, when ill, a mortality rate some 30 per cent greater than that of the non-obese suffering from the same condition.

Treatment

While the reasons for becoming obese may be argued, there can be no doubt about the principle of treatment—the calorie intake must be reduced to become less than the energy expenditure. Weight loss is bound to follow.

Diet. A dietary history should be taken, and it will often be found that an excess intake of calories in some form can easily be curtailed —this is true for beer-drinking in men, and excessive cups of sugared tea and coffee with cakes at elevenses or social functions in women. Thus it may suffice to eliminate from the diet foods of high calorie content such as alcohol, sugar and fat.

If this approach fails, *a reducing diet* of about 1,000 calories daily is prescribed. It is more important that this should be palatable and acceptable to the patient than that it contain a set regime of carbohydrate, protein and fat. It must be clearly understood that no foods are 'slimming' foods—it is cutting down on the total calorie-intake that matters. Usually a low carbohydrate 1,000 calorie diet is acceptable—it contains 80 G carbohydrate, 60 G protein and 50 G fat—articles such as tinned fruit contain much carbohydrate and should be eliminated, also potatoes, but other vegetables, composed mainly of fibre and water can be taken liberally. Patients should lose about 2 lb (1 Kg) weekly if such a diet is followed conscientiously.

'Crash diets' of 500 calories or no-calories, total starvation, should only be applied in hospital, and then only for limited period to prove to the patient that she is bound to lose weight if she eats less. Patients who reject this aphorism may be reminded that no prisoner who emerged from a concentration camp was fat—all were thin because all were starved. Very low calorie diets, such as three oranges totalling 150 calories daily, can be dangerous, causing potassium loss, heart failure and cellular breakdown with raised uric acid and gout. Vitamin and potassium supplements are necessary, plus allopurinol to lower uric acid production. Body protein is lost as well as fat and the long term results of such regimes are disappointing.

Exercise. Though it requires much exercise to lose 1 lb of weight (for example a walk of 30 miles) walking or cycling for a few miles daily does contribute to gradual weight loss. Moreover there is now evidence that taking exercise 1–2 hours after food channels the calories towards muscle utilization and loss as heat instead of towards the laying down of fat. As noted, exercise may rectify the metabolic abnormality of obesity. Thus regular moderate exercise is to be encouraged in any weight-reducing programme.

Drugs. Bulk-producing agents such as methyl cellulose, which swell on contact with water in the stomach, may give a feeling of satiety but are of little value in practice.

Appetite suppressants. Amphetamine has this action but is also a central nervous system stimulant, raises the blood pressure, and is a drug of addiction. It has been replaced by similar less stimulant drugs which retain the appetite suppressant effect, for example diethylpropion (Tenuate) which can be given as a 75 mg long-acting tablet. Fenfluramine (Ponderax) is a drug of different group, and is sedative rather than stimulant. In addition to an appetite suppressing action, it may have a direct effect on muscle glucose uptake. The dose is 20 mg twice daily before meals. Patients on a reducing diet soon lose their initial feeling of hunger and such drugs are not usually necessary. Their use may be justified if they help the patient to keep to the diet, and they may be given in courses of 4–8 weeks.

Supportive measures. In all cases it is important to set a reduced weight target. The patient should record her weight weekly, and attend for review monthly, when the weight chart will be inspected and the patient congratulated, encouraged or cajoled as necessary. Her will-power (or will-not-power, 'I will not eat') must be supported. Group therapy for weight losers may be helpful, and is popular in U.S.A.

Results of treatment

Where the patient is sufficiently motivated in her desire to lose weight, then co-operation is achieved and the therapy is successful. The overall results of attempted treatment are, however, disappointing—about half the patients fail to return for follow-up after a year and have gained weight by resuming their previous dietary habits. Such patients protest that they 'never eat a thing', but their reliability is no greater than that of alcoholics or heavy smokers—they are hooked on eating. The biscuits in their beside lockers or their nocturnal munching of sweetmeats disprove their assertions.

The reasons for this obtuseness are uncertain, and such patients still merit our sympathy and understanding.

Prevention of obesity

This important aspect of management starts in childhood. Health education, dietary understanding and the cnouragement of adequate exercise should contribute to a lowering of the incidence of obesity with its many undesirable consequences.

Vitamins

A normal mixed diet provides adequate vitamins. Vitamin deficiency can occur from

1. Dietary lack—infants, the elderly, alcoholics and food fads.
2. Failure of absorption—malabsorption syndrome, gastric surgery.
3. Effects of drugs—such as folic acid deficiency due to anti-convulsants.

VITAMIN A (RETINOL)

Vitamin A is found in animal fats and dairy products, fish liver oils and as a provitamin in carrots and tomatoes. It is concerned in copper metabolism, is necessary for the formation of visual purple in the retina and for the maintenance of epithelial tissues including the skin and cornea. Deficiency is rare, but occurs in tropical Africa, causing night blindness, and a serious deficiency causes degeneration of the cornea. Excess intake of vitamin A has occurred in Arctic explorers from eating polar-bear liver, causing raised intracranial pressure with drowsiness, and peeling of the skin.

VITAMIN B COMPLEX

This includes vitamin B_1 (aneurine, thiamine), vitamin B_2 (riboflavine), pyridoxine or vitamin B_6, and nicotinic acid (nicotinamide, vit. B_7). Vitamin B_{12} and folic acid are B group vitamins but are usually considered separately.

Vitamins of B complex are found in meat, eggs and dairy produce (milk is a rich source of riboflavine), and cereal germ and bran (rich in aneurine). The vitamins form part of enzyme systems concerned in carbohydrate metabolism. Vitamin B_1 is added to white bread.

Isolated vitamin B_1 deficiency causes wet beri-beri—cardiac failure with oedema and warm extremities, and neurological upset. This includes Wernicke's encephalopathy, cerebral beri-beri—a confusional state plus signs of brain-stem involvement such as nystagmus and ocular nerve palsies. There is now some doubt about the role of B_1 deficiency in nutritional peripheral neuritis, dry beri-beri, from which the name a-neurine was derived. Such conditions occur in alcoholics and after long illnesses associated with vomiting and poor dietary intake. Treatment is with vitamin B_1 tablets (20–100 mg daily) or injections. Parentrovite, which contains vitamin B complex and vitamin C, is a useful preparation for confusional states or dementia due to vitamin B deficiency.

Vitamin B_2 deficiency may occur in malabsorption states and causes cracks at the corners of the mouth (angular cheilitis) and sore, red tongue. Such findings also occur in nicotinic acid deficiency, which classically causes pellagra—dermatitis, diarrhoea and dementia.

The classical syndromes of deficiency of vitamins of the B complex —beri-beri, Wernicke's encephalopathy and pellagra—are rare in Britain, but findings such as a sore tongue or cracked lips should alert one to the possibility of vitamin B deficiency in alcoholics or the elderly. Vitamin B therapy is of no value unless there is such a deficiency, and there is no indication for adding vitamin B to tetracycline treatment as the sore mouth with the latter is due to thrush infection and not avitaminosis.

Pyridoxine deficiency may complicate isoniazid therapy for tuberculosis due to metabolic intereference, causing peripheral neuritis; deficiency may also cause the rare sideroblastic anaemia.

VITAMIN B_{12}

This is found in liver, meat, eggs and milk.

Dietary deficiency is extremely rare, occurring only in Vegans, a strict vegetarian sect who eat no animal protein whatsoever. Pernicious anaemia is due to lack of vitamin B_{12} from malabsorption following gastric atrophy and lack of intrinsic factor, and malabsorption can also occur after gastric surgery. Treatment is with injections of hydroxocobalamin (Neo-cytamen).

Folic acid

This is found in liver and green vegetables, but may be destroyed in cooking. Dietary deficiency may occur in the elderly, needs are increased in pregnancy, malabsorption may occur in intestinal disease, and anticonvulsant drugs impair its availability for metabolism. The result is a macrocytic anaemia, and possibly dementia in the elderly. Pregnant women are now given supplements of 100 micrograms (plus iron) to prevent deficiency. Oral therapy, 5–15 mg daily usually suffices in treatment, but should only be given after any co-existing vitamin B_{12} deficiency has been corrected, to prevent worsening of subacute combined degeneration.

VITAMIN C (ASCORBIC ACID)

Ascorbic acid is found in fruits, blackcurrants, rose hips, tomatoes and green vegetables. Potatoes contain some vitamin C and as they are a staple article of Western diet, they provide a considerable part of the daily requirement of about 40 mg. Stored potatoes lack the vitamin, so deficiency may be seen in winter and spring before the new crop is available. Elderly people may take little fruit and vegetables, subsisting on tea and toast. In hospital they are still at risk from vitamin C deficiency, for high temperatures and bulk cooking destroy it, and hospital food may be deficient. The old 'gastric diets' also lacked the vitamin. Babies are born with a sufficient reserve of vitamin C for some months and breast milk contains the vitamin. There is little in cow's milk and it is destroyed by pasteurization.

Deficiency results in *scurvy*—purpuric haemorrhages into the skin and mucous membranes. The legs are especially affected; other signs are scaliness of the skin around the hair follicles and the hairs may be 'corkscrewed'. There is bleeding from the gums (and from under the periosteum of the bones in infants), anaemia and general debility. Wounds are slow to heal. Aspirin-induced haematemesis may be commoner in those deficient in ascorbic acid.

Treatment: The best measures are preventive, ensuring dietary adequacy or giving supplements to those at risk, especially infants and the elderly. Scurvy is treated with large doses of ascorbic acid 250 mg four times daily for a week, to saturate the body stores.

Ascorbic acid improves iron absorption, but this action is probably of little importance in practice. Massive doses of ascorbic acid are harmless as the vitamin is water-soluble so that excess is excreted in the urine, and have been tried as a cure for colds. There is, however, no evidence that the vitamin is of value unless a deficiency is present.

VITAMIN D

Natural vitamin D is vitamin D_3, cholecalciferol, found in animal fat and formed in the skin by the action of ultra-violet light. Ultra-violet radiation of certain plant substances produces the synthetic vitamin D_2, calciferol, which has the same actions. Butter and cheese contain vitamin D and egg yolk and fish liver oils are good sources. Otherwise natural foods contain little or no vitamin D. Margarine is fortified with calciferol.

Vitamin D promotes the absorption of calcium and phosphate from the gut and has a direct action on bone, causing laying down of calcium salt on the protein matrix—mineralization. Requirements are greatest in childhood, pregnancy, and lactation, but the previously recommended doses were too high and 10 micrograms (400 units) daily is probably adequate here. The requirement otherwise for adults is uncertain, but may be as little as 2–5 micrograms daily.

Causes of deficiency

1. *Dietary-lack* in infants, and in the elderly (? malabsorption element).

2. *Malabsorption.* The vitamin is fat soluble and requires the presence of bile salts for emulsification. It is absorbed from the jejunum into the lacteals. Malabsorption occurs in biliary cirrhosis, malabsorption syndrome, and from the effect of liquid paraffin.

3. *Lack of sunshine.* Smoky atmospheres screen off the sun's ultra-violet rays but smokeless fuel is allowing these once again to penetrate to our cities. Pigmented skin is less sensitive to ultra-violet than fair skin and deficiency of vitamin D has occurred in the infants of coloured immigrants.

4. *Chronic renal disease.* In uraemia there is resistance to the action of vitamin D; deficiency, and calcium loss, may also occur in rare tubular defects.

Results of deficiency: Rickets and Osteomalacia

Deficiency results in *rickets* in children—defective calcification of the bones with swelling of the matrix tissue at their growing ends, impaired growth, and softening of the shafts causing deformities such as bowing of the legs. There is muscle weakness, abdominal distension and tetany from the low blood calcium.

Vitamin D deficiency in adults results in *osteomalacia*, demineralization and rarefaction of the bones. There are bony pains, and trivial injury may result in fractures of the long bones; tiny symptomless fractures called Looser's zones may be seen on x-ray of the pelvis, which may become grossly deformed later. There is again muscular weakness, and a waddling gait. Osteomalacia may occur in the elderly though *osteoporosis* is commoner—see page 392.

Osteoporosis may be an ageing change with bone thinning, especially affecting the vertebrae and causing loss of height. Its cause and treatability are uncertain. Osteomalacia is, on the other hand, a remediable deficiency state and its recognition is important.

Indications for Vitamin D

In the tropics, where there is adequate sunshine, vitamin D deficiency in children is not common, and in Britain dried milk and cereals for infants contains the added vitamin. Cod liver oil or halibut liver oil can be given to children, but excessive doses are dangerous. Margarine, which is fortified with vitamin D (and vitamin A) provides a cheap and adequate source for those elderly people who cannot afford butter.

In deprivational rickets and osteomalacia, treatment is 10–100 micrograms (400–4,000 units) calciferol daily. Larger doses, 1–2 mg, may be necessary in malabsorption syndrome; in coeliac disease the dose may be reduced or discontinued when response to the gluten-free diet has taken place. In the bone disease of renal failure much larger doses of calciferol may be required.

An adequate calcium intake is also necessary in the treatment of rickets and osteomalacia—milk is a good source, and supplements can be given as Sandocal, one to five effervescent tablets, each equivalent to 400 mg calcium, daily.

Use of vitamin D in hypoparathyroidism. Hypoparathyroidism, lack of parathyroid hormone, can occur spontaneously but more commonly follows damage to the parathyroid glands at thyroidectomy. The blood calcium is low and symptoms include tetany—see below. There is no satisfactory preparation of parathyroid hormone to replace the deficiency. However, vitamin D, given in large 'pharmacological' doses as distinct from the small physiological requirements, acts like parathyroid hormone. The dose is 500 micrograms to 2 milligrams daily, careful watch being kept on the blood calcium.

Excessive intake of vitamin D raises the blood calcium which becomes deposited in the kidneys. Symptoms of hypercalcaemia, discussed below, include malaise, nausea, vomiting, polyuria and thirst, and renal failure follows.

VITAMIN E

This is contained in wheat-germ oil. Deficiency in rats causes infertility but is not known to occur in man.

VITAMIN K ('KOAGULATION VITAMIN')

Vitamin K was originally found in pig liver fat but it is also present in the leaves of plants such as spinach and cabbage, and in many vegetable oils. In addition, it is manufactured by bacteria in the gut. The naturally occurring forms are vitamins K_1 and K_2 which are non-toxic even when given in big doses. The synthetic vitamin menaphthone can induce haemolysis if large doses are used.

Vitamin K is necessary for the *production of prothrombin* and other clotting factors by the liver. Dietary deficiency is unknown, but malabsorption of the vitamin occurs in obstructive jaundice from lack of bile salts, and in conditions such as coeliac syndrome. Deficiency may rarely occur from the prolonged use of oral blood spectrum antibiotics which alter the intestinal flora. Lack of the bowel organisms may be partly responsible for the low prothrombin in haemorrhagic disease of the newborn but immaturity of liver function is the more likely cause. In adults, cirrhosis of the liver impairs prothrombin production. Oral anticoagulants act by competing with vitamin K in the liver, blocking the formation of prothrombin.

Prothrombin deficiency results in a bruising tendency haematuria and failure of the blood to clot.

Treatment: Haemorrhagic disease of the newborn can be prevented by giving vitamin K_1 1·0 mg injection at birth. Prothrombin deficiency in cirrhosis may be helped by vitamin K_1 10 mg, preferably by injection, and this route is necessary in obstructive jaundice and malabsorption. Oral anticoagulant overdosage rapidly responds to vitamin K which here can be given by mouth.

Vitamin K has been used to treat chilblains, but there is no evidence that it is effective.

Because a small quantity of vitamins are necessary for health, it is not right to assume that a large quantity must be ever better. Only rarely, as in the case of vitamin D in hypoparathyroidism, have vitamins been found to have an action apart from that in replacing a deficiency. There is no evidence that taking 'added vitamins' (or amino acids) as a 'tonic' is of any value. Many such preparations are taken needlessly and at great expense. As water soluble vitamins such as B and C are excreted in the urine, an excessive dose will do no harm. However, the fat soluble vitamins cannot be excreted, and overdosage with vitamin A or vitamin D is, as noted, dangerous.

Minerals

The minerals sodium and potassium, which are important electrolytes (that is, become charged particles or ions in solution) are considered in the next chapter.

Calcium

Milk and dairy products are rich sources of calcium. An average diet contains 1–2 G calcium daily. Only about a tenth of this is absorbed, balanced by a similar excretion in the urine. Absorption is dependent on vitamin D, and is higher in growing children where calcium is required for the bones, and in pregnant and lactating women. Absorption is also increased where there is excessive bone destruction and loss of calcium in the urine as in hyperparathyroidism, where demineralization and fractures occur if absorption does not keep pace with demand.

There has been a suggestion that osteoporosis in the elderly follows longstanding calcium deficiency from post-menopausal urinary losses and malabsorption later. The understanding of calcium balance has become complicated by the discovery of the hormone calcitonin (produced mainly by the thyroid), which may maintain the calcium content of the bones.

Tetany. Hypocalcaemia, lowering of the blood calcium, occurs in hypoparathyroidism and to a lesser degree in vitamin D deficiency—rickets and osteomalacia. States of alkalosis decrease the solubility of calcium in the blood, so that hypocalcaemic symptoms may follow prolonged vomiting with loss of hydrochloric acid, or overbreathing, which washes out carbon dioxide and carbonic acid. Hypocalcaemia causes increased excitability of the nerves and results in *tetany*. There is numbness and tingling in fingers, toes or around the lips, and a characteristic spasm at the hands and feet, carpopedal spasm. Thus the wrists and metacarpo-phalangeal joints are held in flexion, with the fingers in extension. The sign may be provoked by pressure on the arm with a sphygmomanometer cuff, Trousseau's sign. Tapping over the facial nerve in front of the ear elicits twitching of the lips and muscles of the face, Chvostek's sign. There may be spasm of the muscles of the larynx, with prolonged 'crowing' inspiration, dyspnoea and cyanosis. Convulsions, and epileptic attacks in those predisposed to them, may be precipitated. Emergency treatment of tetany is with 10 per cent calcium gluconate solution, 5–20 ml slowly intravenously, or intramuscularly.

Prolonged hypocalcaemia causes muscle weakness, a coarse, dry skin, calcium deposits in the cornea, and raised intracranial pressure with convulsions or precipitation of epilepsy. Treatment is that of the cause. Oral calcium supplements are given with vitamin D in deficiency states and may be required for a longer period where there is malabsorption—calcium lactate-gluconate may be prescribed as the preparation Sandocal, one effervescent tablet in water three times daily. Calcium supplements are often prescribed in osteoporosis but there is no proof of their value given orally—intravenous therapy is being evaluated.

Hypercalcaemia occurs in vitamin D intoxication, hyperparathyroidism, bone diseases such as myelomatosis, and sometimes in carcinomatosis and sarcoidosis. Symptoms include lassitude, anorexia, nausea, vomiting, polyuria, thirst and renal failure follows. Oral phosphate may be helpful where the cause cannot be eliminated.

Magnesium

Magnesium is required in small quantities; its actions have some similarities to those of calcium.

Iron

Iron is necessary for the formation of haemoglobin and is considered under Diseases of the Blood, page 196. It will be recalled that iron is found in meat and coloured foods—there is little in milk. While dietary deficiency can occur in women whose needs are increased by menstruation and pregnancy, and while malabsorption may follow gastrectomy, it is important to exclude blood loss as the cause of so-called iron-deficiency anaemia.

Excessive iron intake can occur with the use of iron cooking pots and from cheap native alcoholic drinks and wines. Excessive absorption occurs in the condition haemochromatosis, bronzed diabetes.

Iron poisoning occurs in children who may be attracted by the bright colours of some iron tablets and swallow them, causing gastric irritation and later convulsions. Treatment is gastric lavage and desferrioxamine, a 'chelating' agent which binds the iron.

Copper

Traces are necessary for blood formation and possibly for nerve function. In Wilson's disease, hepato-lenticular degeneration, copper becomes deposited in the liver and basal ganglia of the brain; penicillamine, a chelating agent, is used in treatment.

Iodine

Tiny quantities are necessary for normal thyroid function and formation of the thyroid hormone thyroxine. Deficiency is one cause of goitre, thyroid swelling. Iodine is present in sea foods. Inland soils may be iodine-deficient and goitre occurs in such areas. Iodized salt may be used to prevent such deficiency.

Fluorine

A concentration of one part per million in the water supply lowers the incidence of dental caries. Excessive doses cause fluorosis, a hardening of the bones.

Parenteral nutrition

Wherever possible, food should be taken by the natural route, through the mouth. If the patient cannot swallow, then feeding by nasogastric tube is the next best method. 'Complan' provides a balanced source of nutrients.

There are few situations where intravenous feeding is necessary—examples are severe anorexia nervosa (a psychiatric disturbance where food is refused), some cases of renal failure, and following severe burns or abdominal operations. Strong solutions of glucose (dextrose) are irritant to the veins, fructose less so, or 30 per cent sorbitol can be used. An alternative source of calories is a fat emulsion such as Intralipid. Protein can be given as the casein preparation Aminosol, or as amino-acids in Trophysan or Vamin. There is a risk of venous thrombosis and sepsis and careful sterile precautions are necessary when such intravenous preparations are used.

11

Body water, electrolytes and acid-base balance

Physiology

Man has evolved from primitive forms of water life. He is no longer dependent on an aquatic external environment but the metabolism of his cells still occurs in a medium of water and dissolved salts. Each cell is a little sac of fluid suspended in a surrounding of fluid. The volume and composition of the body fluids must be kept constant despite wide fluctuations in intake and metabolism.

WATER

The body has three sources of water—the water drunk, the water present in food, and the water formed by the metabolic oxidation of food. Water is lost in the urine, in the faeces, and by evaporation from the skin and exhaled air from the lungs. The daily balance is as follows:

Water intake		Water output	
Water drunk	1,500 ml	Urine	1,500 ml
Water in food	500–1,000 ml	Faeces	100 ml
Metabolic water	200– 500 ml	Skin evaporation	500 ml
		Lungs	400 ml
Total	2·5 L	Total	2·5 L

The evaporation from skin and exhaled air represents an obligatory litre of water per day; if the ½–1 L necessary for adequate urinary excretion is added, then basal requirements are about 2 L daily. Much higher intakes may be required in hot climates and in fevers, when skin losses are greatly increased.

A 70 kg (11 stone) man is 60 per cent water—about 42 L. Of this, 27 L is intracellular and 15 L extracellular—3 L in circulation in the plasma and 12 L interstitial water and lymph bathing the cells.

ELECTROLYTES

Salts such as sodium chloride when dissolved in water dissociate into particles derived from their molecules. Thus sodium chloride dissociates into sodium, Na, and chloride, Cl. These particles are called ions and carry an electrical charge—hence the salts from which they are formed are called *electrolytes*. Important salts or electrolytes in the body fluids are sodium chloride, sodium bicarbonate and potassium chloride. Sodium and potassium ions carry a positive charge and as they are attracted towards the negative pole or cathode in an electrical circuit, are called cations. Chloride and bicarbonate ions are negatively charged, are attracted to the positive anode and are called anions. In a solution, the number of positively charged cations must equal the number of negatively charged anions to maintain electro-chemical normality.

TONICITY AND OSMOLALITY

The strength, tonicity or osmolality of a solution depends on the total number of particles dissolved in it—the main contribution is from the cations and anions derived drom the electrolytes, and there is a small contribution from non-dissociated molecules such as glucose.

In general terms, water will pass from a more dilute solution on one side of a membrane to a more concentrated solution on the other in an attempt to equalize the concentration on both sides of the membrane—the concentrated solution exerts an osmotic force which *attracts* water. The tonicity or osmolality of the body fluids bathing the cells has to be kept constant and equal to that inside the cells, otherwise these lose or attract water and break up or burst—just as added fluid of the wrong concentration to the bloodstream will cause the red corpuscles to haemolyse.

Sodium is the dominant ion responsible for the maintenance of the extra-cellular fluid volume, that is, for the retention of water. Potassium is the dominant intra-cellular ion. The cell membrane uses energy to keep sodium out of, and to keep potassium in, the cell. In the blood vessels, the osmotic force exerted by the plasma proteins, especially albumin, helps to maintain the circulating fluid volume.

The volume of fluid in the body depends partly on the stimulus of a rise in tonicity affecting a centre in the hypothalamus, causing release of posterior pituitary anti-diuretic hormone and therefore water-retention, and partly on special volume receptors in the circulation—these may act via the renin-aldosterone mechanism regulating sodium loss. The sensation of thirst is one regulator of intake, but the control of the body fluids is largely dependent on the kidneys, which vary the excretion of water and salts to maintain normality.

The composition of the body fluids. Although the quantity of sodium and potassium in a solution can be expressed in terms of weight such as milligrams, it is more convenient to work in terms of the numbers of ions present, expressed as milli-equivalents (mEq) per litre (or milli-normals (mN), numerically the same). The ionic balance of extra-cellular fluid is as follows:

Positive Ions (*Cations*)		*Negative Ions* (*Anions*)	
	mEq/L		mEq/L
Sodium (Na)	140	Chloride (Cl)	100
Potassium (K)	4·5	Bicarbonate (HCO_3)	25
Calcium (Ca), Magnesium (Mg) and others	5·5	Phosphate (PO_4) and others (incl. plasma protein)	25
	150		150

The osmolality roughly equals the sum of these, actually 285 milli-Osmols per litre. This strength of solution is clinically 'normal' and 'normal saline', which contains 9 G NaCl per litre, is isotonic with it. This clinical use of the term normal is different from its use in chemistry—a chemically normal solution has an entirely different strength, based on gram equivalent weights.

ELECTROLYTE BALANCE

Under basal conditions, very little dietary salt, sodium chloride, is necessary, for the kidneys can, if required, secrete a urine almost free of sodium and chloride, and no salt is lost in the normal insensitive evaporation of water from the skin. Thus 1–2 G salt daily is sufficient, except where losses are great, as in visible sweating and in high fevers

Natural foods contain little sodium, but man has developed a taste for salt, preserved and canned meats and sausages containing large amounts. Thus the dietary intake is very variable, from 5–20 G daily of sodium chloride, averaging 12 G which corresponds to 160 mEq sodium. This is usually much in excess of needs, the kidneys excreting the excess.

The kidneys cannot conserve potassium—there is an obligatory daily loss in the urine (unlike sodium). Animal and plant cells are rich in potassium and therefore most natural foods contain it—fruit juices are a rich source. The normal potassium intake is about 6 G potassium chloride, equivalent to 70 mEq potassium, daily.

Sampling the blood gives an indication of the fluid and electrolyte balance of the patient—the packed cell volume (haematocrit) sodium, potassium and chloride being easily estimated. As noted above, the amount of sodium in the body determines the volume of the extra-cellular fluid. The ease of blood sampling should not lead us to forget about the intra-cellular compartment which cannot easily be measured in clinical practice—body potassium deficiency may not be reflected in serum tests.

ACID-BASE BALANCE

Tissue respiration results in the production of carbon dioxide which goes to form carbonic acid and this is duly excreted as carbon dioxide by the lung. Exercise, protein and fat breakdown also result in the production of acids. Thus metabolic processes are acid-forming, that is they result in the production of *hydrogen-ions*.

The acidity of a solution depends on the number of hydrogen-ions it contains. This is commonly expressed in a rather confusing logarithmic scale, the pH scale. It should be understood that a very small change in pH represents a big difference in hydrogen-ion concentration. Chemical neutrality is pH 7, the pH of water. Acids have a pH lower than 7, alkalis a pH higher than 7. The pH of plasma has to be maintained at 7·4, just on the alkaline side. Metabolic processes add hydrogen ions and would tend to shift the pH downwards, the state of acidosis. This tendency is resisted by the presence of 'buffer systems' in the blood which bind hydrogen-ions harmlessly until they can be excreted as carbon dioxide by the lungs, or by the kidney tubules. An important and readily measurable buffer system is the bicarbonate system. Not only do the kidneys excrete hydrogen-ions they also reconstitute bicarbonate buffer and return it to the bloodstream. While the urinary pH is a guide to the hydrogen-ion concentration in the body if the kidneys are working normally, blood measurements are more accurate and are now an essential part of the management of acid-base disturbances. It may be helpful to be aware of the following relationship:

pH (normal 7·4) is proportional to

$$\frac{\text{plasma bicarbonate}}{\text{dissolved carbon dioxide}} \quad \frac{(\text{HCO}_3)}{(\text{pCO}_2)} \quad \frac{(\text{normal 25 mEq/L})}{(\text{normal 40 mm Hg})}$$

A tendency for the pH to fall, that is, a state of acidosis, is recognized by a fall in the plasma bicarbonate ('buffer base deficit'), or a rise in the carbon dioxide, expressed as a pressure in millimetres of mercury. The former occurs in diabetic keto-acidosis and renal failure, the latter in the respiratory acidosis of respiratory failure.

For the preservation of a normal acid-base balance, the body needs a sufficient supply of water and electrolytes, a normal cardiac output, and adequately functioning lungs and kidneys.

Disturbances of water and electrolyte balance

WATER DEFICIENCY

A deficiency purely of water is usually due to insufficient intake—in desert conditions, inability to swallow, or in comas. Water deficiency can also follow urinary losses in diabetes mellitus and diabetes insipidus (lack of posterior pituitary anti-diuretic hormone).

As a result, the tonicity of the extra-cellular fluid tends to rise, and water moves out from the cells into the extra-cellular fluid. The intra-cellular dehydration causes the symptom of *thirst* in the conscious patient, the tongue is dry, and the urine decreased in amount but very concentrated, of high specific gravity.

Water deprivation can usually be remedied by oral fluids, but intravenous 5 per cent dextrose, which is isotonic with plasma, may be required, especially in the more complicated water deficiencies discussed below.

PURE SALT DEPLETION

Salt losses occur with severe sweating in the tropics and in heavy manual workers in hot conditions such as foundries. Symptoms include muscle cramps and weakness. In pure salt depletion the sodium concentration in the plasma (and extra-cellular fluids) falls and the urine flow might be increased to maintain it. The lowered extra-cellular fluid tonicity of sodium depletion results in water passing from the circulation into the cells to equalize the osmotic pressure. Thus there is a lack of fluid in circulation and a fall in blood pressure, but as there is cellular over-hydration the patient is not thirsty.

In Addison's disease, under-activity of the adrenal cortex, the serum sodium is low due to movement into the cells and urinary losses from lack of cortisol (hydrocortisone) and aldosterone. Excessive use of diuretics also causes sodium depletion, but the lowered serum sodium concentration sometimes found in advanced cardiac failure is associated with a high total body sodium, cellular function being defective.

In clinical practice pure water or salt deficiency states are rare—usually the deficiency is a combined one, giving the picture called dehydration.

THE CLINICAL PICTURE OF DEHYDRATION

The clinical state of dehydration is a result of water and salt deficiency, usually from abnormal losses. The extra-cellular fluid becomes depleted but for a time plasma volume can be maintained. Once the deficiency has reached several litres, the blood volume is reduced and the circulation to the kidneys impaired, leading to acidosis and uraemia.

Causes—insufficient intake of fluids as in coma or, more commonly, excessive losses of fluids from the body, for example:

severe vomiting and diarrhoea; also paralytic ileus, a complication of intestinal obstruction of operation when fluid is poured into the gut and lost to the circulation;

sweating especially in fevers in hot climates;

following polyuria in diabetes mellitus or chronic renal failure;

severe burns—here the loss is of serum from skin oozing.

Severe haemorrhage produces pallor and collapse, a different picture, but dehydration may be a complication, especially in haematemesis.

Symptoms and signs—these occur with a deficiency of about 3 L.

Thirst is usual, but may be absent if the deficiency is mainly of salt. The patient is weak and lethargic, the tongue dry, the skin inelastic and slack, remaining in a fold when pinched up. The eyes may be sunken. The pulse rises, the blood pressure falls and coma may result.

The output of urine is markedly reduced, it is concentrated (high specific gravity) if the kidneys are healthy. With renal failure and acidosis, there is vomiting and deep sighing respirations—acidotic breathing, air hunger.

Management

1. *Observations and investigations.* The nature and extent of the fluid loss, and the urine volume must be noted—an input-output chart must be kept, plus record of pulse, blood pressure and weight if possible.

Other *urine tests* include specific gravity, urea and sodium concentration—the Fantus test for chloride is unreliable.

Blood tests. The haemoglobin and haematocrit are raised in dehydration and the blood urea may be raised. The sodium and other electrolyte levels are variable, often unhelpful in diagnosis, but are a guide to therapy.

2. *Treatment.*

(*a*) *Mild dehydration*—if the patient is not vomiting, fluids can be given by mouth or by feeds of 200–400 ml three-hourly by nasogastric tube.

When the patient has been rehydrated yet still requires tube feeding for a few days, for example after a stroke, his needs for 2 L fluid and 2,000 calories daily can be met by spaced feeds including 2 oz (60 G) Complan, which gives 650 calories, and an egg (80 calories) in 300 ml milk (200 calories).

(*b*) *Moderate and severe dehydration*—here the fluid deficit is 4 L or more and even in a conscious patient it is difficult to replace this amount orally. Thus intravenous fluids are required. The object is to supply adequate fluids to allow the kidneys to adjust the body water and electrolyte composition to normal.

Types of i.v. fluid

5 *per cent dextrose (glucose) in water*—this is isotonic with plasma and is a means of giving water, the dextrose being metabolized; 1 L yields only 200 calories so the nutritional contribution is insignificant.

0·9 *per cent sodium chloride in water, normal saline*—isotonic, and its sodium content approximating to that of the extra-cellular fluid.

Refinements include various strengths of saline in dextrose solution (dextrose-saline) and alkalinizing solutions containing bicarbonate or lactate which is metabolized to bicarbonate. Potassium additions are required for the losses in diarrhoea or polyuria.

It is usual to start the drip with normal saline, provided the serum sodium level is not elevated, when 5 per cent dextrose may be used (but not at first in diabetic keto-acidosis). Initially 1 L may be required hourly. The rate depends on the clinical and biochemical response and the establishment of a urine flow—it may be necessary to pass a catheter to confirm this, for it is dangerous to push fluids in oliguria and renal failure.

Once rehydration has been achieved, the basic requirement is for 2 L of fluid per 24 hours, which can be given as 500 ml 5 per cent dextrose alternating with 500 ml normal saline every six hours. More is required if losses are continuing. If there is oliguric renal failure, fluid must be restricted to 500 ml per 24 hours plus the previous day's output.

Complications of intravenous infusions include infection, thrombosis and over-hydration (described below). Other fluids used are noted at the end of the chapter.

OVER-HYDRATION

In health, it is almost impossible to drink too much fluid—the kidneys will excrete the excess. Over-hydration usually results from excessive intravenous fluids, especially in patients with poor circulation and failing kidneys.

Symptoms include lethargy, anorexia and vomiting. The venous pressure is raised, and jugular venous pulsation may be seen in the neck. Fluid accumulates in the lungs, causing breathlessness and crepitations—'moist' sounds heard with the stethoscope over the lung bases. Peripheral oedema develops and there may be hypertension, especially in association with renal failure.

The development of such a state can be prevented by proper fluid balance charts, weighing the patient, and monitoring the central venous pressure by a cannula passed into the great veins and connected to a manometer, when intravenous infusions are given.

Where over-hydration exists, diuretics may be necessary, or peritoneal dialysis or haemo-dialysis if there is renal failure.

OEDEMA

Oedema is due to the accumulation of excess fluid in the interstitial space.

Causes:

A. Local

1. Increased permeability of small blood vessels as in trauma, burns, inflammation and infection, and allergy (angioneurotic oedema).
2. Lymphatic obstruction—in carcinoma and in tropical filariasis.
3. Venous obstruction—thrombosis, pressure of tumours.

In inflammatory oedema, the fluid may be an exudate and of high protein content. In lymphatic oedema, the fluid may also be rich in protein. In venous obstruction, the oedema fluid is a transudate of water and salts forced from the circulation.

B. Generalized—here the oedema fluid is a transudate of salt and water.

1. *Cardiac failure.* Here there is too much fluid both in the circulation and in the tissues. The mechanism is uncertain, but deranged volume receptors in the circulation may act through posterior pituitary anti-diuretic hormone secretion to cause water retention by the kidneys; in addition, a reduced renal blood flow results in sodium retention, and aldosterone secretion may worsen this. Thus there is salt and water retention.

In cardiac failure the additional factor of the raised venous pressure aggravates oedema formation in dependent regions.

2. *Hypoproteinaemic states*

nephrotic syndrome;
cirrhosis of the liver;
malnutrition ('famine oedema'); severe malabsorption.

In these conditions the plasma protein, especially albumin, is lowered. This results in lowered plasma osmotic pressure, the force which attracts water into solution. When it is lowered, water passes from the blood vessels into the tissues. The tendency for the circulating blood volume to fall causes excess aldosterone secretion which acts on the renal tubules to cause salt and water retention, worsening the tissue oedema.

3. *Acute glomerulonephritis.* The puffiness of the face and peripheral oedema were previously ascribed to diffuse capillary damage, but in fact the oedema fluid is again a transudate, and results from sodium and water retention related to the renal disorder.

4. *Toxaemia of pregnancy* (oedema, albuminuria, hypertension and fits) has a similar basis.

5. *Corticosteroid* (*e.g. cortisone*) *overdosage*, and sometimes in Cushing's syndrome.

The oedema following over-hydration has been described above.

Thus there is too much water in the body in these states of oedema —whether this occurs in cardiac failure, nephrotic sydrome or cirrhosis, it always indicates that there has been sodium retention. Sodium 'holds on to' water, and oedema follows. Thus, similar diuretic therapy is applicable to all.

Clinical presentation of oedema

There is swelling on the affected part, and the skin 'pits' on pressure with the finger tip due to the subcutaneous fluid. In chronic lymphatic obstruction, however, the pitting may not be marked, the affected tissues tending to become brawny and thickened. Venous obstruction in the great veins associated with a carcinoma of the lung causes a thickening of the tissues in the neck ('collar sign') with fullness and suffusion of the face. Venous thrombosis in the legs, which may have caused no symptoms, may be followed by ankle oedema.

In generalized cases, oedema accumulates in the dependent parts of the body and where the skin is lax. Thus, ankle swelling is often the first sign.

The patient with cardiac failure is breathless from pulmonary oedema and prefers to sleep propped up, so that a pad of oedema may form above the sacrum.

In the hypoproteinaemic states such as nephrotic syndrome, and in acute glomerulonephritis, the patient can lie flat without discomfort, so oedema may gather about the face, hands and arms.

Effusions occur into the pleural and peritoneal cavities, but ascites tends to be more severe in cirrhosis, where there is a raised portal venous pressure.

Important factors in diagnosis are the mode of onset, accompanying clinical features and the examination of the urine—heavy albuminuria in nephrotic syndrome, red cells and oliguria in acute glomerulonephritis. Further investigations include plasma proteins, urea and electrolytes.

Management of oedema

Localized types. The oedema of lymphatic obstruction is usually resistant to diuretic drugs; operations have been devised to drain the fluid, but treatment is generally unsatisfactory.

In ankle oedema following leg vein thrombosis, prolonged standing or sitting with the legs dependent should be avoided, and venous return may be aided by muscular activity and elastic supporting bandages or hosiery.

Generalized oedema

Observations include weighing the patient, keeping an input-output chart, and noting the blood pressure.

General measures. In cardiac oedema the patient is more comfortable propped up, or sitting in a chair. When the cardiac output has improved with treatment, it becomes possible to raise the legs to the horizontal to allow mobilization of the oedema. A bed cage takes the weight of the bed-clothes off the legs and is helpful.

The causative condition should be treated, and diuretics are applicable in most cases.

Diuretics. As explained, oedema is due to salt and water retention. Frusemide (Lasix) and ethacrynic acid (Edecrin) are potent diuretics, acting rapidly by mouth or by injection; the thiazides such as bendrofluazide, and chlorthalidone (Hygroton) are given by mouth—all promote renal sodium and water excretion, but also cause potassium loss, and potassium chloride supplements must be given. Spironolactone (Aldactone-A) is a less powerful diuretic which acts by competing with aldosterone in the renal rubules and causes sodium and water loss without potassium loss, an action shared with amiloride (Midamor)—these are useful supplementary diuretics.

With these diuretics, the patient can now be allowed a reasonable fluid intake and only in the oedema of cirrhosis is there need for rigid salt restriction. Failure to respond to diuretics may occur in cardiac and renal failure with raised blood urea—in the former, intravenous aminophylline may improve the circulation to the kidneys and allow the diuretics to work; in these states, restricted water intake may be necessary.

Once oedema has been controlled, maintenance doses of diuretics are continued, guided by the patient's weight.

Mechanical methods of removing oedema fluid, such as Southey's tubes, and paracentesis are now rarely required.

DISTURBANCES OF POTASSIUM BALANCE

Potassium is the important intracellular cation. The serum level is a relatively insensitive index of the intracellular level. Disturbance of the balance between intra- and extra-cellular levels contributes to the symptoms in depletion or excess.

HYPOKALAEMIA

This means abnormally low serum potassium, and indicates that a severe degree of intra-cellular depletion has occurred.

Causes

1. Loss from gastro-intestinal tract, especially diarrhoea, in diseases such as cholera and severe ulcerative colitis; also abuse of purgatives.

2. Renal losses and polyuria resulting from

    i Prolonged use of diuretics.
    ii Polyuria following acute renal failure.
    iii Use of forced diuretic therapy in aspirin poisoning.

Hypokalaemia itself worsens polyuria, and causes alkalosis.

3. Cardiac failure.

4. Cirrhosis. Potassium loss is here associated with disturbed cell function, and will be worsened by diuretic therapy unless supplements are given.

5. Diabetic keto-acidosis—loss from the cells and into the urine has occurred early, and in the recovery stages blood levels of potassium may be even lower.

6. Excess aldosterone secretion (Conn's syndrome) and after prolonged use of corticosteroids such as cortisone.

Symptoms and signs—apathy, fatigue, confusion, muscle weakness, intestinal slowing and ileus (paralysis) with abdominal distension, and polyuria. There are E.C.G. changes, cardiac arrhythmias such as extrasystoles, and increased sensitivity to digoxin, so that overdosage may occur. There is risk of cardiac failure.

Treatment. Potassium chloride is given by mouth as tablets such as Slow-K, each containing 8 mEqK, dose 1–3 tablets, three times daily, or as effervescent preparations such as Sando-K or Kloref. Fresh orange juice and black treacle are rich sources of potassium.

In severe depletion, and where intravenous infusions are being given, one or two 5 ml ampoules of 20 per cent potassium chloride (each contains 1 G KCl, that is 13 mEqK) are added to the solution in the infusion bottle. The rate of giving potassium is 3–20 mEq per hour, with careful biochemical control. Potassium chloride solution must never be injected directly into a vein.

HYPERKALAEMIA

Hyperkalaemia is excessive potassium in the blood (normal serum potassium is 4·5 mEq/L) but it need not indicate a high intracellular level.

Causes. Renal failure is the commonest cause the kidneys failing to excrete potassium. In acute renal failure there is oliguria and as the causative condition is usually associated with tissue damage and release of potassium from the cells, the level in the blood rises rapidly. In chronic renal failure the kidneys may excrete potassium normally until the late stages, when hyperkalaemia occurs.

Poor renal function and cellular breakdown cause hyperkalaemia in some cases of diabetic keto-acidosis, and states of circulatory failure and anoxia.

The serum potassium level is raised in Addison's disease from cortisol (hydrocortisone) lack, but the sodium deficiency is more important here.

Symptoms and signs—muscle weakness, and E.C.G. changes (tall T waves); when the serum potassium reaches 7 mEq/L, there is a danger of asystole and cardiac arrest.

Treatment. In conditions carrying the risk of hyperkalaemia, the serum potassium levels must be frequently checked. In renal failure, preventive measures include a high calorie diet to minimise endogenous tissue breakdown, and the use of potassium-exchanging polysterene resins such as Calcium Resonium 15 G by mouth or retention enema. Peritoneal dialysis or haemodialysis may be necessary, and the underlying condition must be treated.

The emergency treatment of hyperkalaemia is 10–20 ml of 10 per cent calcium gluconate injected slowly intravenously, and infusion of 10 per cent dextrose solution with insulin, which helps to move potassium back into the cells.

Disturbances of acid-base balance

ACIDOSIS

This is a tendency for the blood to become more acid, or rather less alkaline, than normal, from an excess of hydrogen ions. The pH is lowered from its normal 7·4, but seldom falls below 7·2—neutral is pH 7 as explained. It will be recalled that the body has two routes for getting rid of acids—the lungs blowing off carbon dioxide from carbonic acid, and the kidneys excreting hydrogen ions; the kidneys also reconstitute bicarbonate, returning it to the circulation.

Acidosis is classified as (*a*) respiratory or (*b*) non-respiratory.

(*a*) *Respiratory acidosis* is due to impaired excretion of carbon dioxide in respiratory failure—in conditions such as chronic bronchitis and emphysema with superadded infection, and less commonly in the respiratory depression of poisoning or following respiratory muscle paralysis (in these states anoxia is more dominant). Thus the CO_2 dissolved in the blood, the pCO_2, is raised above the normal 40 mm Hg, the condition called hypercapnia.

The causative condition is usually associated with symptoms such as dyspnoea and cyanosis from anoxia, and the CO_2 retention contributes to the restlessness, confusion, disturbance of consciousness, and tremor.

In treatment, it will be recalled that it is dangerous to give oxygen at high concentration or intermittently in respiratory failure with CO_2 retention. The respiratory centre has become dependent on the stimulus of hypoxia to maintain ventilation and if the patient is given too much oxygen he will stop breathing—a flow rate of 2 L oxygen per minute using nasal catheters, Edinburgh mask or Ventimask delivers 30 per cent oxygen in the inspired 'air', which is satisfactory. Drugs such as nikethamide have only a temporary stimulant effect on the respiratory centre. Intubation and artificial ventilation may be required.

(*b*) *Non-respiratory acidosis* (*metabolic acidosis*).

Causes

i *Diabetic keto-acidosis*—the ketone bodies are themselves acids.

ii *Renal failure.*

Also rare conditions such as renal tubular acidosis, and following ureteric implantation into the colon which may impair renal tubular function.

iii Conditions associated with *water and salt depletion* impairing renal function, such as prolonged vomiting or diarrhoea with *loss of intestinal secretions* including bicarbonate, or high fevers with lack of fluid intake, i.e. clinical dehydration.

iv *Cardiac arrest* and circulatory failure.

Symptoms and signs. There is lethargy, weakness and vomiting, and the raised hydrogen ion concentration stimulates the respiratory centre causing deep sighing 'acidotic' respiration or 'air hunger' (Kussmaul breathing) in an attempt to get rid of the excess acids as carbon dioxide from the lungs. Finally the patient lapses into unconsciousness.

Investigations include the blood pH and bicarbonate which are lowered: there is a 'base deficit'. Haemoglobin, haematocrit, urea, sugar and electrolytes are also measured.

Treatment. Treatment is that of the primary cause. If there is good renal function, acidosis will be corrected by supplying adequate fluids and sodium. Intravenous therapy is required in severe cases. Fluids which supply alkali (base) to speed correction include:

One-sixth Molar ($\frac{1}{6}$ M) *sodium lactate*—the lactate is metabolized to bicarbonate thus supplying base.

Solutions containing *sodium bicarbonate*—8·4 per cent contains 1 mEq bicarbonate per 1 ml, is very hypertonic, but may be infused directly in 50–100 ml quantities in cardiac arrest and life-threatening acidosis, or added to an existing infusion solution. 4·2 per cent, 2·74 per cent, 1·43 per cent and 1·26 per cent bicarbonate solutions are also available—the latter is isotonic and used in forced alkaline diuretic therapy for aspirin poisoning.

Using such solutions, a calculated base deficit can be replaced, but attempts at rapid correction are dangerous, and the clinical progress of the patient is the best guide to therapy. Fluid balance charts are essential, an adequate urinary output being a favourable sign for recovery.

ALKALOSIS

This is the opposite of acidosis—in alkalosis the blood is too alkaline, with a rise in pH. Alkalosis is not so common but again may be respiratory or non-respiratory.

Respiratory alkalosis is caused by over-breathing with loss of carbon dioxide and carbonic acid. Over-breathing occurs in anxiety, hysteria (an uncommon condition) and occasionally following damage to the respiratory centre in the brain stem. In the early stages of aspirin poisoning over-breathing is due to stimulation of the respiratory centre by the salicylate, and this may cause alkalosis; in the later stages, there is acidosis from dehydration and circulatory collapse resulting in 'acidotic respiration', air hunger.

Non-respiratory alkalosis.

Causes

i Following prolonged vomiting or aspiration of gastric

contents, with loss of hydrochloric acid, as may occur in pyloric stenosis.

   ii Excessive intake of alkalis such as sodium bicarbonate taken to relieve the pain of peptic ulcer—antacids such as magnesium trisilicate are not absorbed and do not carry the risk of causing alkalosis.

   iii As a consequence of potassium depletion, where hydrogen ions pass into the cells and are also lost in the urine.

Symptoms and signs of alkalosis. Calcium is more soluble in an acid solution. Thus alkalosis decreases the amount of ionised calcium in the blood causing increased excitability of the nerves and muscles. There are paraesthesiae (tingling feelings, pins and needles), tetany, clouding of consciousness and convulsions. Tetany is described on page 242, and includes spasm of the fingers and muscles of the larynx, and twitching of the face.

The diagnosis is confirmed by the clinical history and tests such as raised plasma bicarbonate and pH.

Treatment. In the respiratory alkalosis of anxiety or hysteria, restraining the patient from over-breathing with a sedative such as diazepam (Valium), or raising the blood level of CO_2 by rebreathing from a paper bag usually suffices.

In non-respiratory alkalosis, treatment is that of the cause. It is usually sufficient to correct dehydration and electrolyte deficiency, including potassium, by mouth or intravenously. It is not usually necessary to give acidifying substances such as ammonium chloride—given sufficient fluids, sodium and potassium, the kidneys will restore the acid-base balance.

A note on diet and acid-base balance

Fruits contain weak organic acids such as citric acid but do not cause 'acidosis'—indeed their metabolism results in the production of bicarbonate base. The sulphur in some proteins may be metabolized to sulphuric acid, but the acid load is small. It is the body's metabolic processes that cause acid production and the dietary constituents have no major effect on acid-base balance.

Notes on intravenous infusion therapy

Blood transfusion is required to replace losses in severe haemorrhage as in haematemesis or with multiple injuries and fractures. It may also be indicated in the management of leukaemia. Otherwise it is not generally justified to treat anaemias by transfusion—and it may be dangerous to give a blood transfusion in long-standing pernicious anaemia where the heart is flabby and there is danger of circulatory overload. Moreover, response to vitamin B_{12} injections is usually rapid. In an elderly patient with obscure anaemia, cautious transfusion using packed cells may be indicated.

Hazards to the recipient include haemolytic reaction from incompatible blood (from inadequate cross-matching or administrative error), non-specific febrile reactions, transmission of infection especially serum hepatitis, and calcium depletion from the effect of citrate in massive transfusions. Hazards to the donor include pain, thrombosis or sepsis at the site of venepuncture and anaemia if iron reserves are marginal.

Plasma infusion may be given if blood is not immediately available, or if the loss is of serum, as in severe burns. Whole plasma carries the risk of hepatitis; preserved or dried plasma may be safer. Plasma substitutes such as dextran temporarily replace the blood volume before being metabolized to glucose. Low-molecular-weight dextran (dextran-40) has also been claimed to improve capillary flow by lowering the blood viscosity, but large amounts may cause renal tubular damage.

Water and electrolytes are replaced according to the needs of the patient, as described.

5 *per cent dextrose solution* is isotonic and supplies water (and 200 calories, a small amount, per litre) but being acidic, is irritant to veins. 5 *per cent laevulose* (*fructose*) is less irritant and may be metabolized more easily in uraemia, but any advantage is marginal.

0·9 *per cent sodium chloride, normal saline*, is isotonic, and though it contains a slightly higher concentration of sodium than does plasma, and a considerably higher concentration of chloride, it is the most useful stock replacement solution. As explained, 5 per cent dextrose and normal saline can be used alternately in maintenance therapy. A popular alternative is *one-fifth normal saline in dextrose* solution (sodium chloride 0·18 per cent, dextrose 4·3 per cent) also isotonic, and used to give water and sufficient sodium to maintain a low normal intake in a volume of 2–2·5 L daily.

One-sixth Molar sodium lactate is isotonic, and can be used in acidosis. *Sodium bicarbonate solutions*, in strengths varying from 1·26 per cent to 8·4 per cent, the latter being very hypotonic, can also be added to drip infusions. Their use is not always necessary, for the healthy kidneys will correct acid-base balance if the circulation is adequate, and they are provided with water and electrolytes. 8·4 per cent sodium bicarbonate contains 1 mEq bicarbonate per ml, and is used in cardiac arrest.

Potassium chloride is available in ampoules of varying strength— the 20 per cent solution contains 1 G KCl (13 mEqK) in 5 ml; the appropriate quantity is added to the bottle containing an infusion solution such as normal saline, and the rate of administration must be carefully controlled. Potassium chloride solution must never be injected directly into a vein or into the tubing of an intravenous drip.

There are many compound solutions—Hartmann's solution (Ringer-Lactate) which includes calcium, Darrow's solution containing excess potassium, various replacement solutions for diabetic ketoacidosis (coma) and special solutions for forced alkaline diuresis therapy. Their multiplicity is confusing, and most needs can be met by the standard intravenous solutions described above.

Hypertonic solutions such as mannitol 10–20 per cent are used to promote a diuresis in the early stages of acute renal failure and in cerebral oedema, but their osmotic action in raising the circulating blood volume may precipitate cardiac failure.

Hypotonic solutions of saline are given in the condition called hyperosmolar non-ketotic diabetic coma (page 277).

Use of drip infusions as a vehicle for giving drugs

It is now common practice to use a penicillin drip in subacute bacterial endocarditis to avoid the pain of repeated intramuscular injections. Antibiotics can be administered intravenously in septicaemias, either by drip infusion (for example fusidic acid) or by 'bolus' injections into the tubing of an existing drip. Steroids may also be given by such methods. It should be noted that the penicillins, especially ampicillin, lose much of their activity if added to dextrose solutions. There is also the possibility of incompatibility from such infusion cocktails.

Hazards of drips

1. *The risks of cannulating a vein*—discomfort, phlebitis, infection, and air embolus from faulty technique in changing the bottle or letting it run dry—this risk is lessened if collapsible plastic bottles (such as Polyfusor) are used.

2. *Hazards inherent to the solutions infused.*

3. *Circulatory overload and overhydration,* if urinary output is impaired.

4. An induced polyuria may cause *potassium depletion.*

5. *Immobility hazards*—the patient may be afraid to move and runs an increased risk of pneumonia and of leg vein thrombosis with its pulmonary complications.

The importance of nursing care

There has been a great increase in the use of intravenous infusions in recent years and the understanding of fluid requirements has saved many lives. Disposable plastic giving sets and indwelling cannulas mean increased safety and less discomfort for the patient, and less drudgery for the nurse.

More than ever, reassurance and a kind word to the patient, with careful attention to his comfort, care of the mouth and pressure areas are important nursing measures. Accurate charting is essential. Normal eating and drinking should be resumed as soon as possible.

12

Diabetes mellitus

Diabetes mellitus is a disorder of metabolism characterized by a high blood sugar and the passage of large quantities of sugar-containing urine—the word diabetes comes from the Greek 'to pass through' and mellitus is Latin for honey. When the term diabetes is used alone, it refers to diabetes mellitus, a disorder quite distinct from diabetes insipidus, which is due to lack of posterior pituitary anti-diuretic hormone.

Causes of diabetes mellitus

Diabetes is due to a relative or absolute deficiency of insulin action. Insulin is the pancreatic hormone discovered by Banting and Best in Toronto in 1921.

The pancreas has two component parts—the exocrine digestive-enzyme secreting part, and the endocrine part, the islets of Langerhans. Insulin is secreted into the bloodstream by the 'beta' cells of the islets; the 'alpha' cells secrete glucagon. The stimulus to insulin-secretion is a high blood sugar level acting directly on the pancreas, but glucose and amino-acids in the upper intestine after a meal also stimulate insulin secretion indirectly by the action of certain gut hormones on the pancreas.

In diabetes, the secretion of insulin is deranged though the pancreatic tissue may appear normal to the naked eye. In the severe diabetes of the young the beta cells are very defective and there is a lack of insulin production. In older diabetics, who are frequently obese, the plasma insulin may be higher than in a thin, normal person, but there is a deficiency of secretion relative to needs.

Diabetes sometimes runs in families, but the genetic basis is not clear and is probably multifactorial. Thus there may be an inherited defect of islet cell function, especially in young diabetics. However, if one identical twin develops diabetes his fellow twin need not simultaneously manifest the disease, so other factors play a part. Mumps is occasionally associated with diabetes of acute onset, and there is some recent evidence of an association with Coxsackie virus infection, but there is as yet no proof of a virus cause in most cases. There is a raised incidence of auto-immune disease such as pernicious anaemia and myxoedema in diabetics, but the role of auto-immunity as a cause of diabetes is not established.

It was noted that women presenting with diabetes in middle-age frequently gave a history of having large babies (over 4·5 Kg birth weight) and multiple pregnancies. This observation led to the concept of 'pre-diabetes' or diabetes pre-'mellitus', and suggested that there could be a latent period of 10–30 years of metabolic abnormality before overt diabetes with glycosuria appeared. Insulin antagonists, pituitary or adrenal dependent, have been thought to be operative during the latent period. Again, the muscles of the obese may have a metabolic block in glucose uptake (which is sidetracked to the fat depots) which increases insulin demands. Blood vessel abnormalities occur in diabetes, and altered permeability of capillaries might impair insulin passage. All these factors create an increased demand on the pancreas to produce insulin and while this demand may be met for many years, ultimately it results in pancreatic exhaustion and clinical diabetes.

During the long latent period, abnormalities in insulin secretion and glucose tolerance may be detectable, or the hormonal effects of pregnancy and corticosteroid drugs, the effect of sudden gain in weight, or the stress of infection may provoke overt diabetes. Some of the 'complications' of diabetes, especially vascular disease, may develop during the latent period, and the sugar abnormality may be a late one.

Thus, in diabetes, the deficiency of insulin action follows impaired function of the islet cells of the pancreas, which may be genetically defective, or they become exhausted by metabolic or hormonal demands. Insulin is necessary for glucose and amino-acids to *cross cell membranes* and there it is deficient, the body cells *cannot properly utilize carbohydrates, fats and proteins.* The upset in *carbohydrate* metabolism is the obvious manifestation, with high blood glucose and glycosuria, but it is only one aspect of a profound metabolic disturbance.

The above considerations apply to idiopathic, *primary* diabetes.

Diabetes may be *secondary* to known pancreatic disease—it may be transient in acute pancreatitis, or complicate chronic pancreatitis or carcinoma of the pancreas, a condition to be borne in mind in a middle-aged patient who is not improving on treatment of his diabetes. Bronzed diabetes, haemochromatosis, where there is iron deposition and fibrosis of the pancreas associated with cirrhosis of the liver, has already been described. Cirrhosis may itself be associated with hyperglycaemia, and worsens existing diabetes.

Cushing's syndrome, corticosteroid drugs, and the oestrogen content of oral contraceptives can make diabetes manifest. 25 per cent of patients suffering from acromegaly (overactivity of the anterior pituitary with growth hormone excess) have diabetes.

Thiazide and other diuretics may provoke diabetes by damaging the islet cells; the related drug diazoxide is used therapeutically to cause islet cell destruction in patients with an insulin-secreting tumour causing hypoglycaemia.

Adrenaline injection, or the excess of nor-adrenaline in phaeochromocytoma (tumour of the adrenal medulla) causes temporary hyperglycaemia from the breakdown of liver glycogen, and in thyrotoxicosis the blood sugar may be raised by accelerated absorption, but for true diabetes to occur there must be associated insulin deficiency.

INCIDENCE

The highest recorded population incidence is 40 per cent, in the Pima Indians in Arizona aged 45 or older, and there is a high incidence of a type of diabetes in West Africa. Generally, there is an association of diabetes with high calorie intake and obesity. Clinical diabetes exists in about 2 per cent of the population of Britain, but abnormalities of glucose tolerance are much commoner, though the significance of this is uncertain.

Diabetes is rare in infancy, quite common in childhood and adolescence in both sexes, but most commonly presents in patients beyond middle-age, especially women, in Britain.

Clinical types

There are two main groups:

1. *Juvenile, Growth-Onset, Ketotic, 'Insulin-dependent' group.*
   The *onset* is in childhood or young adult life, symptoms are severe

and often acute, the patients are thin, lose weight and are prone to keto-acidosis (excess production of ketone bodies such as acetone and acids from fat-breakdown) and coma. These patients *lack insulin*, and it is essential in treatment—they are insulin-dependent.

2. *Maturity Onset, Adult, Non-ketotic, 'Non-insulin-dependent' group.*

These are middle-aged or elderly people, commonly women, who are or have been obese. It is arguable whether obesity causes diabetes or whether the diabetic diathesis is associated with some forms of obesity. The clinical symptoms may be mild, the condition often presenting as a diabetic 'complication' such as a septic foot sore, and ketosis is unusual.

At some time, the unduly large food intake of these patients caused pancreatic stimulation and plenty of insulin was produced, but ultimately the pancreas cannot quite keep up with the demand, and symptoms result. The treatment therefore is dietary restriction to produce weight loss, when the pancreas can once again cope. In a proportion of patients, the pancreas may remain unable to produce quite enough insulin, but responds to stimulation with an oral sulphonylurea drug such as chlorpropamide. Where carbohydrate restriction is not in itself sufficient, therefore, middle-age diabetics may be treated with oral drugs or insulin injections, but, if misused, these will result in a gain in weight and further impairment of pancreatic function and metabolism.

It should be noted that there is an additional small group of elderly patients, often in their seventies, who are of average weight, or thin, and present with the 'juvenile' type of diabetes and ketosis. They, too, require insulin, a dose of 40–50 units daily, the average daily pancreatic secretion, frequently sufficing. A similar 'replacement' dose is required in haemochromatosis and pancreatic atrophy.

Symptoms and signs

The diabetic patient *cannot utilize* glucose. It therefore builds up in the bloodstream, hyperglycaemia, and is excreted in the urine. As the kidney cannot pass lump sugar it has to dissolve the glucose in lots of water, so there is polyuria. The excessive water-loss causes severe thirst, and dehydration if the patient does not slake his thirst. There is loss of weight despite a good appetite, and muscular weakness. Irritation and pruritus (itching) occurs at the vulva or glans penis.

In the severe diabetes of the young, the body breaks down fats instead of sugar in an attempt to maintain energy processes. These breakdown products are the 'ketone bodies' acetone and keto-acids, which build up in the blood (and spill into the urine) and are toxic to the brain. Ketosis or keto-acidosis is one form of acidosis. The patient becomes drowsy and ill with vomiting, dehydration, and air-hunger, his breath also smelling of acetone. Left untreated, he will lapse into coma—diabetic coma.

Complications

Diabetic keto-acidosis and coma are considered below.

The long-term complications may be the mode of presentation of diabetes in the maturity-onset group, symptoms such as polyuria, thirst and weight-loss being elicited only on questioning the patient, or glycosuria being found on routine examination.

VASCULAR DISEASE

Diabetics are prone to develop arteriosclerosis (atherosclerosis), the degenerative disease of the lining of the arteries, related probably to the disturbed lipid (fat) metabolism. In diabetic women, the incidence of atherosclerosis becomes as high as that in men, the protection afforded by being of female sex disappearing. There is a raised incidence of coronary and cerebral arterial disease, and involvement of the leg arteries is very common—the presentation is similar to that in the non-diabetic, including symptoms such as intermittent claudication, but the distal arteries may be more affected in the diabetic, leading to gangrene of the toes and feet.

Thickening of the capillaries has been described in diabetes, with the suggestion that diabetes may be a disease of small blood vessels. Though this is disputed, it is true that capillary changes may affect the retinae and the kidneys, as described below.

EYE DISEASE

Retinopathy is the most serious ocular complication of diabetes, and the single most common cause of blind registration among the middle-aged in Britain. Some years after the diagnosis of diabetes, little aneurysms and haemorrhages related to the retinal capillaries and veins become visible with the ophthalmoscope, and sometimes 'exudates' are seen. These may involve an important part of the retina, causing visual impairment. Even more important are growths of 'new vessels' in severe retinopathy which break down causing haemorrhage into the vitreous of the eye or retinal destruction and blindness.

Lens changes include temporary refractive upset from disturbance in hydration, causing visual blurring until diabetic control is achieved. Rarely, acute cataract occurs in the young. The slowly-growing cataract of the elderly may occur earlier and advance more rapidly in the diabetic.

RENAL DISEASE

There are capillary changes in the renal glomeruli (first described by Kimmelstiel and Wilson, whose names are sometimes applied to diabetic kidney disease). The capillaries become abnormally permeable, resulting in proteinuria, usually slight, but occasionally severe, with nephrotic syndrome and oedema, progressing to renal destruction and uraemia.

Lesions of the renal papillae are described, and while pyelonephritis has been said to be commoner in diabetics, bacterial counts have shown no increase compared with normals.

NEUROPATHY

Peripheral neuritis or neuropathy may occur in poorly controlled diabetes, with pains and paraesthesiae (pins-and-needles) and sensory loss; the patient may burn or injure his feet without being aware of it. There is loss of vibration sensation, tested with the tuning fork at the ankles; loss of reflexes causes absent ankle and knee jerks; there may be muscular weakness.

Involvement of the autonomic nervous system may cause diarrhoea (often nocturnal), postural hypotension, and impotence.

INFECTIONS

Pruritus and vulval irritation are due to infection with the fungus candida (monilia) albicans, thrush, which may feed on the sugar deposited from the urine.

Skin sepsis and carbuncles, often staphylococcal, are common, and like any infection their presence may provoke the symptoms of diabetes or impair its control. A specific necrosis of the skin of the lower legs may also occur.

Lung infections, especially tuberculosis, are commoner in the uncontrolled diabetic.

Ulceration and infection with risk of gangrene of the *feet*, associated with arterial disease and neuropathy, is further considered below.

Confirming the diagnosis of diabetes—urine and blood tests

The diagnosis is confirmed by finding glucose in the urine and a raised blood glucose level.

URINE TESTS

Glucose (*a*) *Qualitative tests*—Clinistix, Tes-tape, and compound strips such as Bili-Labstix — the test area on these strips is specific for glucose, but unreliable as to the amount present.

(*b*) *Quantitative.* Clinitest tablets have replaced Benedict's and Fehling's tests, but are based on the same principle, the test being positive with substances that reduce copper sulphate (which is blue) to metallic copper. Such reducing substances include glucose, lactose (which may be found in the urine in late pregnancy and lactation), and vitamin C. Having established the presence of glucose with a preliminary strip test, the Clinitest test allows an estimation of its quantity, thus:

> orange-red, 2%   — urine full of sugar
> yellow-brown, 1% — considerable sugar
> green, $\frac{1}{2}$%   — slight sugar
> blue, nil   — no sugar.

In the management of diabetes, it is important to test specimens freshly produced by the kidneys and corresponding to the blood at the time; thus a true 'morning urine' is obtained by voiding the bladder on wakening and discarding this urine (which has lain in the bladder all night), then passing a fresh specimen half to one hour later for test.

Ketones are detected by the Acetest tablet or Ketostix strip. These are very sensitive, and if positive, the ferric chloride test should be applied. Ten per cent ferric chloride is added to the urine: a reddish-purple colour occurs with aceto-acetic acid and indicates a serious degree of ketosis. This test is also positive with salicylate (aspirin) excess, but boiling a further urine sample allows differentiation, ketones being destroyed but salicylate persisting.

In severe diabetes the urine, though pale, is of *high specific gravity* from its glucose content.

BLOOD TESTS

The sugar in the blood is, of course, glucose so that the terms blood sugar and blood glucose are synonymous. The methods of estimation vary, and capillary blood, obtained by finger or ear-lobe prick, has a slightly higher glucose content than venous blood, but the following remarks are generally applicable.

In health the fasting blood glucose is less than 100 mg per 100 ml and even after food seldom rises above 120 ml per 100 ml. In most people, glucose does not appear in the urine until the blood glucose is over 180 mg per 100 ml, the renal threshold for glucose. Some normal people have a low renal threshold and a 'renal leak' for glucose, renal glycosuria. In the elderly, the renal threshold may be raised.

In the presence of other clinical signs, a casual blood glucose level of over 200 mg per 100 ml confirms the diagnosis of diabetes without need for further tests.

In doubtful cases, a glucose tolerance test is carried out. The patient takes his meals normally the day before, but has nothing to eat on the morning of the test. A fasting blood glucose specimen is taken, then after a drink of 50 G glucose in flavoured water, further specimens for glucose estimation are taken at $\frac{1}{2}$ hour, 1 hour and 2 hours. In diabetes the fasting blood glucose level is usually raised and the subsequent levels, which can be plotted as a graph or 'curve', rise very high, sometimes up to 300 mg per 100 ml and fail to return to the fasting level in 2 hours as in the normal. Opinions differ on interpretation, but a blood glucose level of 180 mg per 100 ml or more at some point during the test and of 120 mg per 100 ml or more at 2 hours imply diabetes.

After a stomach operation such as partial gastrectomy there may be a rapid absorption of glucose causing high blood glucose and glycosuria, and a similar peak may occur in cirrhosis from delayed liver storage of glucose. In intestinal malabsorption, the blood glucose curve is flat.

The Dextrostix strip test is a most useful screening test of the blood glucose level: a drop of blood is placed on the test area, washed off after a minute, and the grey colour compared with the standards on the label, range 45–250 mg per 100 ml. This also allows the diagnosis of hypoglycaemia and hyperglycaemia, the exact figures being available later from the laboratory specimens.

Tests for the insulin activity in the blood using a radioactive immuno-assay method are valuable in research, but not yet applicable in clinical practice.

Disturbed lipid metabolism in diabetes may sometimes be detectable as a raised serum cholesterol but again, such tests are not generally helpful.

The blood and urine glucose tests are the only practicable ones we have at the moment for the diagnosis and control of diabetes.

The treatment of diabetes

The aims of treatment are the control of blood and urine sugar levels, the maintenance of normal weight and activity, and the prevention of complications if possible.

There are three important aspects:

1. *Diet.*
2. *Insulin*—necessary for the 'juvenile' group.
3. *Oral hypoglycaemic drugs*—may prevent the need for insulin injections in maturity—onset diabetics who fail to respond to diet alone.

1. DIET IN DIABETES

(a) Maturity onset, non-insulin dependent group

Here the problem is usually one of obesity, and dietary restriction, especially of carbohydrates, is necessary. In theory, no diabetic should be overweight, but in practice control of diabetes in the obese sometimes follows carbohydrate restriction alone, before there is any reduction in weight. The causes and treatment of obesity in general are described in Chapter 10, Nutritional Disorders. The principles of treatment in the obese, diabetic patient are the same—the patient should eat less and cut her calorie intake. Avoidance of sugar and excessive carbohydrates (and beer in many male patients) may suffice, or trimming the carbohydrate intake to 120 G daily, or the 1,000 calorie 80 G carbohydrate diet described, may be necessary.

(b) Juvenile, growth onset, insulin-dependent group

Here the patient is usually of normal weight or thin and the emphasis is on regulation, especially carbohydrate regulation, in the diet. A dietary history should be taken so that it can be ascertained if the patient takes a reasonably balanced intake of carbohydrate, protein and fat, and understands dietetic principles. No diet should be 'imposed' until this information has been considered.

If the patient is of average weight and is to continue his daily work, then clearly he requires the same number of calories. Sugar and excess carbohydrate cause large swings in the blood glucose level and are to be avoided. Some cut in carbohydrate intake may be required, and to compensate for the calorie loss, more protein is given; increasing the fat intake, especially animal fat, may be undesirable. Normal carbohydrate intakes vary from 150–400 G daily, a heavy labourer requiring more than a person in a sedentary occupation. A proportional cut to a figure of 200–250 G daily may be advised; diet schemes are based on 10 G carbohydrate units or 'portions', the protein and fat content of the diet being left to look after itself. The dietician may give advice on the varieties of foods, and their carbohydrate equivalent, suitable to the patient's palate.

However, the timing and apportioning of the food intake is as important as the minutiae of the type of diet and undue restriction is unwise in the young and burdensome in the elderly. Patients on insulin should have a meal within half an hour of their injections, and at regular intervals during the day; a snack at bedtime is desirable, and long periods without food are to be avoided in view of the risk of hypoglycaemia.

2. INSULIN

Insulin is a protein, and while it has been synthesized, at present it is prepared from animal pancreas, ox or pig, and it must be given by injection. Short-acting types include soluble (regular) insulin, Actrapid insulin (pig) and Nuso (ox) insulin. Actrapid and Nuso insulins are neutral, unlike soluble which is acid, and pig insulin more closely resembles the human insulin molecule, but any advantages are marginal. Longer-acting insulins include Insulin Zinc Suspension (Lente, itself a mixture of semilente and ultralente), Rapitard, Isophane insulin (N.P.H.), and Protamine Zinc insulin (P.Z.I.); Globin insulin is now seldom used. The commonly used insulin concentrations are 40 units per ml and 80 units per ml. The British Standard insulin syringe is of 1 ml or 2 ml size, and calibrated in 'marks' for the old 20 unit per ml strength of insulin. One 'mark' on this syringe equals 2 units of 40 unit per ml insulin, and 4 units of 80 unit strength insulin. Dosage is conveniently prescribed in multiples of 4 units.

Insulin injections are necessary in all young diabetics, in those of maturity onset not responding to diet or oral drugs, and in a proportion of elderly yet ketosis-prone diabetics.

The patient should be admitted to hospital for stabilization and instruction, but should be encouraged to be up and about. Soluble, Actrapid or Nuso insulin is given before breakfast, lunch and evening meal according to the blood and urine sugar tests—a 'sliding-scale' dosage such as 20–28 units for a 'red' urine test with Clinitest, 16 units for yellow, 8 for green and 8 or nil if blue can be used initially. Control can subsequently be maintained on a twice-daily soluble (or similar type) insulin regime. If total requirements are small, less than 40 units daily, it may be convenient to switch to a single injection, given before breakfast, of a longer acting insulin such as Lente or Isophane. Soluble insulin can be combined with Isophane or Protamine zinc insulin to allow better control during the morning but if P.Z.I. is to be added to soluble insulin already drawn up into the syringe, which is quite permissible, allowance must be made for some of the soluble becoming 'protaminized' on contact, diminishing its early action. However, a twice-daily insulin regime often gives the best control.

Diabetics, including older children, should be taught to give their own injections subcutaneously into the thigh; a temporary redness at the sites of injection may occur, settling over a few weeks, and other complications are unusual. Glass syringes should be kept in spirit or a clean closed container and boiled weekly. Disposable syringes and needles are often more satisfactory, provided their marking is clearly understood—most errors in insulin dosage stem from confusion over strength, units and marks. Diabetics on insulin must carry a card or identity-disc clearly specifying dosage.

Instability or 'brittleness' of control is frequently due to insulin overdosage, resulting in hypoglycaemia during the night. The body overcompensates with a swing to hyperglycaemia, so that the early morning urine test shows sugar and an increased dose of insulin is mistakenly given, worsening the situation. The remedy in this situation is reduction and adjustment in timing of the insulin dose and dietary adjustment.

3. ORAL HYPOGLYCAEMIC DRUGS

The sulphonylurea drugs, which include tolbutamide, chlorpropamide, and glibenclamide, stimulate release of insulin from the pancreas and may be successful in controlling diabetes in the maturity-onset group of patients who continue to show hyperglycaemia and glycosuria despite dietary measures and weight reduction. These drugs are not applicable in young diabetics or those prone to ketosis. A report from the U.S.A. has suggested that the use of tolbutamide has been followed by an increased incidence of cardio-vascular complications of diabetes, but this is not the British experience with sulphonylureas. Thus, chlorpropamide 100–500 mg daily after breakfast has proved a relatively trouble-free and useful drug, obviating the need for insulin injections and making life much easier for a large group of middle-aged and elderly diabetics.

The biguanides, phenformin and metformin, act by stimulating glucose uptake in the peripheral muscles, but they may also decrease intestinal glucose absorption. Long-acting phenformin capsules of 50 mg twice daily may allow control of diabetes of maturity-onset type, and a biguanide may be justified in the obese as the drug does not stimulate insulin production as does a sulphonylurea. However, used alone, a biguanide is not consistently effective. Combined with a sulphonylurea it may make oral treatment possible, avoiding the need for insulin injections in a small group of patients.

Acute complications of diabetes and their treatment

HYPOGLYCAEMIA

This is really a *complication of therapy*, too much insulin causing an excessive drop in the blood glucose level. The rare islet-cell tumour or insulinoma of the pancreas produces similar symptoms. The onset may follow unaccustomed exertion or activity, or a missed meal. There is *sudden* weakness, unsteadiness, dizzy feelings, with tremulousness and sweating from outpouring of adrenaline as the body attempts to raise the blood glucose by breaking down liver glycogen. The patient may become disorientated and violent before collapsing in coma. Symptoms may be less obvious during sleep, and of less dramatic onset in patients receiving excessive oral sulphonylurea drugs.

Treatment

Diabetics should carry sugar or sweets such as barley sugar to take quickly at the onset of symptoms. It may be wise to induce a slight attack of hypoglycaemia in the initial management of diabetes, so that the patient recognizes the condition should it occur subsequently.

If the patient cannot swallow or is unconscious, glucagon 1 mg by intramuscular injection will raise the blood glucose sufficiently for arousal and for sugar to be taken by mouth. Alternatively, 10–20 ml

25 per cent or 50 per cent dextrose solution is injected slowly intravenously. When the patient has come round, he must be given some food to prevent relapse, and adjustment in insulin-dose or timing of meals may be required.

When called in emergency to a diabetic who is behaving peculiarly or whose consciousness is disturbed, it should be assumed that the case is one of hypoglycaemia and the above measures should be carried out without delay. In the unlikely event of the case actually being one of diabetic ketosis and coma, then no harm will result. On the other hand, if a hypoglycaemic patient is given insulin, the consequences can be disastrous.

DIABETIC KETO-ACIDOSIS (KETOSIS) AND COMA

Diabetic ketosis is a condition of gradual onset, though a young diabetic may present in this way. In a known diabetic, ketosis follows a period of inadequate insulin dosage, and this may have followed infection or stress, which create an increased insulin requirement.

Due to the lack of insulin, the body cannot utilize glucose and burns fats instead with the production of ketones—acetone and the keto-acids, which are toxic to the brain. The patient is dehydrated and thirsty, the tongue is dry, often there is abdominal pain simulating appendicitis or an 'acute abdomen', and vomiting. The breathing is deep and sighing (acidotic or Kussmaul breathing, air hunger) in an attempt to excrete the acids as carbon dioxide from the lungs. The blood pressure falls, and the level of consciousness deteriorates with coma and death if the condition goes untreated.

There will have been a stage of polyuria, though oliguria may have followed. The urine is full of glucose and ketones, positive with Acetest and the ferric chloride test.

Dextrostix finger-prick blood test is useful in confirming a blood glucose greater than 175 mg per 100 ml, pending the laboratory results. These show a very high blood glucose, acidosis (reported as 'low serum bicarbonate' or 'low pH') and electrolyte (sodium and potassium) disturbance often with raised blood urea.

Treatment

Hospital management is essential, it may be necessary to pass a catheter to obtain urine specimens, repeated blood sampling is necessary, and in all but the mildest cases intravenous fluids are required.

1. *Soluble insulin* (or Actrapid or Nuso) is given, 50 units intramuscularly, and 50 units intravenously (or into the drip). These large doses are needed as ketotic patients are insulin-resistant. Further doses will be required hourly or two-hourly depending on the blood glucose levels.

2. *Intravenous fluids.* The drip can be started with normal saline, 0·9 per cent sodium chloride, but in severe acidosis it may be preferable to use isotonic sodium bicarbonate solution or one-sixth Molar sodium lactate, which is alkalinizing. Two litres of fluid may be given in the first hour and ½–1 L hourly subsequently depending on the urine output and blood biochemistry results. As the blood glucose level falls, 5 per cent dextrose solution may be given, potassium chloride being added if necessary; subsequently, oral potassium supplements are generally indicated. (See also Chapter 11, Water and Electrolytes.)

In severe hypotension, blood or plasma may be required.

3. *Gastric aspiration* is required if there is stomach dilatation or vomiting with risk of inhalation of stomach contents.

4. *With recovery of consciousness* and replacement of the fluid deficit, it becomes possible to give frequent small fluid feeds by mouth, each containing about 20 G carbohydrate. A gradual return to a suitable diet and stabilization with insulin injections is then possible.

5. *It is important to seek a precipitating cause* of the ketotic state such as a chest or urinary infection, so that antibacterial drugs can be used if appropriate, but their indiscriminate use in states of coma raises rather than lowers the incidence of complications such as pneumonia.

HYPEROSMOLAR NON-KETOTIC DIABETIC COMA
This is a relatively rare type of coma occurring in elderly diabetics whose diabetes had been previously considered mild. Precipitating factors include cerebral ischaemia, and high sugar intake without adequate fluids, but the cause is uncertain. There is a history of polyuria and thirst, and urine containing glucose but no ketones, and the patient lapses into coma. The blood glucose is extremely high and the fluid deficit contributes to the hypertonic, hyperosmolar state. Treatment is with insulin and hypotonic fluids intravenously, but the prognosis is generally poor.

Treatment of long-term complications

Diabetic neuropathy improves with good control of the diabetes.

Vascular complications may be present at the time of diagnosis and though their relation to the blood sugar is uncertain, it is generally agreed that good control is desirable in an attempt to halt their progress.

THE DIABETIC FOOT

The skin may be abraded unknown to the patient, due to the sensory loss of neuropathy, and pressure sores and ulcers occur from shoes that are too tight. Due to the arterial insufficiency, wounds tend to heal poorly or to become ulcerated, with risk of infection and gangrene. With good control of the diabetes, conservative measures including rest, avoidance of direct heating, careful wound toilet and antibacterial drugs if appropriate, results are often more successful than initially expected. Patience is rewarded by satisfactory healing, or the spontaneous separation of a necrotic toe. If, however, there is continued pain and spreading infection, surgical measures, including amputation (preferably below the level of the knee) become indicated.

Thus care of the feet is important in diabetics—careful nail trimming, avoiding injury, keeping the skin clean, and frequent changes of socks or stockings. The services of a *chiropodist* should be available for elderly patients.

DIABETIC RETINOPATHY

This may advance rapidly in young diabetics, threatening vision. Pituitary factors, possibly growth hormone may be related to it, and pituitary ablation (destruction) using radioactive yttrium seeds implanted via the trans-nasal route may prevent advancement of the retinopathy, but of course hormone replacements become necessary. Photo-coagulation of the affected retinal vessels, using a high energy light beam (laser) is a somewhat less drastic method of treatment, and is currently being evaluated.

DIABETIC KIDNEY DISEASE (NEPHROPATHY)

Proteinuria may be mild for many years, or gross, with nephrotic syndrome. In later stages proteinuria decreases as the renal nephrons are destroyed, but ultimately there is renal failure with rising blood urea. Insulin requirements may decrease and dietetic adjustment, including protein restriction, may be required, treatment following the lines of that described under Chronic Renal Failure.

The diabetic life

Most diabetics can lead full and normal lives but those on insulin are not allowed to drive public service vehicles. Occupations involving working at heights, such as steeplejacking or bridge building are undesirable in case of hypoglycaemic attacks, but otherwise restrictions need be few.

Attendance at a Diabetic Clinic is generally helpful in maintaining good control and the sense of discipline required for best management. Clinic attendance allows early recognition of complications and the help of the ophthalmologist and the chiropodist is readily available. The diabetic clinic also aids doctors and nurses in the understanding and management of diabetes, improving patient care and offering opportunity for research to help future patients.

DIABETES, MARRIAGE AND PREGNANCY

The genetic basis of diabetes is not clear. If one parent is diabetic, the offspring has a one in twenty chance of developing diabetes. If both parents are diabetic, the chance of offspring developing the condition is estimated at one in four. The risks in the former case are not therefore unduly high, and having explained them, decisions as to marriage can possibly be left to the couple concerned.

Diabetic women often go through pregnancy uneventfully, though there is an increased incidence of toxaemia and hydramnios (excess fluid around the foetus). The renal threshold and insulin requirement may alter, and close control with blood glucose checks is essential. Admission to hospital is advisable in later weeks, and as the baby is often big, delivery at 38 weeks vaginally following induction of labour, or sometimes by caesarean section is recommended. The foetal mortality is 10 per cent, and even if big, the baby may be immature and liable to respiratory distress syndrome and hypoglycaemia, so that management in a special-care unit is desirable.

SURGERY AND DIABETES

Surgery in the diabetic is not a problem if the patient is under good control, but it is dangerous to submit a ketotic patient to anaesthetic or operation. It should be remembered that diabetic ketosis may present as an apparent 'acute abdomen' and it is *absolutely essential to check the urine for sugar and ketones in all patients* admitted to, or attending hospital.

Diabetics should preferably be admitted to hospital two days before a planned operation and if on a long-acting insulin, this should be changed to a short-acting insulin such as soluble insulin, given in suitable doses on the morning and evening before operation. On the morning of operation, insulin and breakfast are omitted, the blood glucose checked, and the patient is taken to theatre early on the list. Co-operation between physician, anaesthetist and surgeon is essential, and some prefer to have the patient on a slow-running intravenous drip of 5 per cent dextrose, to avoid the risk of hypoglycaemia should there have been any delayed insulin effect—it is unwise to give glucose by mouth before an anaesthetic for fear of vomiting and inhalation. On return from theatre the patient is given a dose of short-acting insulin which can be repeated later in the day depending on urine and blood glucose tests, and on the intake of fluids or foods being allowed.

Diabetics on dietary therapy only or oral drugs may be managed along similar lines, it often sufficing simply to stop the oral drug on the morning of operation. Urine and blood glucose levels should, however be checked as the stress of operation often demands temporary insulin therapy.

Diabetes and the future

Diabetes has been said to be 'not so much a disease, more a way of life'. Its understanding has led, in most cases, to a normal life for those suffering from the disease. The problems of the vascular and eye complications remain to be solved. Glucuse tolerance tests and insulin assays provide help in the early recognition of diabetes; abnormalities in such tests appear to be commoner in some patients with arterial disease who are not clinically diabetic. A knowledge of the mechanisms of insulin release holds promise for the early detection of the diabetic abnormality, with hope of cure and even prevention of diabetes in the future.

13

Disorders of the nervous system

The nerve pathways and their disorders

THE CEREBRUM

The highest centres of the brain, both anatomically and in terms of the special intellectual functions that distinguish man from the lower animals, are contained in the cerebrum with its left and right hemispheres. These consist of a cortex of grey matter containing the nerve cells or neurones, and the deeper white matter containing the nerve fibres. There are special areas of the cortex concerned with different functions—thus the motor area which governs control of movements, is anterior to the central sulcus or fissure, the sensory area is posterior to it. In general, the left hemisphere is responsible for the right side of the body and vice versa, due to a crossing of the nerve tracts to the opposite side lower in the brain or spinal cord. The speech centre is in the left side of the brain in right-handed people and in most left-handed people, lying below the motor area. Hearing is appreciated in the temporal lobe. Thought processes are dependent on an intact speech and language mechanism—we think in terms of speech. Vision is appreciated in the occipital lobes posteriorly. The function of a large part of the frontal lobe is uncertain, but it may be responsible for behaviour and personality traits.

Consciousness is the awareness of self and environment, but the cortex is concerned with the elaboration of consciousness, with functions such as thought, reasoning and judgement, in the light of experience and memory (which may be stored in the temporal lobe), rather than with the state of consciousness itself. The state of consciousness is dependent on the activity of the central reticular formation, an electrical 'core' which spreads up from the brain stem to activate the cerebrum. Depression of the reticular formation rather than of the cortex is responsible for impairment of consciousness—thus sleeping drugs and states such as uraemia and anoxia act on the reticular formation to depress the level of consciousness and produce coma. Natural sleep may depend in part on the function of the reticular formation, and is of two types—deep sleep necessary for restoration of bodily efficiency, and lighter sleep with dreaming and rapid eye movements (R.E.M. sleep), necessary for restoration of brain function.

THE MOTOR TRACTS

(a) The pyramidal tract or so-called 'upper motor neurone' starts in the motor cortex, the fibres passing into the internal capsule and descending through the brain stem to cross to the opposite side in the medulla. They continue down the spinal cord to end round the anterior horn cells. From these, the lower motor neurone fibres pass out from the cord in the anterior root, which unites with the posterior (sensory or afferent) root in the intervertebral foramen. This mixed nerve root goes to form a peripheral nerve, its motor fibres liberating acetylcholine and causing muscular contraction.

(b) At the base of the brain are certain nuclei called the basal ganglia which also participate in muscular control with their own descending fibres. This is the extra-pyramidal system dysfunction of which causes the tremor and rigidity of Parkinson's disease.

BRAIN STEM AND CEREBELLUM

The brain stem consists of mid-brain, pons, and medulla, and from it pass out the cranial nerves. Centres controlling respiration and blood pressure are situated in the brain stem. Behind it is the cerebellum, concerned in muscle balance and posture, which is also dependent on nuclei called the vestibular nuclei which receive signals from the balance organs in the ear via the auditory nerve.

THE SENSORY TRACTS

The nerve fibres conveying sensation pass into the spinal cord through the posterior roots. Those carrying pain and temperature cross and ascend near the front of the cord. Much of touch sense, and that of the position of joints and muscles, and vibration sense, passes up posterior columns and crosses in the medulla. Sensation is 'collected' in the thalamus at the base of the brain, and from here

fibres pass upwards through the internal capsule behind the motor
fibres to reach the cells in the sensory cortex. Some fibres concerned in muscle sensation pass from the brain stem to the cerebellum,
and there are many connections with other nuclei.

THE REFLEXES

The spinal reflex arc consists of the sensory fibres which receive
information from the periphery and pass it via the posterior root
into the spinal cord, where a connector neurone passes it to the
anterior horn cells, from which the stimulus passes out to cause
muscular contraction.

Damage to the reflex arc at any part of its course results in loss of a
'*deep (or tendon) reflex*' such as the knee jerk, normally produced by
contraction of the quadriceps muscle following the sensory stimulus
of a tap on the patellar tendon with the tendon hammer.

The activity of the reflex arc and its lower motor neurone fibres is
influenced by the upper motor neurone.

A lower motor neurone lesion is characterized by muscle weakness
or flaccid paralysis followed by wasting, and loss of the tendon reflexes.
Groups of muscles in a limb rather than the whole limb are involved.

A classical lower motor neurone lesion used to be seen in infantile
paralysis, anterior poliomyelitis, but this is now rare due to preventive vaccination. Lesions of individual peripheral nerves, e.g.
after injury, cause the same picture. With multiple peripheral
nerve involvement, peripheral neuritis (neuropathy), there is a
more symmetrical paralysis, and of course sensory loss as well.

An upper motor neurone lesion is characterized by muscular weakness, that is paresis, or paralysis, tending to affect the whole of one or
more limbs. There is an increase in muscle tone causing rigidity or
spasticity, and exaggerated tendon reflexes, e.g. excessively brisk
knee and ankle lerks; these may keep jerking after the stimulus
is withdrawn, the phenomenon called clonus. There may also be abnormality of 'superficial' reflexes with an 'extensor plantar response'
(Babinski's sign) where the big toe goes upwards and the other
toes fan outwards and upwards when the lateral border of the sole
of the foot is stroked, instead of the normal downward 'flexor' movement. An upper motor neurone lesion is also associated with absent
abdominal reflexes—that is, stroking the skin of the abdomen fails
to elicit the normal contraction of the muscles of the abdominal wall.

An upper motor neurone lesion of one limb is called a monoplegia,
but much more common is a hemiplegia—a paralysis of one side of

the body including the lower half of the face, the arm, and the leg, classically caused by a stroke (haemorrhage or ischaemia) affecting the internal capsule containing the pyramidal tract. Paralysis of both legs is called paraplegia. This is usually due to a bilateral pyramidal tract lesion in the spinal cord, resulting in a spastic paraplegia. This occurs following a period of 'spinal shock' and flaccidity if the cord has been completely severed as in injuries and fractures of the vertebrae, but in neurological disorders such as multiple (disseminated) sclerosis there is spasticity from the start. Associated bladder disturbance is described below.

EFFECTS OF LESIONS IN THE BRAIN AND NERVE TRACTS

A lesion affecting the left internal capsule causes a right hemiplegia or hemiparesis, and if larger, loss of sensation, on the right side. A more extensive lesion will spread backwards to involve fibres radiating from the optic nerves and tracts, causing loss of the right field of vision. Any lesion of the pyramidal tract in the left internal capsule may also involve speech fibres, causing expressive dysphasia—difficulty in finding the word. Larger lesions affecting the hearing area or its fibres cause receptive language difficulties, and the patient is incoherent and confused.

Small areas of destruction of the cerebral cortex may cause apraxia, a disorder of the motor act—thus the patient may have normal power and be able to hold a box of matches, but he is incapable of striking a light; similarly, agnosia is a disorder of sensory appreciation—crude sensation such as pain and touch is retained, but the patient is unable to state the nature of an object placed in his hand.

Apart from the sensations such as pain, temperature and touch reaching consciousness, the sensory fibres convey information on muscle tone and balance, proprioception, and disturbance results in ataxia, an incoordination of muscular movement. Ataxia may result from destruction of the posterior columns of the spinal cord, as in tabes dorsalis or locomotor ataxia, a form of neurosyphilis, resulting in a reeling or drunken gait. Incoordination of movement also occurs in lesions of the cerebellum or its connections in the brain stem as in multiple sclerosis, so that the patient 'overshoots the mark' when trying to grasp an object and has a tremor, called intention tremor, as he is about to reach it. *Nystagmus* can be regarded as an intention tremor of the eyes when fixing on an object, due to incoordination of the external ocular muscles; it occurs in vestibular (ear) as well as in cerebellar lesions.

THE AUTONOMIC NERVOUS SYSTEM

This has two parts, the *sympathetic* and the *parasympathetic*.

The sympathetic nerves pass out from the spinal cord to relay at ganglia adjacent to the vertebral column, from which fibres pass to organs such as the heart, intestine, adrenal glands and to the blood vessels. These fibres liberate adrenaline or noradrenaline as their chemical transmitter, to effect the 'fight or flight' reaction for an emergency; the sympathetic nerves maintain the tone of blood vessels, and if severed, hypotension results. A branch originating at the root of the neck runs up over the carotid artery to enter the skull and send fibres to cause dilatation of the pupil. A lesion of this nerve in any part of its course results in a small pupil, drooping of the eyelid and lack of sweating on that side of the face, Horner's syndrome.

The parasympathetic system sends fibres out along the third cranial nerve to supply the muscles constricting the pupil and the muscles of accommodation of the lens. The third nerve may be involved in skull fracture or space-occupying lesion of the brain, resulting in a fixed dilated pupil. Parasympathetic fibres pass out in other cranial nerves to supply the salivary glands. The vagus or tenth cranial nerve forms the largest single part of the parasympathetic system and leaves the skull to supply the heart, stomach and most of the alimentary tract. There is also a parasympathetic outflow from the sacral segment of the spinal cord (i.e. from the lower end of the cord just before it terminates opposite the first lumbar vertebra), the nerves emerging at the sacral foramina and supplying the distal half of the colon and rectum, and also the bladder (see below). In general, the parasympathetic system is concerned with the maintenance and restitution of bodily functions and metabolism in the resting phase, when there is no demand for fight or flight. Thus it allows movements and emptying of the alimentary tract and the bladder. The fibres release acetylcholine as their local transmitter to effect muscle action (acetylcholine is also the transmitter at the ordinary voluntary or somatic motor nerves).

Sensory fibres from deep structures such as the intestine and bladder may also pass back in the autonomic nerves and relay to the brain. These reach consciousness in company with the fibres carrying ordinary skin sensation, and visceral pain may be 'referred' to that segment of the skin.

The brain centres controlling the autonomic outflow are uncertain, but probably related to the part called the hypothalamus where the pituitary gland joins the base of the brain. The hypothalamus and its connections are concerned in emotional activity such as happiness or sorrow and tears, sexual feelings, and appetite control. It is probable that there are tracts and transmitter substances in this region of the brain, comparable with the autonomic system in the periphery, and disturbance may be associated with psychiatric and depressive illness.

THE INNERVATION OF THE BLADDER

Fibres from the cerebral cortex which allow voluntary control of micturition and are comparable to the 'upper motor neurone', pass down the spinal cord near the pyramidal tract to end at the spinal bladder centre in the sacral segment of the cord. This bladder centre can be regarded as a part of a reflex arc, similar to that described above, but as the bladder muscle, the detrusor, is smooth 'involuntary' muscle, it is served by autonomic, mainly parasympathetic nerves. Thus the motor fibres to the bladder pass out in the parasympathetic outflow from the lower cord, pass down in the cauda equina, and emerge through the sacral foramina to reach the bladder and stimulate contraction of the detrusor muscle, causing emptying. (Some ordinary motor fibres in the pudendal nerve supply the external sphincter of the bladder, but this is of less importance). Afferent fibres, conveying the sensation of fullness of the bladder use mainly the parasympathetic pathway to reach the cord centre, forming the afferent loop of the reflex arc; some pass upwards in the sensory tract near the front of the spinal cord to convey to the brain the desire to micturate. The voluntary control, descending fibres already described, may permit or prevent the act of micturition by their influence on the bladder centre reflex arc.

Disorders of micturition can therefore result from the following lesions:

1. *Cerebral damage* following a stroke, or senile dementia—resulting in the 'uninhibited' bladder and incontinence, similar to that of an infant before toilet training.

2. *Severing of the spinal cord* or *acute cord compression* is followed by a stage of spinal shock for a few weeks during which the bladder is atonic and distended, and there is overflow incontinence. Later, in some cases there is an 'automatic bladder' which fills to rather less than its usual volume, then empties spontaneously—it may be possible to train such patients to 'void by the clock' every few hours.

3. *Damage to the lower end of the spinal cord* or to the nerves in the cauda equina resulting in separation of the bladder from its spinal centre, causing an 'autonomous', disorganized bladder. Voluntary muscle when separated from its nerve supply by a lower motor neurone lesion becomes paralysed and flaccid. However, the bladder muscle is smooth, involuntary muscle which responds directly to being stretched, resulting in a tense, hypertonic bladder contracting when only a small volume of urine is present, but functioning poorly so that the amount of residual urine is high. There is incontinence, and the need to pass urine is not appreciated. This situation may complicate injuries, or occur in multiple sclerosis.

4. *Apart from these neurological lesions, incontinence may result* from bladder infection or tumour, and obstruction at the prostate or from faecal impaction may cause urinary retention. In women, weakness of the muscles of the pelvic floor, sometimes associated with vaginal prolapse, causes 'stress incontinence' on coughing or straining.

Incontinence and nocturnal frequency of micturition in the elderly may be due to diminished bladder capacity associated with the characteristics of the 'uninhibited' bladder described above. The cerebral control may be weakened by any intercurrent infection, and another precipitating factor is becoming confined to bed, so all elderly people should be encouraged to be up and about. While drugs of the atropine series may provoke urinary retention by their anticholinergic property, this property may be utilized to advantage in some patients with a hypertonic bladder (uninhibited or autonomous in type) and incontinence. Thus the drug emepronium (Cetiprin) 100–200 mg at bedtime, or during the day, may increase bladder capacity and improve symptoms of frequency and incontinence, especially in the elderly. The mechanics of bladder function can be investigated by micturating-cystogram x-rays and pressure measurements.

In some patients with urinary incontinence, electrical stimulation of the external (voluntary muscle) bladder sphincter using battery-powered electrodes or pessary allows some control of symptoms.

Catheterization may be required temporarily or permanently and though the latter should be avoided if possible, the availability of disposable plastic catheters, changed weekly and draining into a plastic bag, has eased management especially in women. Infection can be avoided by a high fluid intake, and instillation of antiseptics is not required routinely. Minor bladder infection may not be serious, but an ascending urinary tract infection demands appropriate antibacterial drugs. Permanent transurethral catheterization is much less satisfactory in men, and should generally be avoided. If frequent 'toileting' or changes of trousers is of no avail, it may be possible to attach a condom device to the penis, draining to a portable urinal, or recourse may be required to surgical perineal or suprapubic catheterization.

THE INNERVATION OF THE RECTUM

The innervation of the rectum is similar to that of the bladder, but voluntary control over defaecation is exerted on the external sphincter (striated muscle) of the rectum only, the organ lacking voluntary inhibition. The arrival of faeces from the colon stretches the rectal wall which reflexly stimulates the rectum to contract and expel the faeces. This contraction is not very strong and is generally aided by voluntary efforts with the abdominal and pelvic muscles.

Though some reflex defaecation may continue after neurological lesions and be facilitated by local skin stimulation, the tendency is for all disturbances of rectal innervation to cause retention of faeces and constipation. The administration of purgatives or suppositories may suffice to prevent this, or enemas may be required once or twice weekly if the rectum becomes distended.

The cerebro-spinal fluid (C.S.F.) and meninges (brain membranes). Raised intracranial pressure

The brain and spinal cord are surrounded and cushioned from injury by the cerebro-spinal fluid. The C.S.F. is formed in the choroid plexuses of the ventricles of the brain and passes through the aqueduct to reach the fourth ventricle in the brain stem, opposite the cerebellum, emerging through foramina in the roof of the ventricle to enter the subarachnoid space, spreading upwards over the brain and downwards over the spinal cord. Reabsorption occurs into the great venous sinuses draining blood from the brain.

The brain and spinal cord are closely invested by the membrane called the pia mater, then there is the subarachnoid space containing the C.S.F., and the arachnoid mater is covered by the tough dura mater, separating the brain and cord from the skull and vertebrae. The C.S.F. is sampled by *lumbar puncture*, considered below.

Hydrocephalus is a raised content or pressure of C.S.F. due to obstruction at some part of its flow. This may be present at birth, often associated with a developmental defect of the spine called spina bifida, and causes enlargement of the skull; drainage operations may be helpful. Hydrocephalus may also result from infections and adhesions (e.g. after tuberculous meningitis) or from a tumour obstructing the C.S.F. flow by compression.

Any swelling of the brain substance from inflammation and oedema, or from a 'space occupying lesion' such as a haemorrhage, tumour, or abscess will raise the intracranial pressure, and the C.S.F. pressure, for the skull is a closed box and does not allow expansion. The symptoms of raised intracranial pressure are headache, clouding of consciousness, vomiting and papilloedema ('choking' of the optic disc from the high C.S.F. pressure obstructing the circulation in the optic nerve). It should be stressed that these are usually late effects of neurological disease, and diagnosis should be possible from earlier clinical manifestations. 'Hypertensive encephalopathy' causes a similar picture, sometimes with convulsions, and is due to raised C.S.F. pressure in association with severe hypertension, which can be controlled in the acute stage by the ganglion-blocking drug pentolinium or the diuretic frusemide (Lasix). Diuretics, mannitol infusions, and steroids in massive dosage (e.g. dexamethasone 4 mg intramuscularly 6-hourly) are sometimes tried in the treatment of presumed cerebral oedema.

Concussion is a lay term to describe the clouding of consciousness that may follow head injury. It has been ascribed to multiple small haemorrhages caused by the impact of the mobile brain against the skull, but perhaps it is the reticular formation that is disturbed. Rather than use the word concussion, it is better to define the site of brain injury in anatomical terms if possible, to record the patient's level of consciousness when first seen and note any change, bearing in mind that deterioration may be due to an expanding haemorrhage or haematoma as described below.

The term 'cerebral irritation' is a rather imprecise one covering symptoms such as restlessness, agitation and disorientation, occurring from inflammations or tumour. If accompanied by hallucinations, the condition is called delirium and is considered further under Dementia.

In meningitis the brain membranes are inflamed and irritated; this also occurs from the presence of blood in subarachnoid haemorrhage. The resulting meningeal irritation or 'meningism' causes headache and neck stiffness.

The cerebral circulation

The brain is supplied by the two internal carotid arteries, and the two vertebral arteries.

The internal carotid arteries arise from the common carotids in the neck opposite the thyroid cartilage. Each passes up into the skull and ends by dividing into the anterior and middle cerebral arteries which supply a large part of the brain, branches of the middle cerebral serving the internal capsule.

The vertebral arteries arise from the subclavians at the root of the neck. Each passes up through foramina in the transverse processes of the cervical vertebrae to enter the skull with the spinal cord, giving branches to the medulla and uniting at the pons to form the single basilar artery which gives branches to the brain stem and ends by dividing into the posterior cerebral arteries, supplying the occipital lobes. This arterial system is referred to as the vertebro-basilar system.

The internal carotid and vertebro-basilar systems are united by anastomotic branches arising near their respective terminations, and forming the *Circle of Willis* at the base of the brain above the pituitary fossa. This circle forms a most important link between the internal and vertebro-basilar systems to both sides of the brain so that, if one internal carotid artery is completely obstructed, an adequate circulation to the brain will be maintained. Even if both carotids are blocked, the Circle of Willis may allow sufficient blood to reach the brain provided the vertebro-basilar system is healthy.

The external carotid artery supplies the face and a small branch to the orbit (eye) forms a minor anastomosis with a branch from the anterior cerebral artery. The external carotid system also gives off the middle meningeal artery which lies between the skull and the dura mater—it supplies the bone and not the brain, but a blow at the temple may damage it and lead to an extradural haematoma which presses on the brain.

The venous blood draining the brain runs in vessels many of which are over the cortex between the arachnoid and dura mater before collecting into the venous sinuses. These are channels in the dura mater which unite and drain downwards near the mastoid process into the internal jugular veins and so to the heart. In the newborn, and in the elderly where the veins are fragile, a blow on the head may be followed by a venous subdural haematoma causing delayed cerebral compression.

Venous sinus thrombosis used to be seen as an inflammatory process from septic spread of nasal or mastoid infection with pain, rigors, cranial nerve palsies or signs of raised intracranial pressure from blockage of the venous absorption of the cerebro spinal fluid. However, with early antibacterial drug therapy for such infections, venous sinus thrombosis is now rare.

By far the commonest disease of the cerebral circulation is *arteriosclerosis*, considered below under *Cerebro-vascular Disease*.

Investigations in neurological disorders

Examination of the retina (optic fundus) with the ophthalmoscope

Papilloedema may be seen in raised intracranial pressure and hypertension. In hypertension, arteriosclerosis and diabetes, retinal vessel changes and haemorrhages may be visible. In subarachnoid haemorrhage there may be a small pool of blood at the retina.

Straight x-rays

The skull may be invaded, or show evidence of raised intracranial pressure, in cerebral tumour, but such changes are late. A calcified pineal gland may show a shift from its normal central position due to a space occupying lesion. Chest x-ray should always be carried out, for a brain tumour may be a secondary from bronchogenic carcinoma.

Lumbar puncture

A specimen of cerebro-spinal fluid is obtained by inserting a special needle, under local anaesthesia, into the subarachnoid space below the level where the spinal cord ends (which is opposite the lower border of the first lumbar vertebrae). The needle is usually inserted between the 3rd–4th or 4th–5th lumbar vertebrae with the patient held curled-up in the left lateral position. Lumbar puncture should not generally be carried out if there is papilloedema, for raised intracranial pressure may cause downward 'coning' of the brain against the skull if fluid is taken off from below.

At lumbar puncture, the C.S.F. pressure is measured with a manometer, normal is 50–150 mm of fluid, and there should be a free rise and fall on pressing and releasing each jugular vein in turn, Queckenstedt's test, excluding any blockage. Normal C.S.F.

is crystal clear, contains virtually no cells and has a protein content of less than 40 mg per 100 ml. Its sugar content is lowered in tuberculous meningitis. White cells may be increased in inflammatory conditions and bacteriological culture will confirm infections. The C.S.F. is heavily blood-stained in subarachnoid haemorrhage and sometimes after intracerebral haemorrhage. Xanthochromia is a yellow coloration of the fluid above the red cells in specimens taken hours or days after a haemorrhage. The Lange curve was a means of expressing abnormalities in the C.S.F. protein, but this is now fractionated chemically; abnormalities occur in neurosyphilis, multiple sclerosis and acute ascending polyneuritis.

Echo-encephalography

This is the use of ultrasound to detect displacement of brain structures. The instrument is portable, the test painless, and the result is printed out on a graph.

Electro-encephalography. The E.E.G.

This is a series of recordings of the electrical activity of the brain, using electrodes attached to the head. The instrument is large and expensive, so the test can only be carried out in special centres. Localized abnormalities may be detected over brain softening or tumour. The presence of more general abnormalities may be diagnostically helpful in epilepsy.

Radio isotope brain scanning

Certain radioactive isotopes (e.g. technetium) are selectively taken up by brain tumours, which can be detected by a counter or 'scanner' over the skull. The isotope is injected intravenously and the scanning process is painless.

Cerebral angiography (arteriography)

This is the injection of a dye, opaque to x-rays, into a blood vessel, usually a large artery (arteriography) such as the carotid. Its branches inside the skull can then be seen on x-ray using a cinematograph technique. Aneurysms may be identified, or displacement from space occupying lesion seen. The procedure is carried out in special centres using local or general anaesthesia.

Air encephalography and ventriculography

These techniques involve the injection of air into the spinal subarachnoid space and into the ventricles of the brain respectively. An air encephalogram requires the patient's cooperation and involves some discomfort but may allow detection of a tumour.

Myelography

Here an oil, opaque to x-rays, is injected at lumbar puncture to show the presence of a spinal cord blockage, not a common condition but usually due to tumour.

Thermography

This painless test measures the heat emitted from an area of skin and is sometimes useful in diagnosing internal carotid artery obstruction, following which there are changes in the normal pattern near the orbit.

Nerve conduction studies and electro-myography

These electrical techniques may define peripheral nerve changes and allow differentiation of nerve and muscle disease, replacing the former electrical muscle tests.

Cerebro-vascular disease

Cerebro-vascular disease is the third commonest cause of death in Western countries, being exceeded only by cardiovascular disease and malignancy. It is also a frequent cause of morbidity and long-term disability.

In elderly people the cerebral arteries are very liable to be affected by arteriosclerosis (atherosclerosis) usually as part of more widespread arterial involvement. Arteriosclerosis is a degenerative change of the lining membrane of the artery associated with patchy fatty deposits with tendency to thrombosis and aggregation of platelets on the roughened surface.

The arteriosclerotic change has two effects—it narrows the arterial lumen (which may become completely obstructed), and the plaque is a source of emboli which may impact in a distal, smaller artery, causing ischaemia or infarction at a distance from the main vessel. Arteriosclerosis can occur independently of hypertension, but hypertension worsens it and may cause weakening of the vessel wall with greater risk of haemorrhage.

STROKE, CEREBRO-VASCULAR ACCIDENT, APOPLEXY
A stroke, also referred to as a cerebro-vascular accident, is an abrupt

loss of function of some part of the brain due to an arterial lesion.

The common stroke of the elderly results in hemiplegia, and it was assumed that a branch of the middle cerebral artery serving the internal capsule had been affected by thrombosis, or haemorrhage, or an embolus had travelled from the heart (e.g. a thrombus from the left atrium in mitral stenosis and atrial fibrillation, or a vegetation from the mitral or aortic valve in subacute bacterial endocarditis). While it is generally true that thrombosis or embolism cause an area of ischaemia and possibly cerebral softening or scarring, but with a fair prospect of recovery, haemorrhage is more catastrophic with destruction of brain tissue and often death. However, the differentiation of thrombosis and haemorrhage may be impossible. For example, haemorrhage may occur into an ischaemic area caused by thrombosis, and a tiny haemorrhage may cause only minor symptoms.

More important, however, is the realization that many strokes are due to arterial disease affecting the internal carotid artery in the neck, narrowing its lumen and being a source of emboli. The cerebral circulation should be considered in total. A stroke will only occur if there is lack of blood through anastomotic vessels in the Circle of Willis, that is, if there is arteriosclerosis elsewhere. Generally, however, there are two broad groups of strokes—those in the internal carotid territory, and those from disease in the vertebro-basilar system. The former produce the classical hemiplegia, the latter produce brain-stem lesions.

It is also now realized that many major strokes are preceded by transient ischaemic attacks or 'little (minor) strokes' with impairment of function lasting less than an hour. These little strokes are often due to small emboli from internal carotid artery thrombosis.

Classification of strokes

A. MINOR STROKE (Transient Ischaemic Attack)

This may affect either the carotid territory, that is the larger part of the cerebrum including the internal capsule, or the vertebro-basilar territory, the brain stem.

B. MAJOR STROKE

1. *Cerebral Ischaemia and Infarction*

This may be due to thrombosis, embolism (from the internal carotid artery, or from the heart) or decreased blood flow following severe hypotension.

2. *Haemorrhage*

This may be either a primary intracerebral haemorrhage or a primary subarachnoid haemorrhage.

Primary intracerebral haemorrhage is the classical 'cerebral haemorrhage' already referred to, usually a complication of arteriosclerosis with hypertension, but occasionally occurring in haemorrhagic states such as thrombocytopenic purpura.

Primary subarachnoid haemorrhage is due to rupture of an aneurysm in the Circle of Willis, occurs independently of arteriosclerosis, and therefore occurs in the young as well as the elderly. Subarachnoid haemorrhage is considered separately.

The major stroke, like the minor stroke, can involve either the carotid or vertebro-basilar territory.

Minor strokes

Symptoms and signs

Minor strokes are commonly due to episodes of embolization from internal carotid artery stenosis and thrombosis, and present as transient weakness of the arm and leg on the other side and perhaps blindness affecting the eye on the same side as the lesion. A murmur ('bruit') may be heard with the stethoscope over the narrowed internal carotid artery. Minor episodes may pass unnoticed. Recurrent episodes may contribute to intellectual deterioration in the elderly, arteriosclerotic subject.

If the vertebro-basilar system is involved, there is transient brainstem disturbance with dizziness, cranial nerve palsies and sometimes momentary loss of consciousness with a 'drop attack'. Symptoms may occur in association with cervical spondylosis and narrowing of the intervertebral foramina, impeding the flow through the vertebral arteries. Kinking of the arteries when stooping may provoke an ischaemic episode.

Minor strokes may leave no residual disability, and may not recur for months or years, the prognosis being generally better for those affecting the brain stem. However, minor strokes may be the prelude to a major stroke, and early recognition is important, for treatment at this stage may prevent a catastrophic hemiplegia later.

Treatment

Arteriosclerosis affecting the arteries to the brain may be patchy, but in the elderly it is usually part of a more general disease. In younger patients, those in their forties and fifties, it may be justified to direct treatment to a diseased segment of internal carotid artery, provided arterial disease elsewhere, especially coronary disease, and hypertension have been excluded. In such patients, carotid arteriography is indicated to define the extent of internal carotid narrowing. If localized, surgical treatment such as endarterectomy may be indicated. This is the only 'curative' measure possible for arterial disease causing strokes and it may be noted that it is rarely applicable after an established, major stroke. Even in the earlier, minor stroke cases, the long-term results of carotid artery surgery are uncertain.

Anticoagulants such as warfarin, phenindione or nicoumalone may prevent recurrent embolisation in internal carotid artery thrombosis. Used long-term, with regular checks of prothrombin activity, they may decrease the incidence of further minor strokes. They should not be used in the initial treatment of major stroke in view of the difficulty of distinguishing ischaemic lesions from haemorrhage; moreover, anticoagulants may worsen any haemorrhage into an area of ischaemic softening. The place of fibrinolytic drugs is not yet established.

In vertebro-basilar ischaemia sudden stooping or changes of posture should be avoided.

In *all* strokes, attention should be directed towards conditions which further compromise the blood supply to the brain. Severe hypertension should be treated, but powerful hypotensive drugs may be dangerous, in the elderly, a swing to hypotension resulting in impaired cerebral perfusion and increased ischaemic damage. Coronary or rheumatic heart disease and failure, anaemia and polycythaemia should be diagnosed and treated.

The oestrogen-containing contraceptive 'pill' is associated with increased risk of strokes, and cigarette smoking may also be contributory.

Major strokes—cerebral infarction (thrombosis and embolism) and cerebral haemorrhage

SYMPTOMS AND SIGNS

There is weakness, or paralysis of one side of the body—hemiplegia. The onset is generally sudden but in developing ischaemia and infarction there may be premonitory symptoms or warning signs of minor stroke. Headache is not a frequent complaint, but frontal headache may be due to the dilatation of anastomotic vessels from the external carotid artery near the orbit. With intracerebral haemorrhage, the onset is abrupt and symptoms progress rapidly.

In right hemiplegia, *dysphasia* may occur from involvement of the speech centre but should be distinguished from *dysarthria*, difficulty in articulation from muscle weakness.

Initially there may be transient disturbance of cerebration, or the patient may be found unconscious, from oedema of the infarcted brain and effects on the reticular system. Deepening coma with no response to commands or to painful stimuli (such as rubbing the knuckles on the breastbone, or applying supraorbital pressure), implies a severe lesion from cerebral haemorrhage and destruction of the brain substance. The vital centres in the brain-stem become involved, with stertorous or periodic breathing of Cheyne-Stokes type, the pulse is slow but full, and there is incontinence of urine. In these severe cases, all four limbs may be flaccid, both plantar responses extensor and deterioration may be rapid with death in hours or a day or two.

In the majority of strokes, however, the lesion is an ischaemic rather than a haemorrhagic one, and consciousness is quickly regained or improves over hours or a few days. The paralysis affects the lower half of the face, the arm and the leg, but the limbs may be initially flaccid and remain so, or develop the classical spasticity of the upper motor neurone lesion, with extensor plantar response. Difficulty in swallowing and articulation is usually transient, unless there has been a previous stroke affecting the other side, when the brain-stem nerves remain affected and there is emotional lability ('pseudo-bulbar palsy').

A hemiplegia may be accompanied by loss of sensation on the paralysed side, and if the lesion is more extensive, involvement of the optic radiation causes loss of one half of the visual field—thus a lesion in the left internal capsule can cause right hemiplegia, dysphasia, right hemi-anaesthesia, and right hemianopia—the patient may not be aware of objects on the right side of his body and may ignore that side.

The facial paralysis is usually the first to improve, followed by the leg, then the arm. Sensation returns gradually too and may become normal, though slight visual field defect may remain. However, the important aspect is the return of motor function. Improvement may be obvious in a few days, when the prognosis is good, often with full return of power, including hand and finger movements. In other cases, improvement of paralysis may be delayed for a week or two or be confined to the leg, the arm remaining flaccid or becoming increasingly spastic. Usually, if movement is going to return, it does so within a month, but there are exceptions. Improvement in the power of movement continues over several months.

The prognosis is better in younger patients. In the elderly or those with previous strokes, there is a higher risk of residual hemiplegia, intellectual deterioration or dementia, or persistent incontinence.

INVESTIGATIONS

There is usually little difficulty in distinguishing a stroke from other neurological conditions—a stroke is a vascular occlusion or haemorrhage and therefore of sudden onset, distinct from the gradual onset of symptoms from a cerebral tumour.

The usual observations—level of consciousness, pulse, blood pressure, respiration, temperature, fluid intake and urine output—should be made. Deterioration of consciousness, a slowing pulse and rising blood pressure suggest rising intracranial pressure or cerebral destruction. Hyperpyrexia, with pinpoint pupils, may occur in pontine haemorrhage. The urine may contain sugar, for a lesion spreading to involve the brain-stem near the fourth ventricle can cause hyperglycaemia, though of course existing diabetes must be excluded.

The blood pressure may rise as a result of a stroke, but a previous history of hypertension should be sought. As discussed under Minor Strokes, other conditions may impair the cerebral circulation and an E.C.G. may reveal evidence of myocardial infarction. Atrial fibrillation and mitral valve disease, and subacute bacterial endocarditis, can cause cerebral embolus and stroke. Anaemia and polycythaemia should be excluded.

SPECIAL INVESTIGATIONS

Lumbar puncture may be helpful but is not always essential. It may be necessary if the diagnosis is in doubt and will reveal blood-stained cerebro-spinal fluid if there has been a large cerebral haemorrhage. Otherwise the fluid may be normal. The test is dangerous if there is raised intracranial pressure and papilloedema, for the brain may 'cone' down into the foramen magnum of the skull, causing respiratory arrest and circulatory collapse.

In a few cases, improvement immediately after the stroke may be followed by deterioration of consciousness and a dilated pupil or other evidence of an expanding lesion, a haematoma. If echo-encephalogram suggests a brain 'shift', it may be justified to proceed to cerebral arteriography to confirm the presence of a haematoma, for which surgery with 'burr-hole' may be indicated, aspiration allowing re-expansion of the brain. Some neurologists suggest that such measures should be considered more often in the management of strokes, but they are not usually indicated in the average patient, who tends to be elderly and to have evidence of arterial disease elsewhere.

TREATMENT
The initial treatment is directed to maintaining the essential functions, that is the management of coma. As there is no 'cure' for paralysis, management involves prevention of bedsores and contractures, encouragement of movement when it returns and progressive weight bearing and exercises. No drugs directly influence the established stroke, and the effect of 'vasodilators' is seldom of practical value. The patient and his relatives require understanding and support, and a subsequent programme of rehabilitation frequently allows resumption of normal activity.

(a) Management of coma

1. *Maintenance of the airway*—the patient is generally nursed on his side, that is, the semi-prone position, flat with a low pillow so that the tongue does not fall back and obstruct the pharynx, and to allow secretions to drain from the mouth. Dentures should be removed. A plastic or rubber oro-pharyngeal airway may be required. If respiration still tends to obstruct, the doctor may pass an endotracheal tube. Usually ventilation is maintained without the need for mechanical respirators in coma due to stroke.

2. *Aspiration of secretions* from mouth and throat—using a portable electrical machine or piped suction.

3. *Frequent turning*—the patient should be turned every 2 hours and good care of the skin is essential to prevent pressure sores. Frequent turning or changes of position also lowers the risk of hypostatic pneumonia.

It should be noted that antibiotics should not be used prophylactically—the incidence of pneumonia is actually higher in those so treated. Antibacterial drugs should only be given if there is evidence of infection, in the chest or elsewhere.

4. *Treatment of incontinence*—a Foley plastic self-retaining

catheter should be passed, and continuous drainage may be necessary for a few days. Where incontinence persists, a further period of catheterization, with weekly changes, may be required. A twice-weekly suppository or enema may be necessary to clear the rectum.

5. *Fluid balance and nutrition*—fluids are not generally required for the first 24 hours but if the patient remains unable to swallow, he should be given fluids by nasogastric tube. If the tube cannot be passed, intravenous fluids are necessary.

(b) *Management of paralysis*

The weight of the bedclothes is taken off the legs by use of a cage. The arm and leg on the affected side should be placed in such a position as to prevent deformity should power not ultimately return. There is a tendency for the leg to rotate externally and for foot-drop to occur, but this can be prevented by sandbags, supporting board or plaster of Paris splints, care being taken to avoid pressure sores. The arm should be supported on a pillow with the elbow slightly flexed.

The limbs should be put through the full range of passive movements at least twice daily to preserve joint mobility. As consciousness returns the patient should be encouraged to work his paralysed limbs with his good arm and leg. He may be progressively propped up in bed with pillows and back rest and encouraged to cough and clear his secretions. Deep breathing exercises will also assist re-expansion of the lungs.

The slightest return of voluntary movement is a good sign and the patient should be encouraged to develop it, for example wiggling the toes and attempting to bend the knee. Active movements of the fingers are promoted by a soft rubber ball in the palm.

It is undesirable for any patient to be completely confined to bed for more than 48 hours. As soon as possible after consciousness has returned, the patient should be assisted up and into a chair. This often improves bladder control and catheterization may be dispensed with. The programme now is sitting, standing, walking. It is much easier for the patient to move his limbs if he is sitting in a chair rather than in bed. Active exercises should now be practised with the assistance of the physiotherapist. Although paralysis may still affect the foot, frequently there is sufficient power in the hip muscles to allow the patient to stand with support and within a day or two the quadriceps may be strong enough to allow weight bearing. Balance may have been affected, but tends to improve and the patient is taught to stand and then lower himself into the chair—he may find new ways of performing normal activities.

With support, he becomes able to walk again, increasing his distance every day. The pulpit-type (Zimmer) walking frame promotes confidence, or walking aids such as a stick or tripod can be used. It is much easier to walk properly dressed with trousers, socks and shoes than to struggle in pyjamas and soft slippers. If paralysis and foot-drop persist a toe-spring or caliper will assist walking. A board at each side of the wheel of the bed, against which the patient can place his toes, will enable him to rise from a chair using his arms.

Until power returns to the arm, it may be necessary to cut up food into small pieces. In due course, even if finger or arm movement remains impaired, it is usually possible for the patient to feed himself using a spoon or fork, and devices such as a rubber mat to prevent plates from slipping. He may have to learn a new method of writing. Zips or Velcro fasteners may be easier to manage than buttons. Once a patient can walk he can get to the lavatory and when he can feed himself, he has regained sufficient independence and pride to look forward to returning home.

(c) *Management of speech and visual disturbance*

The severely dysphasic patient is confused and often disorientated, but it is much commoner for dysphasia to be mainly expressive, that is the patient knows his wants but cannot state them. This is distressing to him, and relatives may misunderstand the situation and shout at him, thinking he is deaf or simple, and thus worsening his agitation. The good nurse should be able to interpret the patient's wants at this stage, attending to his food, drink, or toilet requirements and comforts. Usually improvement occurs in days or weeks during which conversation should be practised, and other patients can help. Speech therapy is sometimes required. It should of course be remembered that many elderly patients are deaf in addition—relatives should be questioned as to whether the patient had a hearing aid, and if so he should be encouraged to wear it.

The patient may not see objects on the affected side, so his locker should be placed on his good side and of course the bed should be in such a position that he can see his surroundings, his link with reality, and not be looking at a blank wall. His spectacles should be available, and opportunity can be taken to check if he has any additional visual impairment, as from cataract, so that this can be remedied in due course to improve the chances of successful rehabilitation.

(d) The place of drugs

Sedatives. In the early stages restlessness can be managed with chlorpromazine (Largactil) 25–100 mg 4 to 8 hourly orally or intramuscularly. It should, however, be noted that restlessness may be a sign of a full bladder or a wet bed or be due to inability of the patient to make his wants known—the good nurse will anticipate this situation. Sedatives by day may not be required, but chlorpromazine 50 mg in the evening, or nitrazepam (Mogadon) 5–10 mg may ensure sleep and allow activity and cooperation the next day. Such drugs are not always necessary.

Antibacterial drugs, as has been pointed out, should not be used prophylactically and are only indicated if there is evidence of infection.

Anticoagulants should not be used in the acute stage of established stroke, for they may worsen haemorrhage. They may have a place a few weeks after embolus, and sometimes in internal carotid artery thrombosis, to prevent recurrence.

Treatment of hypertension. High blood pressure may be due to the stroke, and is not necessarily its cause. Thus an initially high reading may settle as acute cerebral oedema disappears, and if the pulse is slow, it may be unwise to use hypotensive drugs. If a very high blood pressure is thought to be worsening the situation, it may be justified to lower the blood pressure with intravenous frusemide or subcutaneous pentolinium. Measures to lower the intracranial pressure, such as massive doses or steroids, or mannitol infusions should not be used as they worsen intracranial bleeding.

(e) Rehabilitation and follow up

The stages of sitting, standing and walking have been stressed already in progressive patient care. The early stages of rehabilitation include using the lavatory, retraining in washing and use of baths, and taking food again. Even if walking is limited, the patient may be able to use his legs or one or both arms to push himself in a wheelchair, the aim being the resumption of independent activity. Apart from physical rehabilitation, mental rehabilitation is most important and, as emphasized, encouragement by nurses, doctors and by the patient's relatives will often tip the balance in favour of recovery.

Occupational therapy may speed the patient's progress in activities such as writing, cooking and housework.

The Day Hospital bridges the gap between the sheltered life in hospital and the exigencies of life at home; weekly attendance allows continuation of physiotherapy and rehabilitation. The *Medical Social Worker* will advise on home circumstances and on *Industrial Rehabilitation* where appropriate.

The majority of patients with a stroke recover, and more than 50 per cent achieve full independence, many of them being able to resume work, and participate in normal social activities and even in sport.

Some patients, especially the elderly or those with a previous history, remain disabled, and their condition is frequently complicated by arteriosclerotic heart disease and failure. In the elderly, dementia and urinary incontinence are the principal handicaps following stroke. However, only a small proportion of patients require permanent hospital care.

Intracranial haemorrhage

The forms of brain haemorrhage are

INTRACEREBRAL HAEMORRHAGE (as in Stroke, described above)
SUBARACHNOID HAEMORRHAGE
EXTRA-DURAL HAEMORRHAGE
SUBDURAL HAEMORRHAGE

SUBARACHNOID HAEMORRHAGE

This is due to rupture of a small aneurysm of one of the arteries of the Circle of Willis at the base of the brain. The aneurysm forms as a result of a developmental defect in the vessel wall, and it manifests in adult life.

Symptoms and signs

Subarachoid haemorrhage occurs in any age group but is commonest in young and middle-aged adults. There may be a warning headache or neckache, which settles. Some days later the patient suffers severe and often agonizing headache and neckache with neck stiffness and there may be sudden loss of consciousness with deep coma and flaccid weakness of all limbs, or some lateralization of signs of paralysis.

Provided the optic discs are not 'choked', indicating raised intra-cranial pressure, diagnosis is confirmed by lumbar puncture which reveals heavily blood-stained cerebro-spinal fluid.

Treatment

Patients are best managed in a special neurosurgical unit, though active measures may be postponed for a day or two by which time the level of consciousness has often improved. *Cerebral arteriography* is now carried out to ascertain the site of the ruptured aneurysm, and surgical ligation may be indicated to prevent recurrence of bleeding, which is very liable to occur in the first few weeks. There is no actual treatment possible for the bleeding itself, and if there is deep coma or evidence of severe cerebral destruction, surgery is not indicated. Surgery is essentially prophylactic, but gives marginally better results than conservative treatment. Even so the mortality of subarachnoid haemorrhage is 40–50 per cent.

EXTRA-DURAL HAEMORRHAGE

This follows a *head injury*, usually with fracture of the temporal bone of the skull, and is due to rupture of the middle meningeal artery. Thus it occurs after road accidents or knocks at sport. The patient may have been transientally stunned, then there is a 'lucid interval', and then deepening coma from the pressure effects of the bleeding displacing the brain—there may be a dilated pupil from involvement of the 3rd cranial nerve. Surgical exploration with burr holes and decompression are indicated.

SUBDURAL HAEMORRHAGE

This is a more slowly developing collection of blood from ruptured veins in the subdural space. It occurs in birth injury, and also in the elderly, possibly because of some shrinkage of brain substance and weakening of the walls of the veins, which rupture after relatively trivial injury. Usually there is a history of a bump on the head, which may have been forgotten, and the skull may or may not have been fractured. Some days or weeks later there is disturbance of consciousness or lateralizing signs, and *the condition may be mistaken for a stroke*. The subdural haemorrhage is one form of 'space occupying lesion' and the treatment is surgical.

Space occupying lesions of the brain

These are:

1. HAEMATOMAS
2. CEREBRAL TUMOURS
3. ABSCESSES

{ The term 'space occupying lesion' is a useful one, for although the nature of the lesions is very different, their effect on the brain, and therefore the clinical presentation, is the same.

Symptoms and signs are due to (*a*) local effects,
(common to all)   (*b*) displacement effects,
                      (*c*) raised intracranial pressure.

(*a*) *local effects*—by destroying the brain substance, the lesion may cause complaints such as difficulty in moving part of a limb, or disorder of the motor act (apraxia). There may be speech disturbance, transient deafness or defective sense of smell. The personality may change with behaviour disorders, e.g. inappropriate urination. There may be focal fits related to disturbance in electrical function.

(*b*) *displacement effects*—a nerve may be displaced and stretched —thus there may be paralysis of the 6th cranial nerve with resultant orbital muscle weakness and double vision (diplopia). A tumour at the cerebello-pontine angle, the 'acoustic neuroma' not only causes deafness and ataxia (disturbance of gait) but also causes loss of the corneal reflex from stretching of the 5th and 7th cranial nerves.

(*c*) *raised intracranial pressure.* The space occupying lesion is inside a closed bony box, the skull, and there are diffuse pressure effects on brain metabolism and disturbance of the normal circulation of the cerebro-spinal fluid. Thus there is headache, vomiting and drowsiness sometimes with slowing of the pulse and of the respiratory rate. The doctor will note papilloedema, or 'choked' optic disc. These are *late* signs.

CONFIRMING THE PRESENCE OF A SPACE-OCCUPYING LESION
It is important to make the diagnosis before there are gross clinical signs, for these indicate that the lesion is advanced, with less chance of successful treatment.

The portable echo-encephalograph causes no discomfort and may demonstrate a 'shift' of brain structures. Skull x-ray may show a displacement of the pineal gland from the mid-line, should the gland be calcified as it often is in middle age; some tumours are calcified. Raised intracranial pressure may cause erosion of the bone near the pituitary fossa—which can itself be enlarged in pituitary tumour. Chest x-ray may show a primary tumour in the lung. Lumbar puncture, contra-indicated if there is papilloedema, may show raised C.S.F. pressure; the fluid may contain red cells in haematoma, or pus cells from an abscess, and its protein content may be raised in these and in tumours, but the test may be normal. Electro-encephalography (E.E.G.) and Radio-Isotope Scan may be useful. The patient may be referred to the neurosurgical unit for angiography or air encephalography.

THE NATURE OF THE LESION AND ITS TREATMENT

Usually there are clinical pointers allowing the differentiation of haematoma, tumour or abscess.

Haematoma follows head injury and may be extradural (arterial) or subdural (venous), or may form in the infarcted brain following a stroke, and surgical removal may be called for.

Cerebral tumour. The symptoms here are of gradual onset, unlike the suddenness of the vascular catastrophe.

Cerebral tumours may be *primary* or *secondary*. The latter are often from the lung (bronchogenic carcinoma in cigarette smokers), sometimes from stomach, prostate or breast, and the prognosis is hopeless.

Primary tumours include the *meningioma*, arising from the meninges, non-malignant, pressing on but not invading the brain, the *neurofibroma*, a non-malignant tumour of the nerve sheath (e.g. the acoustic neuroma, or a spinal nerve neuroma), and the *gliomas*. The gliomas are tumours of the supporting glial tissue, not the neuronal cells. Some gliomas are relatively benign and slow growing. Others are highly malignant and destructive, but unlike malignant tumours elsewhere, they do not metastasise outside the central nervous system.

The nature of a cerebral tumour can often only be established at operation or by biopsy. Surgical removal may be possible. Cerebral tumours are not usually sensitive to x-ray therapy (except some pituitary tumours), and intra-arterial anti-tumour chemotherapy has proved disappointing.

Cerebral abscess is now a rare cause of space occupying lesion. It used to be seen in septic spread from middle ear and mastoid infection. Facial sepsis may cause a septic venous sinus thrombosis and abscess formation. A cerebral abscess may complicate bronchiectasis, a septic embolus having passed from the lung to the brain.

Symptoms include swinging pyrexia, and there may be pus cells in the cerebrospinal fluid and risk of meningitis. Treatment is with appropriate antibacterial drugs, which usually obviate the need for surgical measures.

Infections of the central nervous system

Sepsis causing venous sinus thrombosis, and cerebral abscess have already been described.

The following will now be considered:

MENINGITIS—infection and inflammation of the meninges.

ENCEPHALITIS and ENCEPHALOMYELITIS—encephalitis is infection of the brain, myelitis is inflammation or infection of the spinal cord, and the two are often combined to produce an encephalomyelitis.

POLIOMYELITIS—a virus infection of the anterior horn (motor) cells.

HERPES ZOSTER—a virus infection of the posterior (sensory) nerve root ganglia, the virus being the same as that causing chicken-pox (varicella).

NEUROSYPHILIS—syphilitic (venereal) infection.

TETANUS—caused by the toxin of the Bacillus (Clostridium) tetani.

MENINGITIS

This is an acute inflammation of the meninges, usually bacterial, spread having occurred from a septic process penetrating the skull following injury or operation, or via the bloodstream from a distant focus, e.g. the throat in meningococcal meningitis or the lower respiratory tract in meningitis due to the pneumococcus or the organism called Haemophilus influezae.

Symptoms and signs: Meningococcal meningitis is commonest in young people, especially in closed communities such as barrack rooms which may allow spread of infection from throat or nasal secretions.

The onset is usually acute with headache, neckache and neck stiffness and there may also be inability to straighten the knee when the hip is flexed (Kernig's sign)—due to the inflamed meninges irritating the nerve roots. There is tachycardia, fever, dislike of bright light (photophobia) and clouding of consciousness. Tuberculous meningitis is now rare but complicates miliary tuberculosis, in which the patient has little resistance to the tubercle bacillus. The onset is slower, with vague headache, tiredness and often only slight neck stiffness.

Virus meningitis may complicate mumps. Other viruses more commonly cause an encephalitis rather than a true meningitis, but signs of meningeal irritation may occur.

Fulminating meningococcal meningitis may be accompanied by a severe purpuric rash, haemorrhage into the adrenal glands, and collapse.

Diagnosis is confirmed by lumbar puncture. The cerebrospinal fluid may be under raised pressure, is cloudy due to pus cells in the bacterial cases and the organisms can be cultured from it. In tuberculous meningitis, the C.S.F. sugar is reduced.

Treatment: The patient is put to bed in a quiet room with subdued light. At diagnostic lumbar puncture, 10,000 units of penicillin (penicillin G, benzyl penicillin) may be injected into the subarachnoid space. A sulphonamide drug is given by mouth (e.g. as sulphadimidine 3 G then 1 G 6 hourly, or combined with trimethoprim as Septrin or Bactrim) plus penicillin 1 mega unit 6-hourly by intramuscular injection. This regime will generally cope with meningococcal and pneumococcal infections and should be given until the bacteriology is known. Haemophilus influenzae infection may require the use of chloramphenicol.

If treated early, most cases now recover in a few days.

Tuberculous meningitis, previously invariably fatal, responds well to streptomycin, isoniazid, and para-aminosalicylic-acid therapy.

ENCEPHALITIS AND ENCEPHALOMYELITIS

Epidemics of a disease called encephalitis lethargica ('sleepy sickness', not to be confused with the tropical disease trypanosomiasis or sleeping sickness) occurred in the 1920s. The cause was unknown, but assumed to be a virus. Many years later the condition might be followed by 'post-encephalitic Parkinsonism', a form of Parkinson's disease (shaking palsy). No cases of encephalitis lethargica have been described since 1927 and the disease may have disappeared.

The enteroviruses (or picornaviruses), which include the poliomyelitis, Echo and Coxsackie viruses, are so named because they colonize in the intestinal tract, and are excreted in the faeces. They may spread in the bloodstream to reach the nervous system and cause an encephalitis, an inflammation of the brain cells, or in the case of poliomyelitis the virus tends to localize at the anterior horn cells of the spinal cord. Many such infections are mild and pass unnoticed.

The virus of herpes simplex, which normally causes only 'cold sores' at the mouth, can at times cause a severe encephalitis; similar viruses are responsible for epidemics of encephalitis occuring in the tropics and the Far East.

The childhood fevers—measles, mumps, rubella (German measles) and chicken-pox—may be accompanied or followed by virus invasion of the nervous system resulting in encephalitis or encephalomyelitis and mild meningitis. Encephalomyelitis may also follow glandular fever, and vaccination against measles and smallpox, and here it is probably due to an auto-immune reaction.

Encephalomyelitis is characterized by patchy *demyelination* of the insulating and nutritive myelin sheath that surrounds the nerve fibres in the brain and spinal cord. Demyelination may also involve the peripheral nerves. Similar changes may complicate carcinoma, especially bronchial carcinoma on a 'toxic' or auto-immune basis. More important, however, is the realization that some viruses may lurk quietly in the central nervous system for many years. This is called 'slow' (or 'latent') virus infection. Thus the measles virus may cause cerebral deterioration and dementia in young adult life, and other viruses may cause the pre-senile dementias of middle age. Kuru, a fatal cerebellar disorder, is a slow virus infection occurring in the Fore tribe of New Guinea; they were formerly cannibals, and infection was acquired from eating diseased human brains. It is possible that some demyelinating diseases, a group which includes multiple sclerosis, are caused by slow viruses or allergic reactions to them. Such diseases may be forms of chronic encephalomyelitis.

Symptoms and signs of acute encephalitis and encephalomyelitis

Symptoms are often mild, and the illness transient. In severe cases there is fever, disturbance of cerebration with intellectual disturbance, emotional upset and clouding of consciousness. The patient resents interference. Sleep rhythm may be upset. There is headache, vomiting and a degree of neck stiffness. There may be cranial nerve palsies, signs of long tract involvement in the spinal cord, and additional motor or sensory impairment from peripheral nerve involvement.

At lumbar puncture, the C.S.F. may be normal or show increased cells or protein. A specimen should be sent to the laboratory as quickly as possible (in a vacuum flask containing ice) for virus isolation. The blood may show a rising virus antibody titre. Virus may also be cultured from the stools, in which enteroviruses survive for up to 24 hours at room temperature.

The E.E.G. may show diffuse electrical disturbance of the brain. Brain biopsy may be necessary to establish the diagnosis of herpes simplex encephalitis.

Treatment

The only specific antiviral remedy is idoxuridine for herpes simplex encephalitis.

Steriods such as prednisone are probably indicated for encephalomyelitis following childhood fevers and vaccination. Massive doses may be used in acute encephalitis if there are signs of rapidly developing cerebral oedema, but it should be remembered that steroids may provoke a spread of infection, whether bacterial or viral.

Serious cases demand bed rest and skilled nursing care, with attention to pressure areas and to fluid and toilet requirements. Respiratory failure may require intubation or tracheotomy with use of a mechanical respirator.

Many ill patients make a remarkable recovery, with full return of intellect and normal emotional response, but this may take weeks or months.

RABIES

Rabies is a virus infection which results in a form of encephalitis, usually fatal. The virus is transmitted to humans through bites from infected animals, especially dogs, but bats are also carriers. Strict quarantine measures for imported dogs eradicated rabies in Britain until 1969, when a dog was found to be infected, so quarantine measures have been more strictly imposed. An animal suspected of having rabies must be kept in isolation for a few weeks, and if it dies, its brain must be examined for the virus. A rabid animal is usually aggressive and has a fear of drinking, hydrophobia. If a person is bitten, he must be given an immediate course of anti-rabies vaccinations, otherwise the virus passes up the nerves to reach the brain, symptoms including muscular stiffness, convulsions and paralysis of swallowing. There is only one recorded case of recovery; the treatment included measures used in tetanus—sedatives, tracheotomy and artificial respiration.

POLIOMYELITIS

This is increasingly rare due to effective vaccination. The poliomyelitis virus is of the enterovirus group, colonizing in the intestinal tract and excreted in the faeces. Thus infection is still common in under-developed countries with poor hygiene and primitive sanitation. The virus spreads to the central nervous system, affecting mainly the anterior horn cells of the sinal cord, though the brain stem may also be involved. Thus the condition is also called acute anterior poliomyelitis, or *infantile paralysis*, as it occurred in children, but young adults may be affected if they have no immunity.

Symptoms and signs

There is an initial febrile illness, often with signs of meningeal irritation, followed by paralysis of sudden onset usually affecting one leg or arm. If the phrenic nerve supplying the diaphragm and the nerves to the intercostal muscles are involved, respiration becomes impossible. Involvement of cranial nerves results in difficulty in speaking and swallowing, and the respiratory centre in the medulla can also be affected.

Treatment

This is essentially preventive, oral vaccination preventing the gut infection which is the source of the virus—vaccination is carried out in infancy and again at school.

There is no specific treatment once poliomyelitis has occurred. Rest in the acute stage may limit the extent of paralysis. Later, passive and then active movements are encouraged. In severe cases with respiratory or brain-stem involvement, the treatment is that of respiratory failure with aspiration of secretions, intubation, tracheotomy and artificial respiration.

Long-term management includes physiotherapy for weeks or months. Destroyed nerve cells do not recover and there is wasting of muscle groups: it is therefore imperative to build up those that remain. A caliper may be necessary for foot drop. Where deformity occurs despite preventive measures, orthopaedic correction may be necessary.

HERPES ZOSTER (SHINGLES)

This is a virus infection of the posterior (sensory) nerve root ganglia. The virus is the same as that causing chickenpox in children. Herpes zoster is commonest in the middle aged and elderly, the virus possibly lying dormant in the nervous system. The condition may only appear if the patient is debilitated, or it may accompany an irritative lesion such as a tumour near the nerve root. Usually, however, herpes zoster appears without an obvious precipitating factor. It is of low infectivity, cross infection is uncommon and isolation unnecessary, but children may develop chicken pox from contact with herpes zoster—the reverse is rare.

Symptoms and signs

'Herpes' describes the herpetic or vesicular eruption, and 'zoster' means its band-like distribution along the line of a nerve, often an intercostal nerve. Thus the patient has a painful, itchy vesicular rash commonly at the trunk, but any nerve can be involved. The ophthalmic division of the fifth (trigeminal) cranial nerve may be affected with typical rash on one half of the forehead, and painful redness of the eye.

Treatment

No specific drug treatment is available. Analgesics such as aspirin, pentazocine (Fortral) or stronger drugs including pethidine may be required to relieve pain, which may be very severe and distressing. A drug of dependence such as pethidine should not, of course, be used for more than a few days—many patients have discomfort in the part for weeks or months after the acute stages, and there is danger of addiction in such a situation.

Calamine lotion is soothing and aids drying of the vesicles. An antibiotic may be required should they become infected. Steroids such as prednisone sometimes help in severe cases. Steroid eye-drops may reduce the inflammation, but their use may predispose to other infection with risk of destruction of the cornea.

Usually herpes zoster clears within a week or two. Apart from the use of analgesics, residual discomfort can sometimes be improved by electric vibratory massage.

NEUROSYPHILIS (SYPHILIS OF THE NERVOUS SYSTEM)

This occurs usually some years after the primary infection which, of course, can now be effectively cured with penicillin. Thus neuro-syphilis is relatively rare in Britain but should be watched for in persons such as seamen, and alcoholics, and in immigrants from under-developed countries, where infection is still rife. There has in fact been an increase in the incidence of primary syphilis in some Western countries, including the United States, in recent years, so the late results of infection, such as neurosyphilis, may yet be seen again.

There are three types of neurosyphilis

1. *Meningovascular syphilis* may occur in the primary infection, but usually delayed till secondary (or tertiary) stage a few years later.

2. *Tabes dorsalis* ⎰manifestations of the tertiary stage,
3. *General paralysis of the* ⎱ occurring 10–15 years after initial *insane* (G.P.I.) infection.

1. *Meningovascular syphilis*

The arteries to the brain are inflamed and narrowed causing patchy degeneration of the nerve cells, especially of cortex and brain stem. Thus there may be weakness of a limb and transient cranial nerve palsies, the oculo-motor nerves to the eyes being especially affected. Meningeal irritation gives rise to neck stiffness. Occasionally the spinal cord is involved, causing a *myelitis* with long-tract signs.

2. *Tabes dorsalis*

Here there is a degeneration of the posterior nerve roots and tracts resulting in sensory loss—especially the sensation from muscles and joints. The patient has a characteristic gait called *locomotor ataxia*, walking with legs wide apart and stamping them down in an attempt to know where they are. He is worse on closing his eyes or at night. There may also be shooting- or '*lightning*'-*pains* in the limbs or even the abdomen, simulating an abdominal emergency. Disturbance of bladder sensation causes retention of urine or incontinence. The mid-brain is often affected, causing eye changes—'Argyll Robertson pupils'—the pupils are small, irregular and fail to react to light, but still react to accommodation to a near object. The knee and ankle jerks are absent. In very severe cases the loss of joint sensation is associated with a deformed and swollen yet painless joint called a Charcot's joint.

3. *General Paralysis of the Insane* (G.P.I.)

Here the higher centres in the cerebral cortex and the pyramidal tracts are involved. There is progressive deterioration of intellect with personality change and often grandiose ideas, the patient be-lieving that he has great wealth or power and acting accordingly. This

11—EM

may cause ruination of family and of business. There may a coarse tremor of hands, lips and tongue, and Argyll Robertson pupils. There is increasing paralysis of upper motor neurone type affecting the legs, impeding walking and associated with increased reflexes and extensor plantar responses. However tabes dorsalis and G.P.I. may co-exist, when physical signs may include absent reflexes yet extensor plantar responses. The end result, as the name implies, is paralysis and 'insanity' (dementia).

Neurosyphilis often complicates cardiovascular syphilis. The diagnosis should be suspected in any obscure neurological case and confirmed by tests such as the Wassermann Reaction (W.R.) Reference Laboratory (V.D.R.L.) and Treponemal Immobilization tests (T.P.I.) in the blood and cerebro-spinal fluid, which may also show protein changes recorded as the 'Lange curve'.

Treatment

Courses of penicillin, 1–2 mega units daily by intramuscular injection for two weeks, improve symptoms in meningovascular syphilis and in general paralysis of the insane, and will prevent advancement of tabes dorsalis. Nerve cells and roots do not regenerate, however, so there may be considerable residual disability. Thus it is important to treat syphilis in its primary stage, before neurological complications. It is necessary to make a diplomatic approach to other members of the patient's family, so that blood tests can be done to see if they are infected and treatment instituted if necessary.

TETANUS (LOCKJAW)

The spores of the bacillus (Clostridium tetani) causing tetanus are found in manure, soil and dust. Infection is now uncommon in Britain, horse transport having been replaced by the motor car, but tetanus still occurs in under-developed countries where people live in close contact with their animals and may indeed use dung as a wound dressing. Like the gas gangrene organisms, the tetanus bacilli grow best where the oxygen supply is poor, and infection follows contamination of deep punctures and wounds.

Tetanus is due to a toxin produced by the bacilli in the wound. The toxin travels up the peripheral nerves to reach the central nervous system.

The syptoms and signs of tetanus, its treatment and its prevention are described in Chapter 3 (page 32).

Multiple sclerosis (disseminated sclerosis)

Multiple sclerosis is a chronic disease of the nervous system, almost always arising before the age of forty. It is characterized by remissions and relapses and by the presence of multiple patches of sclerosis scattered throughout the brain and the spinal cord.

Cause

The cause is unknown. The disease affects 1 in 2,000 of the population of Great Britain, is commonest in temperate Northern climates, rare in the tropics and South Africa, and unknown in China and Japan. Multiple sclerosis is a *demyelinating disease*—the myelin sheath, which protects and nourishes the nerve fibre (just as insulation protects an electric cable) is destroyed by some unknown agent. Conduction in the underlying nerve fibre is at first only temporarily affected, and early changes may be reversible, but later, plaques of scar tissue are formed, destroying the nerve fibres.

The demyelination may be due to some form of disseminated encephalomyelitis. It has been suggested that the cause may be an infective agent or virus, possibly a 'slow-virus' similar to that causing Kuru, the cannibal disease of New Guinea referred to on page 309, or an infective agent similar to that causing 'scrapie' in sheep. The agent may be activated by stress, injury, intercurrent infection, or in the puerperium, but usually there is no obvious precipitating factor, and multiple sclerosis may represent a disturbance of immunity.

Symptoms and signs

These are disseminated—scattered both in time and in place. The presenting sign is often a transient weakness of arm or leg or a blurring of vision which clears up. Months or years later there are more permanent signs. The pyramidal tracts are commonly involved causing spastic weakness, becoming fairly symmetrical in both legs. There is no pain, and sensory changes are slight. There is often disturbance of bladder function such as urgency of micturition, incontinence, or retention. Cranial nerve involvement includes the optic nerve causing the visual disturbance and sometimes pallor of the optic disc seen with the ophthalmoscope. The voice may have a peculiar staccato quality. The cerebellum and its connections may be involved, causing disorder of muscle balance and control, and ataxia. There is a fine tremor of the fingers, more marked on movement (intention tremor) and brought out by the 'finger-nose' test, as the patient, starting with hand outstretched, brings in the index finger to touch the tip of the nose. He cannot perform rapid to-and-fro movements of the hands. A similar disturbance of the ocular muscles causes the fine tremor of the eyes called *nystagmus* when attempt is made to fix the gaze on an object held in front.

Some patients with multiple sclerosis appear strangely unconcerned despite the severity of their symptoms, making such symptoms easier to bear. A true euphoria, or elation of mood may occur in a few cases, but depression can also occur.

Course

There may be acute exacerbations of symptoms, settling in early cases and followed by months or even years of remission. In severe cases, there is gradual deterioration over the years, the patient becoming paraplegic (paralysed in both legs) and incontinent, unable to get out of bed without help, and prone to urinary and chest infections and to pressure sores.

Further investigations

Lumbar puncture. In half the cases of multiple sclerosis, the cerebrospinal fluid shows an increase in the gammaglobulin fraction of the protein.

Further investigations, apart from routine ones such as urine testing, blood count and chest x-ray, are seldom required, but myelography may be indicated in the occasional patient with purely pyramidal tract signs, to exclude a tumour or other lesion causing compression of the spinal cord.

Treatment

(a) Drugs

In acute exacerbations, *A.C.T.H.* (adrenocorticotrophic hormone, corticotrophin) may produce a remission. It may be given as long-acting A.C.T.H. gel, initially an injection of 80 units daily; other slow release preparations include A.C.T.H. zinc or methyl cellulose complexes, or the synthetic product tetracosactrin may be used. A.C.T.H. is continued at reduced dose for 3 or 4 weeks. It is of no value given beyond this time, but a further course can be given for any subsequent relapse. Though A.C.T.H. has a steroid-like action, corticosteroid drugs such as prednisone are less effective.

No known drug has any curative effect. Diazepam (Valium) may have some relaxing effect in patients with severe spastic signs. Antidepressive drugs such as amitriptyline (Tryptizol) may be indicated.

(b) General management

It is important to maintain an attitude of hope—quite often, as we have seen, the symptoms are mild, may not recur for many years and may cause little disability. In their search for a cure, patients are often tempted to seek advice from quacks, and they must be protected against the possible dangers and financial losses incurred by such consultations. It is therefore vital to maintain the patient's confidence.

What to tell him depends very much on his personal circumstances, but it may be wise to give a full explanation to his relatives. To the patient, it may be sufficient to refer to the condition as 'neuritis', yet it may be wrong to withhold the diagnosis when it is becoming clear there is increasing disability and difficulty at work.

Most patients become adjusted to their disorder. Short courses of physiotherapy may improve morale and strengthen the unaffected muscles, but spastic limbs will not be helped. Walking should be encouraged wherever possible, though a wheelchair or adapted motor car may become necessary, enabling the patient to lead a reasonably full life. *The Multiple Sclerosis Society* may help, and is at 4 Tachbrook Street, London, S.W.1.

In the later stages, intrathecal phenol may relieve painful spasticity. The management of the bed-ridden patient includes frequent turning, care of the skin, attention to pressure areas, assistance in feeding and care of the bowels and bladder. Catheterization may be required, with frequent bacteriological checks of the urine to allow prompt detection and treatment of infection. Deep breathing exercises may prevent chest infections. Such infections may be the terminal event, but skilled nursing allows the patient many years of reasonably comfortable life.

Faints, dizzy turns and blackouts

FAINTING (SYNCOPE)
This is transient loss of consciousness due to inadequate cerebral bloodflow.

The simple faint (vasovagal attack)

This occurs in *healthy people*, usually the young, and is a feeling of light headedness which is followed by collapse—the person has some *warning* of an impending faint.

Causes: Precipitating factors may be psychogenic—emotion, an unpleasant sight, fear of an injection, or the presence of severe pain (cardiac pain, renal 'colic'). These result in vagal stimulation with lowered peripheral resistance and pooling of blood, causing reduced venous return and cardiac output. The heart is also slowed. Prolonged standing in the erect posture in a hot climate also causes venous pooling, with the same result.

Symptoms and signs include pallor, sweating, feeling of sickness and swimming in the head then loss of consciousness and collapse. The fainting person seldom falls heavily and injury is rare unlike fits, in which injury is common. In fainting, the pulse is slow and the blood pressure lowered, but as soon as the person is flat, the cerebral circulation improves and consciousness returns in a few seconds.

Treatment is therefore to let the patient lie down, loosening tight clothing around the neck, until there is spontaneous recovery.

Cardiac syncope

This occurs in the older age groups, and usually there is a known history of heart disease. Fainting occurs on effort in patients whose hearts cannot meet the demand for blood created by exercise, and there is temporary cerebral anoxia—this may occur in aortic stenosis or mitral stenosis.

Stokes-Adams attacks are sudden episodes of cerebral anoxia following heart block, with return of consciousness and facial flushing when the ventricle restarts. The onset of atrial fibrillation or other arrhythmia may also cause temporary cerebral ischaemia. In myocardial infarction, the lowered cardiac output may cause collapse, but usually the dominant symptom is severe chest pain, making the diagnosis obvious.

Carotid-sinus syncope is due to pressure of a tight collar stimulating the carotid sinus nerves with resultant reflex hypotension, but is probably rare.

Cough syncope ('cough drop') occurs when a patient, frequently a chronic bronchitic, coughs so much that he impedes the venous return to the heart, resulting in collapse.

'DIZZY TURNS'

This term is commonly used by patients, and it is important to define what they mean. A 'dizzy turn' may refer to a feeling of light headedness as part of a faint, or a sense of unsteadiness or giddiness related to temporary disturbance of balance, or it may mean ataxia.

Vertigo is a feeling of spinning or tilting of the surroundings, or of the self. True vertigo occurs in disorders of the labyrinth of the inner ear (the labyrinth comprises the vestibule and semicircular canals), or of the vestibular division of the eighth cranial (auditory) nerve, or of its connections in the brain stem, which may be affected in vertebrobasilar ischaemia.

BLACKOUTS AND DROP-ATTACKS

These again are loose terms. The word blackout should really apply to loss of vision, but it is more frequently used by a patient to describe an episode of unconsciousness or collapse—the cause of which may be a simple faint, a small stroke, a hypoglycaemic attack, or even epilepsy (fit).

By a 'drop-attack' the patient may mean sudden weakness of the legs, or a fall to the ground with momentary loss of consciousness. *Sudden* loss of consciousness always suggests epilepsy, but drop-attacks may be due to brain-stem ischaemia. The vertebral arteries are encroached on by arthritis of the cervical spine (cervical spondylosis) and attacks may occur from further narrowing due to kinking of the vessels when stooping. Again, in the elderly with rigid arteries and impaired blood pressure control, suddenly assuming the erect posture after recumbency may precipitate a drop-attack.

Narcolepsy is attacks of extreme sleepiness and is rare, as is cataplexy, a sudden loss of muscle tone usually precipitated by strong emotion.

In all these disorders, and even more so if the complaint is of 'fits' (see below, Epilepsy), it is essential to seek the patients relatives or to get an eye-witness account of the attack—its speed of onset and the circumstances, and the appearance of the patient during it. As a rule, a faint is a condition in which the patient has a premonitory feeling of something about to happen, and faints are common in adolescence. With an epileptic fit, however, any aura or premonition is in fact rare, the onset is sudden, and the patient is quite unaware of what is happening.

Epilepsy

Epilepsy is a group of conditions characterized by recurrent attacks of disordered brain function called seizures or *fits*. Fits are of sudden onset and each is usually short in duration, lasting only a matter of minutes. The word 'ictus', meaning a blow, may be used to avoid the term fit, the occurrence of which used to be ascribed to the presence of evil spirits.

Cause

Epilepsy results from disordered electrical activity of the brain. The fit is due to an abnormal electrical focus firing off a discharge with resultant disturbance of cerebration and usually loss of consciousness.

TYPES OF EPILEPSY

Symptomatic Epilepsy

Here there is some definable irritant focus, and the epilepsy is a *symptom* of the underlying disorder. Thus epilepsy may follow damage to the brain at birth, or head injury, or indicate the presence of a space-occupying lesion such as tumour, abscess or haematoma, or result from a scar of the brain after a stroke

Idiopathic epilepsy

In the vast majority of cases of epilepsy, no reason for the electrical instability can be discovered—thus 80 per cent of the patients belong to this idiopathic group.

The incidence of known epilepsy is 5 per 1,000 of the population but the condition may go unrecognized, and many people have an epileptic attack at some time during their lives. There is a familial tendency, the incidence of epilepsy in the children being slightly higher if one parent is affected, and considerably higher if both parents have known epilepsy.

Factors precipitating an attack include fatigue and stress over-hydration, anoxia and metabolic causes such as uraemia, hypoglycaemia and hypocalcaemia. Fits also occur in severe toxaemia of pregnancy—eclampsia. In children, fevers are said to precipitate attacks, but sometimes it is the attack that causes the fever and not the reverse. A flickering television screen may provoke a fit, the stroboscopic effect. More often, no precipitating cause can be recognized.

Idiopathic epilepsy is of two main types:

1. *Petit mal*
2. *Grand mal*

Additional types include Jacksonian attacks and psycho-motor epilepsy.

PETIT MAL—MINOR EPILEPSY

This arises in children or adolescents and never starts in adult life. The abnormal focus is a central, deep-seated one. The attacks or fits consist of a transitory interruption of consciousness, without any convulsive element. The patient simply stops what he is doing or saying and may stare vacantly into space for a few seconds before resuming his previous activity. He seldom, if ever, falls, and he has no realization that anything abnormal has occurred. Attacks may occur once every few weeks or months, or there may be several in one day.

If the condition is not recognized in a schoolchild, he may be chastised for his inattention in class. Diagnosis should be possible from a description of the attacks, and can be confirmed by the electroencephalogram, which shows a characteristic spike-and-wave pattern.

Treatment

The drug of choice is ethosuximide (Zarontin), 0·5–1·5 G daily.

Ethosuximide should probably be given for 6–12 months or longer if attacks recur. However, as petit mal attacks tend to become less frequent with the approach of adult life, the drug may not be required long-term. Sometimes petit mal is associated with grand mal, and as ethosuximide may worsen convulsive seizures, it may be combined with phenobarbitone.

GRAND MAL—MAJOR EPILEPSY

This commonly begins between the ages of 7 and 17. Attacks starting in adult life should raise the suspicion of a lesion such as a tumour, but very often no such cause can be found. The classical major attack may be caused by a deep seated central focus or a more superficial focus in the cortex, the abnormal electrical activity spreading to cause a generalized effect.

Despite statements to the contrary, a major fit is seldom preceded by any *aura* or premonition. If, however, an aura occurs, its nature may help to localize the site of the abnormal focus. Thus the fit is almost always of sudden onset and has three stages:

The major fit

1. *Tonic stage.* The patient may cry out, consciousness is suddenly lost and he falls to the ground. All the muscles are in rigid spasm, so he falls heavily and may bump his head or otherwise injure himself. The limbs are extended, the jaw clenched and the tongue may be bitten. Respiration ceases, resulting in cyanosis. The tonic stage lasts for about half a minute.

2. *Clonic stage.* Muscle twitching often starts at the fingers or around the mouth, then the limb muscles contract and relax causing jerking movements. These movements spread becoming violent and convulsive, the arms and legs thrashing about with risk of further injury, but breathing is resumed. The muscle jerkings involve the jaw and mouth, so the tongue may be bitten again and with foaming of the saliva the patient froths at the mouth. There may be incontinence of urine. The clonic stage lasts for 1–3 minutes after which the movements gradually cease.

3. *Sleepy stage.* The patient now passes into a deep sleep or coma, remaining unrousable for a few minutes or up to an hour. During this and the clonic stage the pupils and reflexes may be abnormal with extensor plantar responses. The patient may subsequently feel drowsy and sometimes complains of headache. He has no idea what has happened to him. Occasionally there is a period of post-epileptic automatism during which the patient may carry out some action of which he is unaware, and though this may have medico-legal implications, criminal acts are rare.

Status epilepticus

This is the occurrence of a series of major fits, the patient passing from one fit to another without regaining consciousness. Status epilepticus is a dangerous condition as the patient may become hyperpyrexial, and the periods of anoxia may precipitate brain damage.

Jacksonian fits

These are fits that begin unilaterally and usually the term is applied to motor seizures. They start as twitchings or jerky movements of one part of the body and may spread to involve a limb. With further spread, the fit becomes similar to the clonic stage of the major fit, with or without loss of consciousness.

The importance of a Jacksonian fit is that it pin-points the site of the epileptic focus. Thus if the fit begins as jerking of the right hand, the focus is in the left precentral area of the cortex. Such localization should lead to a search for an organic lesion, such as a tumour, which may be irritating that part of the brain.

Jacksonian fits can be sensory as well as motor, an abnormal feeling occurring in part of the body, spreading to involve other parts.

Psycho-motor epilepsy

This type of epilepsy commonly arises in the temporal lobe, which may be scarred after birth injury, so it is not necessarily 'idiopathic'. A warning of aura is common in psycho-motor epilepsy and consists of 'psychic' symptoms—feelings of unreality, or of previous experience (déjà-vu), auditory or visual hallucinations, a sense of an unpleasant smell, these psychic symptoms being shortly followed by a motor element, but twitching or jerking is not as marked as in the classical major fit.

Epilepsy in the elderly

Fits may be related to arteriosclerosis and previous strokes and may present as behaviour disturbances or episodes of bed-wetting.

Further investigations in grand mal

It is essential to obtain an eye-witness account of the fit and usually this allows diagnosis.

Electroencephalography. The E.E.G. may be helpful in showing an electrical abnormality of the brain, which may be of localizing value, or it may be generalized. However, the tracing may be normal, and though provocative tests can be applied, the E.E.G. in Grand Mal is really an *aid to*, the clinical diagnosis.

Most cases of epilepsy are idiopathic, but the fact that the condition may be a symptom of an underlaying lesion such as a tumour should be borne in mind, especially where fits start in adult life. Usually it suffices to carry out the normal clinical examination, including ophthalmoscopy and urine testing, check blood count and blood sugar, and have x-rays of chest and skull. Echo-encephalography and isotope scan may be carried out if a space-occupying lesion is suspected. Lumbar puncture need not be done routinely but a raised C.S.F. protein would heighten a suspicion of tumour.

An important investigation is *periodic review* of the patient, recurrence of fits, lateralizing signs or blurring of the optic discs (papilloedema) being indications that the epilepsy is not, in fact, the usual, i.e. idiopathic, type.

Treatment of the major fit

The only treatment of the major fit is to prevent the patient hurting himself until the attack is over. It may be possible to remove his dentures or to place a soft padded tongue depressor in his mouth to prevent him biting his tongue. Tight clothing should be loosened and the patient allowed to lie down until spontaneous recovery occurs.

Treatment of status epilepticus

1. Diazepam (Valium) 10 mg slowly intravenously, or paraldehyde 5–10 ml intramuscularly.
2. Insertion of airway and correct positioning to ensure ventilation.
3. Tepid sponging if hyperpyrexia occurs.
4. In intractable cases, it may be necessary to anaesthetise the patient with intravenous thiopentone, ventilation being maintained artificially through an endotracheal tube if necessary.

Usually the fits become less intense within an hour or two, the patient goes into a deep sleep and recovery ensues.

The drug treatment of grand mal

Phenobarbitone remains the drug of choice for preventing seizures. The dose is 30 mg two or three times daily. Phenytoin (Epanutin) 100 mg three times daily may be added if fits are not controlled on phenobarbitone alone. Primidone (Mysoline) and sulthiame (Ospolot) may also be useful, especially in the more localized types of fit.

Drug treatment should be given for at least a year after the last fit, but treatment for several years or even life-long may be necessary.

General measures and follow-up

The public has an unfounded fear of epilepsy. It should be explained to the patient that his condition is simply due to an electrical over-activity and that his brain is otherwise normal. Most epileptics are of normal intelligence—only a few children, usually those with brain damage from birth, are backward or have personality defects and need special schooling.

Epileptics should not work at heights or with dangerous machinery such as circular saws. Generally, however, restrictions need be few, and the patient should be encouraged to lead a normal life—indeed, a fit rarely occurs when he is actually engaged in vigorous activity. The condition must be declared in driving licence application, but the licence may now be granted if the applicant has remained free of attacks for three years, whether or not he is on medication.

The inheritance of epilepsy is in dispute for, although a person may have an epileptic electrical abnormality, he may never have a fit. If one parent is epileptic, the incidence in the offspring is about 5 per cent, but of course the condition may be mild. Thus epilepsy in one partner is no bar to marriage, but epileptics should probably not intermarry.

Migraine

Migraine is recurrent attacks of headache, often in bouts for a week or two, then there may be freedom for months. Migraine begins in adolescence, often there is a family history and attacks tend to be less severe after middle-age. Sufferers are often tense, worrying types. A common time for an attack is Sunday morning after breakfast in bed, for the patient worries that he has not justified this pleasure. Attacks may occur pre-menstrually, possibly due to fluid retention.

Symptoms and signs: The attack has three phases:

1. *the 'aura'*—this is due to spasm of intracranial arteries and may present as flashing lights or visual upset minutes or even some hours before the next stage. Occasionally there is weakness of a limb or one side (hemiplegic migraine).

2. *The headache*—this is due to dilatation of extracranial arteries, causing irritation of pain-sensitive nerve endings. Thus the headache is often localised to the region of the superficial temporal artery or one part of the head, and it is usually the same part that is involved in each attack. The headache may be so severe that the patient has to lie down in a dark room to gain relief.

3. *Nausea and vomiting*—may complicate or follow the headache. The vomit may of course contain bile, hence the term 'bilious attack'—but the trouble is in the cranial arteries and not in the biliary tract.

Treatment

Sometimes it is sufficient for the patient to lie down and take simple analgesics such as aspirin or paracetamol at the onset of an attack. The drug ergotamine is specific, but must be given *early* to prevent the painful dilatation of the arteries. Thus sufferers can be taught to inject themselves, dose 0·5–1·0 mg, or tablet or aerosol preparations can be used (Femergin, Cafergot, Migril). Excessive use of ergotamine is however dangerous as it causes arterial constriction, which may lead to gangrene of the finger tips.

Methysergide can be used in the interim treatment of migraine to prevent attacks, but, used long-term, side-effects include retroperitoneal fibrosis.

'Periodic migrainous neuralgia' is a similar condition, but commoner in men, and associated with extremely severe headaches (which may waken the patient from sleep), salivation lacrimation and often tenderness over part of the face. Bouts ('cluster-headaches') may occur every few months or there may be complete freedom for many years. Ergotamine is again effective.

Parkinson's disease (paralysis agitans)

Parkinson's disease is a chronic and progressive disease due to degenerative changes in the basal ganglia of the brain, and is a common condition in the middle-aged and elderly. It is named after James Parkinson, who in 1817 described the clinical picture, calling the disease 'the Shaking Palsy'.

Cause

In all types, there are degenerative changes in the basal ganglia, the nuclei at the base of the brain or their connections, which form part of the extra-pyramidal system concerned in normal muscle tone. The part called the substantia nigra is especially affected, losing its dark colour—it becomes depigmented. This is associated with depletion of a substance called dopamine, a neurological chemical transmitter. Although it is related to adrenaline, the effect of dopamine is inhibitory and not excitatory. Dopamine regulates the function of the extrapyramidal system, and lack of it results in the increased muscle tone of parkinsonism.

Types

Parkinson's disease proper, idiopathic parkinsonism

The cause of the degenerative change in the basal ganglia is here unknown. This is the common form of parkinsonism, the disease developing insidiously between the ages of 50 and 65, being commoner in men, and there is a slight familial tendency.

Arteriosclerotic parkinsonism

Here the degenerative changes are vascular in origin. The condition occurs in the elderly and is accompanied by other evidence of cerebral arteriosclerosis. There may be a history of strokes, and signs of pyramidal tract, as well as extra-pyramidal involvement, and sometimes a degree of dementia.

Post-encephalitic parkinsonism

This appeared up to thirty years after encephalitis lethargica, epidemics of which occurred from 1917 to 1927. Thus the onset was at an earlier age than in the other forms of parkinsonism. These patients are now elderly, and comprise a small proportion of all those suffering from parkinsonism. The post-encephalitic type is often accompanied by emotional and autonomic disturbance, and periodic upset of eye movements, oculogyric crises.

Drug-induced parkinsonism

Phenothiazine drugs such as chlorpromazine (Largactil), and methyldopa (Aldomet), and reserpine may induce parkinsonism by interfering with the action of dopamine or other neuro-chemical transmitters.

Carbon monoxide poisoning may also be followed by parkinsonism from effects on the basal ganglia.

Symptoms and signs

These comprise tremor, rigidity, poverty of movement, and sometimes *emotional change*.

The tremor is often the presenting sign, and is described as a 'pill-rolling' movement or shake of the fingers. The tremor becomes more marked if the patient is engaged by the examiner in conversation, or if he is emotionally upset. It may disappear on performing a voluntary movement and is absent during sleep. The patient may sit on his hands to prevent the distressing shake being seen by others. The tremor may be unilateral or both hands may be affected, one more than the other. The arms, legs and even the neck may be involved.

There is a rigidity of the muscles; the patient has difficulty holding a pen and his writing becomes smaller. The muscular rigidity causes a 'poverty of movement', with lack of blinking and a loss of the normal facial expression, producing a 'mask-like' facies. The patient walks with short, shuffling steps, does not swing his arms, and becomes stooped—the diagnosis is often obvious when he enters the room. His voice becomes low and monotonous and all movements are performed slowly. He chews his food slowly, but swallowing is little impaired as it is only the voluntary muscles that are involved. Though the muscles have increased tone, there are no reflex changes and no true paralysis, rather a restriction of movement. Bladder function is preserved. A useful sign is the glabellar tap sign—when the forehead of the patient with parkinsonism is tapped, he keeps on blinking, unlike the normal person.

In idiopathic parkinsonism, Parkinson's disease, the intellect is preserved and the patient can continue to read and participate in business and social affairs. However, he may become depressed with advancement of symptoms over the years, tending to shun company and sitting expressionless in a chair.

In arteriosclerotic parkinsonism, there may be repeated small strokes and associated urinary incontinence and progressive dementia.

Patients with advanced parkinsonism tend to become progressively immobile, taking to their beds if allowed to do so and dying of intercurrent infection.

Treatment
Drugs

Levodopa (*L·Dopa*) is now the drug of choice, and acts by increasing the content of dopamine in the basal ganglia. The initial dose is 250 mg given by mouth, gradually building up over a period of weeks to a maintenance dose of 1–5 G daily, depending on tolerance. Side-effects include gastric irritation and hypotension—if these occur, the dose is reduced and then progressively increased again. The drug benefits more than half those affected with parkinsonism, being especially useful in the idiopathic type. Rigidity is improved, movements become much freer, and there is a general improvement in well-being. The long-term results are not known. Tremor is but little improved.

Amantadine (Symmetrel), initially tried as an anti-viral agent in influenza, also benefits a proportion of patients, and can be used in those intolerant of levodopa; the dosage is simple, 100 mg once or twice daily, and no side effects have been reported. Amantadine is less effective than levodopa, but the drugs can be given together.

Atropine-like drugs. These probably act by their anti-cholinergic effect, which interferes with neurochemical transmission in the basal ganglia. A series of drugs has been developed, their principal effect again being to improve the rigidity rather than the tremor of parkinsonism. Though they have less tendency than atropine itself to cause drying of the mouth and visual upset, these will occur if the dose is pushed. These drugs include orphenadrine (Disipal), which has the advantage of a euphoriant (mood elevating) effect and benzhexol (Artane). Antihistamine drugs are also of some value.

Antidepressives such as imipramine (Tofranil) or amitriptyline (Tryptizol) may be indicated.

Surgery

This is the only measure that will benefit the tremor, and it may improve rigidity in addition. It is indicated in patients with severe unilateral tremor, but it can be carried out, one side at a time, in those with bilateral incapacitating tremor if their condition is otherwise good. The method is called stereotaxic surgery, and involves destruction, usually by electrocoagulation, of a small area of the thalamus having connections with the basal ganglia. The surgical lesion is made in the brain on the opposite side to the limbs affected and if successful, the tremor is completely abolished.

General measures

It is most important to encourage patients with Parkinson's disease to remain mobile and continue their daily duties as far as possible. Levodopa gives considerable assistance in achieving this. Sometimes short courses of physiotherapy with active exercises permit walking in a patient who would otherwise sit in a chair, and attendance at a Day Hospital or Centre may be helpful. If intercurrent illness demands bed rest, its duration should be as short as possible—it is important to get the patient ambulant. He requires time to take his meals, and may require to be fed. Care of the mouth, skin, bowels and bladder is important; coughing to clear secretions and deep breathing exercises may prevent pneumonia, to which patients are prone. Infections demand the use of appropriate antibacterial drugs.

Other disorders of the basal ganglia

Rheumatic (Sydenham's) chorea occurs in children as a complication of rheumatic fever, but is now rare. There are rapid purposeless movements of the face, tongue (Jack-in-the-box tongue) and limbs, with emotional upset, and there may be cardiac involvement. A period of bed rest with sedation, and penicillin for the underlying streptococcal throat infection are indicated.

Huntington's chorea is a disorder of dominant-type inheritance—that is, half the children of a sufferer may be affected, but symptoms are delayed until adult life. There are irregular purposeless movements for which the drug reserpine is of some benefit, but there is an accompanying dementia and the course is a downhill one over a few years.

Wilson's disease, hepato-lenticular degeneration, is due to excessive copper deposition in the tissues, especially the liver, causing cirrhosis, and the basal ganglia. Deposits in the cornea cause a brown Kayser-Fleischer ring. Symptoms include tremor, rigidity and dysarthria. Treatment includes penicillamine, a 'chelating' agent which binds and removes the excessive copper and may benefit a condition otherwise fatal in a few years.

Athetosis is a description for writhing, purposeless movements due to disorder of the basal ganglia. This and other abnormal movements may complicate cerebrovascular disease but their cause is often unknown.

Some disorders of the cranial nerves

The *first (olfactory) cranial nerve* may be damaged in fractures of the base of the skull, leading to loss of the sense of smell (anosmia). Anosmia may also follow virus infections, and disturbance of the sense of smell may result from deep seated lesions in the brain, sometimes associated with temporal lobe epilepsy.

Second (optic) nerve—conveys the impulses of vision from the retina to the occipital lobe of the cortex, where they are appreciated as sight. Each nerve runs backwards to the optic chiasma (near the pituitary gland) where the inner fibres from each eye cross to the opposite side and pass backwards in the optic tract and optic radiation. This part is commonly involved by a stroke, for it is just behind the internal capsule of the brain. A stroke affecting the left optic radiation causes a failure of sight from the left halves of both retinae producing a right visual field defect—the patient cannot see objects on his right side. The right arm and leg will also be affected by the stroke. Tumours in the region of the pituitary gland may encroach on the optic chiasma causing visual field defects.

The optic nerve head can be seen as the 'optic disc' with the ophthalmoscope. It may be affected by hypertension, and by raised intracranial pressure causing blurring or papilloedema, though vision need not be affected at this stage.

The optic nerve may be involved, just behind the eyeball ('retro-bulbar neuritis'), by conditions including disseminated sclerosis, syphilis, vitamin B group deficiency—especially vitamin B_{12} deficiency (pernicious anaemia) in association with excessive tobacco smoking (tobacco amblyopia), and in methanol (wood alcohol) poisoning. In such conditions there may be patchy loss of the visual fields; these blind spots or 'scotomas' are detectable by the instrument called the perimeter. Later there may be optic atrophy, seen with the ophthalmoscope as pallor of the disc.

The *third, fourth and sixth cranial nerves* supply the muscles to the eyeballs. Paralysis may cause squint, or there may be double vision (diplopia) as binocular vision depends on the axes of the eyes being completely parallel. Transient paralysis may occur in multiple sclerosis and in diabetes mellitus.

The third nerve (oculo-motor nerve) also carries autonomic (parasympathetic) fibres to the muscles constricting the pupil, and the muscles of accommodation of the lens. A space-occupying lesion may cause irritation and then paralysis of this nerve, with a fixed dilated pupil on the affected side. Pupillary inequalities and changes are important signs of rising intracranial pressure or of an expanding lesion such as a haematoma after head injury. Argyll Robertson pupils—bilaterally small and failing to react to light—are found in tabes dorsalis and G.P.I. from syphilitic involvement of the third nerve nuclei.

A fixed small pupil may occur in *Horner's syndrome*, from paralysis of the sympathetic nerve supply and resultant over-activity of the parasympathetic constrictor fibres. The sympathetic fibres arise in the neck and are involved by a neoplastic process such as carcinoma of the lung.

The *fifth (trigeminal) nerve* is mainly sensory from the face, and has three divisions—the upper or ophthalmic supplying part of the forehead and eye, the middle supplying the skin over the maxilla or upper jaw, and the lower or mandibular division supplying the lower jaw. Herpes zoster commonly occurs in the ophthalmic division, causing pain and vesicular eruption over the part.

TRIGEMINAL NEURALGIA

Trigeminal neuralgia is a condition usually affecting the maxillary division. The patient, often elderly, has bouts of severe knife-like pain often brought on by trivial stimuli such as a cold wind, or simply touching the face. The cause probably lies in the central connections of the nerve. The drug carbamazepine (Tegretol) often relieves the condition, rendering unnecessary neurosurgical procedures such as injection of alcohol into the nerve, or root section.

The *seventh (facial) nerve* supplies the muscles to the face, which it reaches after traversing a bony canal related to the middle ear and mastoid process—infections here used to caused facial paralysis.

BELLS PALSY

Bell's palsy is a paralysis due to inflammation of the facial nerve, of unknown cause, within its bony canal. There is sagging of the facial muscles, inability to close the eye and to chew properly on the affected side. While mild cases often clear up spontaneously within a week or ten days, injections of A.C.T.H. are now generally recommended as soon as the diagnosis is made. This drug limits the inflammatory oedema, and by preventing undue compression of the nerve may speed return of normal function, and obviate the permanent paralysis that used to be seen in a few cases.

The *eighth (auditory) nerve* has two sections, the *acoustic* concerned with hearing, and the *vestibular* concerned with bodily position in space and equilibrium and, through its connections with the brain stem and cerebellum, with balance. Disorders of the inner ear and its vestibular connections may cause bouts of *vertigo* (spinning of objects or of self) and *vomiting*, worse when the head is moved. Mild epidemics of this condition, *Vestibular neuronitis*, presumed to be viral, may occur and the patient lies stock-still in bed afraid to move for fear of precipitating an attack. Drugs such as prochlorperazine (Stemetil) and cinnarizine (Stugeron) may be helpful. Motion sickness occurs in those who have an abnormally sensitive balance organ, and the best preventive is hyoscine 0·6 mg an hour before the journey.

A tumour called an acoustic neuroma involves the nerve at the cerebello-pontine angle and in addition to deafness and vertigo, encroachment on the fifth and seventh nerves causes loss of the corneal reflex so that the eye fails to blink when the cornea is touched. The cerebral spinal fluid protein content is raised. Operative removal may be possible.

MÉNIÈRE'S DISEASE

Ménière's disease occurs in the elderly—there is increasing deafness, tinnitus (noises in the ear) and paroxisms of vertigo and vomiting. The cause probably lies in the inner ear and operative destruction with ultrasound is sometimes justified.

Excessive doses of the drugs streptomycin and gentamicin, especially in those where renal failure impedes excretion, may cause an irreversible destruction of the vestibular division of the eighth nerve, and was tried in the treatment of Ménière's disease.

The *ninth (glosso-pharyngeal) nerve* includes sensory fibres from the back of the tongue and mouth, some motor fibres to the pharynx and secretory fibres to the parotid gland, one of the salivary glands. It is rarely involved alone.

The *tenth* or *vagus nerve*, in addition to forming the largest part of the parasympathetic division of the autonomic nervous system, supplies the muscles of the pharynx and larynx. The nuclei of the vagus and other cranial nerves in the medulla each receive fibres from both pyramidal tracts. While a lower motor neurone lesion will of course cause paralysis, symptoms of which may be slight in unilateral cases, a lesion of the upper motor neurone confined to one side will not result in paralysis, though there may be transient weakness. Involvement of the nuclei of both vagus nerves may occur in bulbar paralysis or following bilateral strokes, and there is dysphagia, dysarthria and inability to cough. The fibres of the vagus which serve the vocal chord have a long course in the recurrent laryngeal nerve, which on the left side arises from the vagus at the root of the lung. This nerve is liable to be involved by tumours of the lung or mediastinum in its long ascent to reach the vocal chord, paralysis of one side of which may point to such a lesion. The parasympathetic fibres, which constitute the bulk of the vagus, have a wide distribution to the heart, stomach, small intestine and part of the large intestine. Surgical section, *vagotomy*, reduces gastric acid secretion and is used in the treatment of peptic ulcer.

The *eleventh (accessory) nerve* carries motor fibres to the muscles of the shoulder and is rarely involved in isolation.

The *twelfth (hypoglossal) nerve* supplies the muscles of the tongue. Following a stroke, the tongue may be temporarily paralysed on the hemiplegic side and when protruded will be pushed over to that side by the unopposed action of the muscles of its other half. In motor neurone disease, the tongue is sometimes contracted and stiff.

Headache

Headache is a common symptom which generally has no serious cause, but it can be associated with organic disorder. The brain itself is insensitive to pain but intracranial structures such as the arteries and meninges are pain-sensitive, and traction on certain parts causes pain. The extra-cranial arteries are also pain-sensitive. Spasm of the cervical muscles also results in pain.

CAUSES OF HEADACHE

Vascular

The headache accompanying fever is probably due to dilatation of intracranial arteries. Migraine headache is due to dilatation of extra-cranial arteries in the external carotid system. The same mechanism explains the headache that may occur with internal carotid artery thrombosis, though most patients with strokes do not complain of headache. Headache may occur in cerebral haemorrhage before consciousness is lost—in subarachnoid haemorrhage there is severe occipital headache and neck stiffness, and there may have been premonitory neck-ache from leakage of the aneurysm a few days earlier.

Temporal (cranial) arteritis is one of the connective-tissue, auto-immune diseases and is an inflammation of the arteries of the skull, with headache and tenderness at the temple, usually unilaterally. The condition may involve the retinal arteries, leading to blindness and it is commonest in elderly men. The E.S.R. is raised. Treatment is with steroids such as prednisone.

Headache on wakening may occur in hypertension, but in fact headache is not a common complaint in hypertension, and is only severe in advanced cases.

Tumour and raised intracranial pressure

Tumour may cause headache, its site being of localizing value. It is dull in character, rarely severe and tends to occur early in the day.

Though raised intracranial pressure from any cause can produce a generalized headache, its intensity need not be related to the height of the pressure, and sometimes there is no headache.

Inflammation and irritation

Meningitis and encephalitis can cause severe headache. There is also neck-ache and neck stiffness. Occipital headache and neck stiffness occurs also in subarachnoid haemorrhage.

Sinusitis—stuffy, headachy feelings and tenderness over the affected part.

Eye causes—'eye-strain' from refractive errors may cause evening headaches, but this is probably uncommon. More important is glaucoma—raised intra-ocular pressure, with risk of loss of vision, and often accompanying vomiting—as a cause of headache in the elderly.

Cervical spondylosis—tension headache

This is a form of arthritis affecting the cervical spine. There is associated muscle spasm with pain and tenderness at the neck, often spreading to cause a generalized headache. Symptoms are worse in tense, anxious patients, their state probably contributing to increase muscle tension—tension headache. Such a headache may complicate that of migraine.

Depression

Depression and psychogenic factors lie behind many chronic or recurrent headaches, muscle tension making the symptoms worse. It is of course, important to exclude any of the above organic causes.

TREATMENT

Treatment is that of the cause. Aspirin may be used symptomatically, but may provoke haematemesis and its long-term use causes anaemia from gastric blood loss. Phenacetin in excess may actually cause headache, and as its long-term use is associated with renal damage, it has been largely replaced by other drugs, such as paracetamol, a phenacetin derivative. However, paracetamol can itself cause hepatic damage taken in excess. Thus the occasional use of such analgesics to relieve a headache may be justified, but their long-term use is undesirable.

Disorders of sleep

The state of consciousness, of being awake, is due to the activity of the central reticular formation, acting like a beacon from the base of the brain. When the activity of this system is lowered, sleep results.

It is not known why the activity is lowered at night—regulation must depend on some internal 'clock' which controls this, and other bodily rhythms—perhaps from the hypothalamus. There are two types of sleep, deep sleep, and a lighter type of sleep associated with dreaming and rapid eye movements—deep sleep may be required to restore physical function, rapid-eye-movement (R.E.M.) sleep to restore mental function. The E.E.G. shows characteristic patterns during sleep. Sleep deprivation causes irritability and slight memory upset with impaired concentration, but these disappear when normal sleep can be resumed. Lack of sleep is not in itself serious, but people tend to worry if they do not have a good night's sleep, and this anxiety is usually the cause of symptoms attributed to the lack of sleep.

Disorders of the hypothalamus, as in encephalitis or tumour involvement, may cause disturbance of sleep rhythm, so that the patient turns night into day. New and unfamiliar ward surroundings often upset elderly patients making them confused, with sleepless nights until they become used to their environment, when a normal sleep rhythm becomes re-established.

Difficulty in sleeping may occur with pain or respiratory embarrassment, but the most common reasons are anxiety, when there is difficulty in getting off to sleep, and depressive illness. In depression, the patient may wake in the early hours of the morning and cannot get back to sleep. Early waking may result from the taking of alcohol the previous evening.

Management

It was traditional to prescribe sleeping drugs for patients in hospital and some may feel cheated if these are withheld. Moreover, many middle-aged people are accustomed to taking sleeping drugs, often for no good reason. There is no justification for the widespread use of such drugs in or out of hospital.

Attention to *simple points in patient care* is preferable—a quiet ward, a comfortable bed with a soft pillow of accustomed height and warm feet, with bed socks if desired—all contribute to a good night's sleep. Many people sleep better if they have a warm drink and light snack shortly before retiring, but of course a full bladder will disturb sleep.

It is illogical to prescribe a potentially harmful drug for a condition that is not serious. If drugs have to be used to procure sleep, then their use should be temporary. Barbiturates are cheap, effective and widely prescribed, but carry a risk of misuse and over-dosage, especially in patients who are depressed. Chloral hydrate is effective and its unpleasant taste may contribute to its safety—there are several proprietary preparations which are more palatable. Attempts have been made to produce drugs without the 'hangover' effect and overdosage risks of the barbiturates—the former aim has not really been achieved, but the latter hazard has been minimized by drugs such as nitrazepam (Mogadon).

A good night's sleep may contribute to recovery—and it is best if sleep comes naturally.

Coma

Coma is an abnormal state of depression of consciouness.

ASSESSING THE DEPTH OF COMA
The degree of loss of consciousness is graded thus:

(i) Drowsy but responds to commands.
(ii) Unconscious but responds to mild stimuli—e.g. pinching the skin.
(iii) Unconscious and responds only to maximal painful stimuli— e.g. rubbing the sternum with the clenched fist, or pressing on the supraorbital ridges.
(iv) Unconscious and completely unresponsive to stimuli.

The size or reaction of the pupils, and the state of the limb reflexes are *not* good guides to the depth of coma. Avoid using words such as torpor or stupor—they mean different things to different people. What is required is a statement of the depth of the coma, as described.

PROCEDURE WHEN CONFRONTED WITH A PATIENT IN COMA
1. *Take immediate steps to maintain life*
clear the airway, remove dentures, turn the patient on his side and support the chin; insert airway if available.
if breathing has stopped, apply mouth to mouth respiration (or Ambu bag).
feel for the pulse or listen for the heart beat—if absent, raise the legs, give a sharp thump on the chest, call for assistance; if still no heart beat, apply cardiac massage and proceed with

artificial respiration; take E.C.G. if available, and consider immediate electrical defibrillation if defibrillator is to hand.

2. *Take stock of the general situation* if breathing is established and the heart beating—the condition is no longer desperate and it is important to avoid panic. Look for circumstantial evidence—seek witnesses or relatives, look for tablets, preserve any vomit or urine.

3. *Consider the likely causes and proceed with treatment.*

COMMON CAUSES OF COMA AND CLUES TO THEM

(i) *Injury*—circumstances, bruising of skull, bleeding from nose or ears implies fracture; transitory loss of consciousness followed by deeper coma suggests expanding haemtoma— extradural or subdural haemorrhage; pupils here may be unequal.

(ii) *Cerebro-vascular accident*—stroke with hemiplegia.
                                   subarachnoid haemorrhage (neck stiffness).
Cardio-vascular causes are less likely but consider Stokes-Adams attack.

(iii) *Epilepsy*—usually convulsions, plus history.

(iv) *Poisoning*—barbiturates: patient deeply 'asleep'.
                  alcohol; breath may smell.
Aspirin alone does not cause loss of consciousness.

(v) *Hypoglycaemia* in diabetics—sudden onset, sweating—give sugar if able to swallow, glucagon 1 mg by intramuscular injection if not. Or inject 25 per cent Dextrose solution intravenously.

(vi) *Diabetic Coma—Ketosis*—gradual onset, dry tongue, 'air-hunger', urine contains sugar and ketones; blood (finger-prick) Dextrostix test shows high glucose, over 175 mg/100 ml.

Coma in infections such as meningitis is of gradual onset, as is that in uraemia and hepatic coma and here there is a history of disease. Endocrine causes such as myxoedema, Addison's disease (hypoadrenalism) and hypopituitarism are rare, usually follow neglect of treatment.

Bear in mind *hypothermia in the elderly* as a cause of coma— living alone, cold house, may have infection; cold skin, rectal temperature below 95°F (35°C).

GENERAL MANAGEMENT OF COMA

The care of a patient in coma is described under Cerebrovascular disease, a very common cause—the importance of maintaining the airway usually by nursing on the side, with frequent turning to avoid bed-sores and allow aeration of the lungs, care of the mouth, bladder and bowel, and attention to fluid requirements cannot be over-emphasized.

Successful management is a tribute to good nursing care.

The management of specific causes of coma is considered in the appropriate sections of the book.

Spinal cord compression

The spinal cord runs from the foramen magnum of the skull, where it is continuous with the medulla, and ends at the lower level of the first lumbar vertebra. In its course, it gives off and receives the motor and sensory nerve roots, being protected in front by the bodies of the vertebrae (separated by the discs) and surrounded by the neural arches of the vertebrae behind.

CAUSES OF SPINAL CORD DAMAGE

1. *Compression*
    (a) *Trauma*—following crush fractures, or fracture-dislocation of the vertebrae.
    (b) *Vertebral disease* and spontaneous fracture, as in tumour, myeloma, or tuberculosis affecting one or more vertebrae, causing their sudden collapse.
    (c) *Prolapsed intervertebral disc* in the cervical (or dorsal) spine— usually the associated *cervical spondylosis* causes earlier signs, however.
    (d) *Tumour*—*primary*—rare—may be inside the cord, or affect the meninges or nerve root, pushing on the cord; neurofibroma is one such tumour, is benign, and may occur as part of neurofibromatosis, von Recklinghausen's disease, with skin modules and patchy brown pigmentation.
        Secondary—metastases from carcinoma (lung, breast, prostate) or deposits in a reticulosis such as Hodgkin's disease.
    (e) *Extra-dural abscess*—often staphylococcal from sepsis elsewhere, which may not be obvious.

2. *Arteriosclerosis*

Thrombosis of the anterior spinal artery (a single vessel formed by a branch from each vertebral artery) which serves the upper and anterior part of the cord. It may be affected by any of the above lesions.

3. *Transverse myelitis*—as part of encephalomyelitis, or in meningo-vascular syphilis.

EFFECTS

Transection of the cord above the fourth cervical level is incompatible with life. Transection at a lower level affects the *long tracts* thus:

(i) *Pyramidal tracts*—causes paralysis below the lesion; quadriplegia is paralysis of arms and legs, the more common paraplegia is paralysis of the legs.

(ii) *Ascending sensory tracts*—results in complete loss of sensation below the lesion.

(iii) *Tracts controlling bladder* and rectum—causes disturbance of micturition and sometimes of defaecation.

(iv) *Nuclei of the sympathetic in the cord*—affection causes hypotension and loss of sweating.

Spinal cord compression has the same effects, to varying degree. The unusual event of a lesion affecting the cord unilaterally may cause an upper motor neurone type paralysis on the same side, with loss of pain and temperature sensation on the other side, as the latter fibres cross on entering the cord (Brown-Séquard Syndrome). In addition to these long tract effects, spinal cord compression may be associated with pain and sensory disturbance (including hyperalgesia, increased susceptibility to pain) at the site of the lesion. This may be of localizing value in a slowly developing lesion, but is over-shadowed by the acute long tract effects if the lesion is a sudden one.

ACUTE SPINAL CORD DAMAGE OR COMPRESSION

This is usually due to injury or sudden collapse of a diseased vertebrae, the damage is severe and the cord lesion irreversible.

Immediately after the event, there is a period of spinal shock which gradually passes off over 3–6 weeks. During the period of spinal shock, there is flaccid paralysis of the muscles below the level of the injury, as well as sensory loss with liability to sores and ulcers, retention of urine and circulatory disturbance, including hypotension and cold or blue skin. As the state of spinal shock passes off, reflex activity returns to the limbs and slight stimulus may provoke painful spasm. Due to the pyramidal tract involvement, the limbs become spastic—spastic paraplegia, with brisk jerks and extensor plantar responses and of course there is no return of voluntary power, nor of sensation. The bladder regains some tone and empties automatically when slightly distended.

Management of the paraplegic is carried out in special centres. During the stage of spinal shock, attention to the position of the limbs, frequent turning and catheterization are required. When the bladder regains some tone training to 'void by the clock' helped by pressure on the suprapubic muscles may allow some degree of urinary continence, and a portable urinal may be used. Faecal retention and incontinence can usually be obviated by a suppository or enema twice weekly. Subsequent rehabilitation often allows the patient some measure of independence.

GRADUAL SPINAL CORD COMPRESSION

This may present as spastic weakness in the legs, usually symmetrically, from bilateral pyramidal tract involvement with upper-motor-neurone lesion signs including brisk jerks and extensor plantar responses. There is varying sensory loss. There may be urgency of micturition or incontinence, and it is surprising that the patient may sometimes not complain of this, but admit to it only on questioning.

Usually there are some localizing features at the site of the lesion —pain and tenderness over a vertebra, or root or girdle pain from irritation of the nerve roots, sometimes with a band of hyperalgesia, so that pin-prick is felt more severely than normally. Root pain is worsened by coughing or straining.

In addition, there may be evidence of a lesion such as a primary tumour elsewhere.

Further investigations

X-ray of spine (which may show vertebral involvement).

Lumbar puncture: blockage of the C.S.F. circulation may be revealed by compressing each jugular vein in turn (Queckenstedt's test), when the normal rise and fall of C.S.F. pressure will be absent. Complete blockage, Froin's syndrome, causes yellow C.S.F. with a high protein content, so that it may actually coagulate.

Myelography (injection of radio-opaque oil into the subarachnoid space at lumbar puncture) will localize the level and may indicate the nature of the spinal block.

It is not always wise to carry out lumbar puncture, for removing the C.S.F. below a block may render it difficult to enter the subarachnoid space for myelography.

Treatment

Patients with suspected spinal cord compression should be transferred to a neurosurgical unit for further investigation and treatment. The development of disturbances of micturition makes such transfer urgent for at this stage damage to the cord may be irreversible.

Surgical measures such as laminectomy (removal of the neural arch of a vertebra) or drainage of an abscess may take the pressure off the cord and allow rapid improvement in symptoms. It may also be possible to remove a tumour, with complete recovery if the tumour is benign.

X-ray therapy may be of value in some primary malignant tumours or metastases, and in reticuloses such as Hodgkin's disease.

In the few cases where the spinal cord damage is in fact a myelitis, appropriate drug therapy is indicated (e.g. penicillin for meningovascular syphilis, steroids for allergic encephalomyelitis).

In patients whose spinal cord lesion is not amenable to such measures, or in whom irreversible damage to the long tracts has occurred, treatment is that of the paraplegic patient with good nursing, frequent turning, care of the bladder and bowel, and rehabilitation where possible. Patients with advanced malignant disease will require analgesics, including the proper use of opiates to prevent pain and suffering.

Other disorders of the spinal cord

SYRINGOMYELIA

This is a rare disorder and is due to a dilatation of the central canal of the spinal cord, usually in the cervical region. The word syringomyelia has the same derivation as syringe, meaning a pipe or tube.

Syringomyelia presents in young adults as loss of pain and temperature sensation in the fingertips. These fibres cross in the mid-line, but the fibres supplying touch sensation are on the surface of the cord and are not involved. The patient may burn his fingers without realising it. Later, motor fibres are involved with muscular weakness.

The condition was ascribed to some developmental abnormality with cyst formation in the cord, and there may be associated congenital defects. Recently it has been realized that the cord dilatation may be due to a high internal cerebro-spinal fluid pressure, drainage being obstructed by developmental faults at the foramen magnum of the skull.

Myelography may therefore be indicated to reveal such a lesion, and surgical correction may be possible in some cases of an otherwise incurable condition.

SUBACUTE COMBINED DEGENERATION OF THE SPINAL CORD

This is due to vitamin B_{12} deficiency. There is degeneration of the pyramidal tracts, causing spastic paralysis, and of the posterior columns, causing sensory loss and ataxia. (There may also be some degeneration of the peripheral nerves.)

Usually the condition is seen only in those with advanced pernicious anaemia, but sometimes it occurs before there are gross blood changes. Physical signs include loss of vibration sense and extensor plantar responses. Any suspicion of such a condition should lead to testing the serum B_{12} level, which will be low. Treatment with injections of hydroxocobalamin (Neo-cytamen) will prevent deterioration, but will not affect existing cord damage. (Folic acid should not be used in treatment, for while it may have a beneficial effect on the anaemia, it may mask and indeed contribute to deterioration of the cord lesions.)

MOTOR NEURONE DISEASE

This is a relatively rare condition, of unknown cause, occurring in middle-aged men (women are seldom affected).

There is progressive degeneration of the anterior horn cells of the spinal cord, and of similar motor neurones in the brain stem. The small muscles of the hands are usually first affected, then the arm and shoulder muscles with weakness, wasting and atrophy. This part of the condition is called progressive muscular atrophy. The wasting muscles show a tremor or twitching of their fibres called fasciculation or fibrillation. Brain stem affection causes progressive bulbar palsy with dysphagia and drooling of saliva, dysarthria, and inability to cough. Secretions and food may be inhaled, with danger of pneumonia.

The condition also includes degeneration of the pyramidal tracts in the cord, amyotrophic lateral sclerosis causing spastic weakness and ultimately paralysis of the legs. Thus in motor neurone disease there is a combination of muscle wasting, mainly in the arms from the lower motor neurone element, and spastic weakness in the legs from pyramidal tract, upper motor neurone, involvement. There are no sensory changes. Disturbance of bladder control is unusual until the later stages.

There is no effective treatment, and it is therefore important to differentiate treatable conditions such as cervical spondylosis, described below.

In motor neurone disease there is progressive deterioration over a few years. The final result of this distressing condition may be a bedridden patient, in whom intellect and insight are retained but who succumbs to pressure sores, urinary infection, or, more commonly, pneumonia.

FRIEDREICH'S ATAXIA (HEREDITARY SPINO-CEREBELLAR ATAXIA)

This is one of a group of rare inherited disorders; its genetic basis is not understood. There is degeneration of the posterior columns of the cord, the lateral columns, and tracts leading to the cerebellum, and the optic nerves may be affected.

Symptoms appear before the age of twenty, the presenting complaint being unsteadiness in walking—ataxia, followed by weakness in the legs and clumsiness of the hands. Associated defects include club-foot and scoliosis (curvature of the spine), and there may be degeneration of the heart muscle with E.C.G. changes.

The disease is a slowly progressive one, the patient becoming increasingly ataxic and paralysed over the years, and there is no effective treatment.

PERONEAL MUSCULAR ATROPHY (CHARCOT-MARIE-TOOTH'S DISEASE)

This rare condition is usually inherited as a dominant, but sporadic cases also occur. The disease begins in children or adolescents and is more common in boys.

There is atrophy of anterior horn cells and their peripheral nerve fibres, leading to weakness, paralysis and wasting of the muscles of the legs and lower thirds of the thighs. As the name implies, the peroneal muscles are first to be affected, causing foot drop and a high 'stepping' gait. The arm muscles may be affected. Sometimes the sensory tracts are involved with varying degree of loss of sensation over the affected muscles. Despite the muscle wasting, power in the limbs may be quite well preserved, so that a reasonably active life is possible. Progression of the disease is very gradual, and spontaneous arrest can occur. There is no effective treatment but calipers and other appliances may aid mobility.

A NOTE ON INHERITED NEUROPATHIES AND MUSCULAR
DYSTROPHY

Peroneal muscular atrophy is one of a group of rare inherited neuropathies, a term applied to any disturbance of nerve function, whether arising in the nerve cell or peripherally. In some of these conditions, an underlying metabolic or enzyme defect has been recognized. Such conditions may be difficult to separate from those in the group called muscular dystrophy and indeed, in some of the latter, the underlying abnormality may be in the motor nerve supply rather than in the muscle itself.

Muscular dystrophy (the inherited myopathies), and *myasthenia gravis* (a disorder of the neuromuscular junction) are more conveniently grouped, for clinical purposes, as Disorders of Muscle, and are described in Chapter 15.

Disorders of the nerve roots and peripheral nerves

A nerve fibre can be involved by disease anywhere in its long course from the spinal cord to the periphery. The fault may lie in the nerve cell or its axon (peripheral process), in the insulating myelin sheath, or in the connective tissue binding the fibres to form the nerve trunk. The fault can be the result of many processes—compression and irritation, inflammation, infection, and metabolic or vascular upset. Involvement of the nerve fibre leads to impairment of conduction, whether motor or sensory, and this may be followed by degeneration. If, however, the causative process is reversible then, provided the nerve cell is intact, gradual regeneration of the nerve will occur.

The term neuropathy refers to any disturbance of the nerve or its roots but its clinical use is often restricted to disorders of the peripheral nerves.

'Neuritis' literally means inflammation of a nerve, but as the condition is not always an inflammatory one, and as the word neuritis has rather loose connotations (being synonymous with 'pain' to many people), the term neuropathy is generally preferable.

CLASSIFICATION OF NERVE DISORDERS:

A. *Nerve root disorders*

These include conditions such as tabes dorsalis which are part of a more generalized neurological disease, and we have seen above that spinal cord tumours can cause root involvement. However, the commonest disorder affecting the nerve roots is *degenerative arthritis of the spine*, especially *cervical spondylosis* causing *pains in the arm*, and *lumbar* spine affection causing *sciatica*.

B. *Peripheral nerve disorders*

1. *Entrapment neuropathies*

Here a nerve (or nerves) is trapped by overlying structures, and compressed. The group includes: *cervical outlet syndrome—'cervical rib'*. and *carpal tunnel syndrome (median nerve* compression).

2. *Mononeuropathy*

This is the involvement of one nerve by injury, or by any pathological process.

3. *Peripheral neuropathy—polyneuropathy—peripheral neuritis*

Here there is involvement of the peripheral nerves bilaterally and symmetrically, and as the longest nerve fibres are the most vulnerable to damage, the neuropathy commonly affects the distal parts, such as the feet and legs, with both motor and sensory involvement to varying degree, but to an equal extent in both limbs.

A. **Nerve root disorders. Arthritis of the spine**

THE NATURE OF ARTHRITIS OF THE SPINE—SPONDYLOSIS

The vertebral bodies are separated by the intervertebral discs, tough rubbery structures which contribute to the resilience of the spine. With advancing age the discs tend to dry and 'perish' causing stresses on the spinal joints and resulting in a form of degenerative osteoarthritis or arthrosis, with the formation of little bony outgrowths called 'osteophytes' at the vertebral margins. These encroach on the nerve roots. There is also a varying degree of backward prolapse of the degenerate disc. The whole process is termed 'spondylosis' and, it affects the parts of the spine which have most movement and most wear-and-tear. Thus some degree of spondylosis in the neck region is almost invariable in persons beyond middle-age—this is *cervical spondylosis*. The lumbar spine is also commonly affected but the term arthritis is usually retained to describe the condition here.

CERVICAL SPONDYLOSIS AND ITS EFFECTS

(i) *Nerve root pressure*

In the cervical region spondylosis affects the intervertebral joints from the fifth to the seventh vertebrae and may result in irritation and compression of the nerve roots serving the shoulder and arm, usually more marked on one side.

There may be aching at the neck and movements are restricted. There is muscle spasm and tenderness at this region.

Discomfort, tingling sensation, or pain is felt in the part of the arm served by the affected nerve root or roots, the outer (radial) border of the arm being commonly involved. There may be some diminution of appreciation of light touch or pin-prick within the affected *dermatome*, the area of skin supplied by that nerve, but complete sensory loss is unusual. Motor symptoms such as muscular weakness are usually slight, and any muscle wasting is seldom gross, but there may be some diminution of the tendon reflexes in the arm.

X-rays of the cervical spine will confirm the existence of spondylosis. (It should be noted that cervical spondylosis is common, and may not cause any symptoms.)

Treatment: Immobilization of the neck for a few weeks with a felt or polystyrene collar, neck traction and exercises at the physiotherapy department and local heat are usually helpful, the affected nerve root apparently accustoming itself to the lesion so that symptoms gradually settle.

(ii) *Cervical myelopathy—cord compression*

Sometimes cervical spondylosis is more severe and a backward protruding disc may cause compression of the spinal artery or the cord itself, producing pyramidal tract signs of leg spasticity in addition to the above.

(iii) *Vertebro-basilar ischaemia*

The vertebral arteries pass upwards through foramina in the transverse processes of the cervical vertebrae and may be compressed by the osteophytic outgrowths in spondylosis, or nipped during stooping, resulting in brain-stem ischaemia.

EFFECTS OF ARTHRITIS OF THE LUMBAR SPINE—LUMBAGO AND SCIATICA

The degenerative changes in the lumbar spine may be a cause of low back ache or *lumbago*. Protrusion of a disc may occur acutely after sudden flexion, as in stooping to pick up a heavy bucket. *The first sacral nerve root* is often compressed, it contributes largely to the sciatic nerve. The patient experiences sudden pain down the back of the thigh and leg—'*sciatica*'. There may be loss of the ankle jerk and pain on attempting to raise the leg to a right-angle. Usually rest on a hard bed for two to three weeks suffices in treatment, but surgical removal of the prolapsed disc may be necessary.

B. Disorders of the peripheral nerves

ENTRAPMENT NEUROPATHIES

Cervical outlet syndrome, cervical rib, scalenus anticus or costoclavicular syndrome

All these terms are used to describe a lesion which causes compression of the brachial plexus of nerves at the root of the neck. Usually it is the lowest trunk of the brachial plexus which is involved. The eighth cervical and first thoracic nerves, emerging from the vertebral column, go to form this trunk which lies on the first rib behind the subclavian artery and the scalenus anticus (scalenus anterior) muscle, which are in turn protected in front by the clavicle. An extra, cervical, rib, or anomalies of structures between the first rib and the clavicle cause narrowing of this space, the cervical outlet, resulting in pressure on the nerve trunk.

There is sensory disturbance usually along the inner (ulnar) border of the arm and hand, but, as is the case also in cervical spondylosis, the changes are less discrete than if a single peripheral nerve were involved. Muscle weakness and wasting are also described. Such symptoms might be worsened by drooping of the shoulder girdle or the carrying of heavy weights. Cervical-rib syndrome was blamed for arm pains especially in middle-aged women but it is now believed that the carpal tunnel syndrome is a more usual cause. Thus operations such as removal of cervical ribs are seldom indicated.

(Some symptoms ascribed to cervical rib may really result from narrowing or thrombosis of the compressed *subclavian artery* and ischaemia of the limb. The 'subclavian-steal' syndrome may be referred to here—it is a disturbance of consciousness from vertebro-basilar ischaemia during active use of the arm in the presence of arteriosclerosis of the cerebral arteries. The blood supply to the brain may depend on an adequate vertebral artery supply in such cases, and the demands of the arm muscles during activity result in insufficient blood reaching the brain through the vertebral artery, which is a branch of the subclavian.

The cause of the '*shoulder-hand*' *syndrome*, aching and muscular weakness affecting the left shoulder and hand after myocardial infarction, is uncertain, but may be due to autonomic disturbances of the circulation to the part.)

Carpal tunnel syndrome

The *median nerve* may be compressed as it passes through the fibrous tunnel at the wrist on its way to serve the hand. This causes the *carpal tunnel syndrome*—pain and tingling in the hand and fingers, especially those on the medial side of the hand, often occurring by night. There may also be discomfort more widely felt at the wrist with tenderness over the fibrous tunnel, and wasting of the small muscles at the base of the thumb, some of which are supplied by the median nerve.

The condition is not uncommon in middle-aged women and is sometimes associated with arthritis or undue use of the wrist. It may also occur in pregnancy, from fluid retention and tissue swelling; and in myxoedema (hypothyroidism) and acromegaly (a result of hyperpituitarism).

Treatment. Mild cases may be helped by simple splinting of the wrist to prevent undue movement by night, or by injections of hydrocortisone locally. Surgical division of the fibrous tissue of the 'tunnel' is justified in severe cases, and produces dramatic relief.

Meralgia paraesthetica

The lateral cutaneous nerve of the thigh is sometimes affected by compression at the inguinal ligament causing discomfort or tingling, and a patch of sensory loss, at the outer aspect of the thigh. This sometimes arises after an operation or period of bed rest, and usually clears up spontaneously in a few weeks.

MONONEUROPATHY

This refers to the effects of a lesion of an individual peripheral nerve. It results in localized symptoms related to the distribution of that nerve. The commonest cause is trauma. In the arm, the radial nerve is very liable to be damaged in its long winding course round the humerus—and it may also be affected in the axilla from prolonged hanging of the arm over a chair ('Saturday night' or 'drunkards' paralysis). The radial nerve is mainly motor, and the lesion results in inability to extend the wrist and fingers.

Sometimes diabetes is complicated by an isolated paralysis of the lateral rectus muscle of the eye causing diplopia (double-vision) from a lesion of the sixth cranial nerve, but diabetic neuropathy is more commonly of the symmetrical distal type affecting the legs.

Multiple isolated nerve lesions may occur in leprosy and the connective-tissue diseases when the term mononeuropathy multiplex is applied. If the lesions are sufficiently widespread the condition blends into that of polyneuropathy.

PERIPHERAL NEUROPATHY—POLYNEUROPATHY—PERIPHERAL NEURITIS

As noted, in this group of conditions the peripheral nerves are *symmetrically* involved. The longer the nerve fibre, the more liable it is to be damaged. Thus there are varying degrees of sensory disturbance and muscular weakness in the feet and limbs.

CAUSES

(i) *Toxic*

Lead, arsenic and heavy metals. Lead poisoning (e.g. inhalation of fumes from the burning of car batteries) causes motor-weakness without sensory loss (also constipation, anaemia and a blue-lead-line on the gums).

Triothocresyl phosphate (TOCP) and acrylamide, both used in plastics industry; TOCP was misused as cooking oil and resulted in outbreak in North Africa.

(ii) *Deficiency*

Vitamin B_1 and effects of alcohol; dry beri-beri may be due to multiple dietary deficiencies rather than deficiency of B_1 alone, and occurs in the underdeveloped countries. Alcoholic neuropathy is probably due in similar B vitamin deficiencies, for alcholics tend to neglect their food, but alcohol may have a direct toxic effect on the nerves. The symptoms are usually sensory ones in the legs and there are associated signs of alcoholism, including memory disturbance and cirrhosis of the liver.

Vitamin B_{12}—peripheral neuropathy can occur in pernicious anaemia—it is more common than subacute combined degeneration of the cord, but both conditions may be present.

pyridoxine (vitamin B_6)—deficiency may complicate isoniazid treatment of tuberculosis.

(iii) *Metabolic*

Diabetes; loss of sensation at the feet with tendency to ulcer formation absent vibration sense and reflexes; rarely motor weakness; often improves with good control.

Porphyria; a group of conditions due to disturbance of haemoglobin metabolism or liver defect, inherited, and the type found in South Africa was introduced by one girl during the Boer settlement. The disorders are rare, but the acute intermittent type presents as bouts of abdominal pain, from accompanying autonomic neuropathy, and may be associated with abnormal pigments in the urine which goes dark on standing, and it contains porphobilinogen, detected as for urobilinogen with Ehrlich's reagent or urobilistix. Importance of condition is that it is worsened by barbiturates.

(iv) *Infective and inflammatory*

Acute infective (ascending) polyneuritis—Landry-Guillain-Barré syndrome; occurs after infection especially respiratory infection, or after glandular fever, and may be a disturbance of immunity. May be associated encephalomyelitis.

Leprosy.

Diphtheria—due to toxin—paralysis of palate or limbs; now rare.

(v) *'Connective-tissue' (collagen-vascular) diseases*

probably disorders of immunity, 'auto-immune diseases'—group includes rheumatoid arthritis, but polyarteritis nodosa, an inflammation of arteries and nerves affecting middle aged men, is the usual cause in this group.

(vi) *Carcinoma—carcinomatous neuropathy*

Carcinoma, especially bronchogenic carcinoma, may be associated with distal sensory changes or sometimes a mixed motor and sensory neuropathy. Symptoms may antedate the discovery of the underlying carcinoma and may improve if it can be removed. Cause possibly a toxin produced by the growth.

(vii) *Hereditary neuropathies*—rare.

General clinical features

The sensory disturbance includes complaints such as numbness, paraesthesiae (pins and needles) and pain. On testing, there may be loss of sensation to pain (pin-prick), temperature and touch; this often affects feet and ankles, and sometimes the hands, and is described as 'glove and stocking' anaesthesia. There may be tenderness on squeezing the calf muscles.

The motor weakness affects the distal muscles causing paralysis of dorsiflexion of the feet and 'foot-drop'. The ankle and knee jerks are absent.

Acute ascending polyneuritis often starts as motor paralysis in the legs with loss of reflexes and varying sensory impairment. In severe cases the paralysis ascends to involve the respiratory muscles. The cerebro-spinal fluid may show a very high protein content.

Management of peripheral neuropathy

This will depend on the cause—an accurate history should lead to diagnosis in toxic exposure and alcoholism.

Diabetes will be revealed by testing the urine for sugar—which should, of course, be a routine. Blood examination will generally reveal pernicous anaemia, though serum vitamin B_{12} level should be estimated if there is any doubt, and injections will cure the condition.

Carcinomatous neuropathy occurs in the middle-aged and elderly, and chest x-ray may be helpful.

Although porphyria is rare, the condition can be easily excluded by urine testing. It should be noted that barbiturates can precipitate an attack of acute porphyria, and may have been given inadvertently as an intravenous anaesthetic.

Alcoholic neuropathy will improve on withdrawal of alcohol, and, as in the dietary deficiency cases, vitamin B complex should be given. Parentrovite injections may be used initially. Vitamins of the B group are only of value if a deficiency exists.

Management of severe cases

Especially in acute infective polyneuritis, bed rest may be necessary, for the condition is often a febrile one. Careful nursing is required—the patient is liable to pressure sores and skin care is important. Foot-drop is prevented by the use of a board at the end of the bed, or plaster splints. The limbs should be put through their full range of painless movement daily, and the physiotherapist will supervise active muscle exercises.

Steroids such as prednisone may be indicated in the connective-tissue disorders such as polyarteritis. In severe cases of acute ascending polyneuritis, steroids or corticotrophin (A.C.T.H.) injections may be of value in suppressing the inflammatory process.

Catheterization may be necessary for urinary retention, and such severe cases may have autonomic disturbance causing hypotension.

In very severe cases, the danger is of the paralysis ascending to involve the respiratory muscles. Respiratory impairment exists if the patient cannot count up to twenty after taking a deep breath, but before this stage is reached, the use of a simple spirometer and blood gas analysis will permit this diagnosis. Thus severely ill patients are best managed in a special unit where facilities exist for tracheostomy and mechanical ventilation—see Respiratory Failure, page 97.

Most patients show a gradual improvement; with persisting foot-drop, calipers may allow earlier ambulation. Recovery from motor weakness and sensory loss may take many months but except in cases complicating carcinoma, it is usually complete.

Pain

Pain is a most important, protective sensation. A few people are born with a congenital indifference to pain and they sustain severe trauma unknowingly, often dying in infancy as a result. As doctors and nurses, we have a duty to alleviate pain, but we must also seek, and if possible eliminate, the cause of the pain.

THE PAIN PATHWAY AND ITS LESIONS

There are pain-sensitive nerve endings in the skin. The sensation is transmitted by the spinal nerves to the posterior columns of the spinal cord. There, the pain fibres (as well as those conveying temperature and some touch fibres) are relayed, cross the cord diagonally and ascend anteriorly in the spino-thalamic tract to reach the thalamus. Here, crude pain may be appreciated. From the thalamus, fibres ascend to the sensory cortex, where pain is more finely appreciated and discriminated.

This pathway can therefore be interrupted, and pain abolished, with lesions in the peripheral nerve (as in peripheral neuritis), in the posterior roots of the spinal cord (as in tabes dorsalis), in the ascending tracts by a tumour, at the thalamus, or by a lesion such as a stroke affecting the fibres radiating to the cortex in the internal capsule.

Moreover a lesion at the thalamus may cause a disturbed sensation of pain—so called 'central' or thalamic pain which may be extremely severe, yet without outward explanation. The pain of trigeminal neuralgia may be of this nature.

DEEP AND 'REFERRED PAIN

The mechanism of pain from the deep structures is not clearly understood. The conducting pathways may be in the autonomic nerves, which are otherwise dominantly motor rather than sensory, or even in the somatic 'motor' nerves. Thus sensation from inflamed structures in contact with the diaphragm may be transmitted up the phrenic nerve, the motor nerve to the diaphragm. This nerve arises in the cervical region of the spinal cord and through associations there with the sensory tracts, the sensation from the inflamed structure may be felt in the shoulder tip as pain, the skin of that region. being supplied by nerves running to the same segment of the cord This is called 'referred' pain.

Another example of referred pain is that of myocardial infarction, felt in the chest, upper part of the left arm and sometimes even in the lower jaw—whereupon the patient may remove his denture, believing the pain originates here.

The abdominal viscera are not sensitive to cutting, but distension may be felt as pain referred to the central, umbilical region. Colic means spasmodic abdominal pain, the word being derived from 'colon', distension of which causes such pain. It should, however, be noted that biliary colic and renal colic are not usually spasmodic pains, more often they build up to severe intensity over minutes or an hour, then subside, only to recur.

The visceral layer of the pleura and peritoneum is not pain sensitive—thus the initial pain of appendicitis is a 'distension' one referred centrally. However, the parietal layer of these membranes, that is the layer reflected off the chest or abdominal wall, is pain sensitive. Thus when appendicitis spreads to involve the parietal layer of the peritoneum, a different and more severe pain is felt, and it is well-localized at the right iliac fossa, where there is also tenderness and muscle guarding. Similarly, pneumonia is in itself not painful, but should the inflammation spread to the parietal pleura, there is pain, that of pleurisy, worsened by deep breathing.

Pressure on a nerve or nerve root, can, as we have seen, cause an ache, pain or disturbance of sensation—'pins and needles' are felt when the pressure is taken off a peripheral nerve such as the sciatic nerve after sitting with the legs crossed, but may occur at the time of nerve root pressure. Such feelings of discomfort are referred to the area of distribution of the nerve, motor or sensory, and there may be associated diminution of sensation to pain (such as pin-prick), temperature or touch in the area of skin supplied by the nerve, or in the *dermatome*—the area of skin supplied by a nerve *root*, a more diffuse area.

HEADACHE
See page 334.

CHEMICAL TRANSMITTERS OF PAIN
'Vascular' headache, such of that of migraine which is associated with vasodilatation, may be due to release of chemicals or 'kinins' which specifically affect nerve endings and cause pain. Such chemicals may be the transmitting substances causing other forms of pain.

THE REACTION TO PAIN. EFFECTS OF DEPRESSIVE ILLNESS
The reaction to pain depends not only on its intensity, but on the constitution, personality and background of the patient. There is controversy concerning a person's pain threshold, and it is difficult to measure pain, but it does seem to affect some people more than others. Thus, while myocardial infarction is usually associated with severe crushing chest pain, some patients with major infarction may complain only of vague discomfort. There may, of course, be family or business reasons for belittling the severity of pain.

A complaint of pain may be the patient's way of drawing attention to some form of suffering which he realizes exists, but which he cannot explain in other terms. Failure of the doctor or nurse to appreciate this may result in the patient exaggerating his symptoms in order to emphasize his plight, which may be real.

On the other hand, pain is worse or more difficult to bear in depressive illness, which often presents with complaints of pain.

MANAGEMENT OF PAIN
Pain is a symptom, a protective sympton, and its cause must be sought.

It is dangerous to give a pain relieving drug before the diagnosis is clear, especially in patients with abdominal pain who may be suffer-ing from conditions such as acute appendicitis, perforated peptic ulcer or ruptured ectopic pregnancy—conditions which need immediate surgical attention. Once the course of action has been decided, then one must proceed to alleviate the pain.

It is wrong to allow a patient to continue to suffer pain, the cause of which cannot be eliminated. Severe pain may be harmful and, through effects on the autonomic nervous system, can have adverse action on the heart in myocardial infarction, leading to arrhythmias. Continuous pain is demoralizing and impedes recovery—it should not go unrelieved. If a drug to alleviate the pain has not been prescribed, then this omission should be remedied—no patient should suffer in silence. The fact that the patient may be attached to monitoring devices and on complicated treatment must not blind us to our prime duty to relieve suffering.

(a) Local measures to relieve pain

Rest alleviates pain, especially that of an inflamed joint, as in rheumatic fever and rheumatoid arthritis—bed rest, and local splintage can be considered.

Heat in the form of a hot water bottle, electric paid (dangerous in incontinent patients) or old-fashion kaolin poultice, and wax baths for the rheumatoid hand, is often comforting. An infra-red lamp can be used to produce local heat and is safe provided it is not pushed to produce skin-burning. The effect penetrates a few millimetres. Short-wave diathermy causes heating of deeper tissues between two applied electrodes, and is useful in some forms of arthritis, but requires a skilled physiotherapist because there is no warning of overheating.

It is dangerous to apply any form of heat to an area where the circulation is in jeopardy. The skin becomes heated and its metabolic requirement raised, but if there is insufficient blood to cope with the increase demanded, gangrene will result. Thus heat must not be applied to a painful but ischaemic limb.

Cold. Cold compresses have little effect. Ether or other sprays cause cooling by evaporation, and temporary loss of sensation, anaesthesia at the part.

Local anaesthetics such as procaine or lignocaine may be injected to relieve pain from a joint or ligament.

(b) Drugs in the relief of pain

Mild analgesics (pain relieving drugs). These include aspirin, paracetamol and compounds which may include codeine, itself a mild analgesic. Aspirin may cause haematemesis or blood loss from gastric oozing. Paracetamol may be safer than phenacetin, but excess can be toxic to liver and kidneys.

These drugs may relieve pain through an effect on its peripheral mechanism; they are useful in 'muscular', ligamentous and joint aches and pains, and in headache. Aspirin also has an anti-inflammatory effect.

Stronger analgesics which are also anti-inflammatory and used in rheumatic disorders include phenylbutazone and indomethacin, both gastric irritants and phenylbutazone can be a cause of bone marrow depression.

Dihydrocodeine (DF118) is also intermediate in potency and sometimes effective when aspirin or paracetamol fails, but it causes histamine release and should not be used in allergic conditions or asthma.

Powerful analgesics. The opiates morphine and diamorphine (heroin) are by far the most powerful pain-relieving agents, probably working in the central nerve pathways. They also have a calming effect. They are indicated in conditions causing severe pain such as myocardial infarction and in painful maglignant disease, but they are drugs of dependence (addiction) and should not be used for more than a few days for remediable pain. Morphine depresses respiration and may cause vomiting, and both morphine and heroin have a hypotensive effect and should only be given if the patient can be kept in a reclining position. Pethidine is slightly less potent but may be useful in pain with associated spasm, such as biliary colic. It is also a drug of dependence. Pentazocine (Fortral) is claimed to be as powerful yet non-addictive.

Drugs which diminish the appreciation of pain

These include phenothiazines such as chlorpromazine (Largactil) which affect the cortical reaction to pain, rendering the patient indifferent to it. Such drugs are useful in malignant disease. Carbamazepine may benefit 'thalamic' pain and trigeminal neuralgia.

In some patients, antidepressive drugs such as amitriptyline (Tryptizol) or imipramine (Tofranil) may be applicable.

A note on general anaesthetics

These render the patient unconscious so that he cannot appreciate pain—anaesthesia carries a risk of anoxia and the effects of some damage to brain cells may not always be obvious. Techniques short of complete unconsciousness, are sometimes used. It has been suggested that inhalation of a mixture of 50 per cent nitrous oxide in oxygen provides safe analgesia in some painful conditions.

Hypnosis is occasionally applicable in relieving a pain for which there is no organic cause.

Relief of intractable pain—usually the proper application of the drugs discussed above is sufficient in all but the most severe cases. In painful malignant disease the anticipatory use of morphine and cocaine mixtures, as in the Brompton cocktail often enables the patient to remain relatively symptom free and cheerful. Only rarely need recourse be made to surgical procedures such as section of posterior nerve roots or spino-thalamic 'tractotomy' to destroy pain-carrying fibres.

14

Endocrine disorders

The common endocrine disorders are diabetes mellitus, considered in Chapter 12, and the thyroid diseases thyrotoxicosis and myxoedema described below. The other disorders are comparatively rare.

The endocrine or ductless glands secret hormones, chemical messengers, into the bloodstream. These have an effect on distant tissues or organs. In health, there is a balance of hormone secretion. Thus the pituitary gland secretes adrenocorticotrophic hormone (A.C.T.H.). This stimulates the adrenal cortex to produce cortisol (hydrocortisone). Excess cortisol, however, acts on the pituitary to cause a shutting-off of the secretion of A.C.T.H., so that ultimately the balance is restored.

Similarly, giving hormones as drugs to patients may depress their own secretion if previously normal. On the other hand, patients who are deficient in such hormones will benefit from small, replacement doses.

Thyroid disorders

The thyroid gland consists of a left and right lobe lying against the lower half of the thyroid cartilage, united by a isthmus across the front of the trachea. It secretes the iodine-containing hormone, thyroxine, a metabolic stimulant acting on many tissues. (The thyroid also secretes another hormone called calcitonin which affects calcium metabolism.)

SIMPLE GOITRE
This may be due to iodine deficiency in endemic areas such as Switzerland and parts of Derbyshire; the addition of tiny quantities

of iodine to salt is preventive. However, simple goitre is not always due to iodine deficiency and may have a genetic basis. Again, excessive iodine intake (e.g. from proprietary cough remedies) may actually cause a goitre. Slight thyroid enlargement is common in pregnancy, related to increased iodine demands.

Simple goitre is a soft swelling of the thyroid gland and is commonest in young women. It may be regarded as an attempt by the thyroid to produce enough of its hormone secretion by enlarging. Usually the attempt succeeds, so there is no hormone upset—the patient remains 'euthyroid'. No treatment is generally required, but surgery may be demanded for cosmetic reasons or in the rare case of pressure effects.

THYROTOXICOSIS (HYPERTHYROIDISM, GRAVES' DISEASE, TOXIC GOITRE)

This is overactivity of the thyroid gland, the excess thyroxine causing increased metabolism. The overactivity was previously attributed to excessive production of the thyroid stimulating hormone of the anterior pituitary, but most cases are in fact due to, or associated with, a substance in the blood called 'long acting thyroid stimulator', L.A.T.S. This is an antibody, a globulin formed in lymphocytes, and thyrotoxicosis may therefore be a disturbance of the immune mechanism, an auto-immune disease. Though L.A.T.S. is an antibody, it is unusual among antibodies, for it actually causes a stimulation of the thyroid gland.

Thyrotoxicosis is commoner in women, and a frequent reason for out-patient referral. There is a familial tendency.

Symptoms and signs

The patient complains of excitability, 'nerves' and irritability and may notice that she loses her temper more easily than before. She feels the heat badly and prefers cold weather. The palms are warm and sweaty and there is a tremor of the fingers. The pulse is rapid. The appetite remains good, the patient may say that she eats like a horse, but there is loss of weight from the increased metabolism.

Young women tend to have a diffuse enlargement of the thyroid, and this goitre is usually obvious. With the stethoscope a 'bruit' may be audible over it, from the increased blood flow. There is a varying degree of 'exophthalmos'. Exophthalmos really means protrusion of the eyeball, but the term is used to described prominence of the eyes. The commonest sign is a 'staring' appearance from overactivity of the sympathetic nervous system which supplies a small muscle in the upper lid, causing lid retraction. There is a 'lid lag' on eye movement so that more of the white sclera is seen and the eyes appear prominent. True exophthalmos is less common and may not be clinically obvious. In severe cases there is oedema of the orbit with weakness of the external occular muscles, and vision may be threatened. The severity of exophthalmos is not related to that of the thyrotoxicosis and the cause is uncertain. It may be associated with a reddish swelling over the shins called pretibial myxoedema and occasionally with a type of finger clubbing. Steroids have been tried in the treatment of severe exophthalmos, but surgical decompression of the orbit is sometimes necessary.

Thyrotoxicosis in middle age may present with a nodular type of goitre and in such cases the primary fault may lie in the thyroid gland itself. Eye signs are less common, but cardiac excitability may cause *atrial fibrillation* and occasionally heart failure.

Investigations

The diagnosis is confirmed by:

1. Clinical features such as weight loss and raised sleeping pulse.

2. Raised 'Protein Bound Iodine' (P.B.I.), which corresponds to thyroxine, in the blood.

3. High uptake of radio-active iodine (131_1 or 125_1) over the thyroid gland.

The 'Thyopac' radio-active iodine test may also be carried out on a blood specimen.

The Basal Metabolic Rate (B.M.R.) is raised, but this test has been superseded by the above.

Treatment

1. *Antithyroid drugs*, such as carbimazole or methyl thiouracil, are the treatment of choice in young patients (e.g. carbimazole 10 mg 4 times daily initially), maintenance doses being continued for at least a year. The only important side-effect is agranulocytosis, occurring in the first few weeks of treatment. The patient must be warned to stop the tablets if she develops a sore throat and a white cell count must be done.

Propranolol or similar adrenergic-blocking drug may be added initially to slow the heart rate.

2. *Thyroidectomy*—indicated in recurrences in young women, or in the middle-aged with nodular goitres. It should be an elective

procedure, and a small dose of iodine is given for 10–14 days pre-operatively, which acts as a further thyroid suppressive drug over a short period.

Complications include hypothyroidism, hypoparathyroidism (from inadvertent removal of parathyroids) and vocal chord paralysis from recurrent laryngeal nerve section.

3. *Radio-active iodine.* This can be used in the elderly and to avoid second operations. Suitable doses cause partial destruction of the thyroid gland, but there is a high incidence of late hypothyroidism.

MYXOEDEMA — HYPOTHYROIDISM — UNDERACTIVITY OF THYROID GLAND

In the newborn baby, the thyroid gland may function defectively or be absent. If untreated, there is lack of brain and bodily development or *cretinism*. Early diagnosis is therefore essential, for small doses of thyroxine are curative.

In adults, hypothyroidism usually follows destruction of the thyroid gland by an auto-immune process, and antibodies are detectable in the blood. At some stage there may have been swelling and lymphocyte infiltration of the thyroid—this is called *Hashimoto's disease*—but the condition ends up as atrophy, with complete lack of thyroxine, and the clinical picture called myxoedema.

Symptoms and signs

The condition is commonest in middle-aged women. As the thyroid fails to produce enough thyroxine, the bodily functions generally run down. The patient loses interest in life and becomes slower with coarsening and puffiness of the facial appearance and skin, hence the name myxoedema, but it is not a true oedema. There is a characteristically slow relaxation of the tendon reflexes which may allow early diagnosis in suspected cases. If untreated, patients become increasingly sluggish, have a husky voice like a running-down gramophone record, feel the cold badly and curl-up in bed with only their nose and eyes peeping out—the 'snug-sign'. The pulse is slow, and there may be pericardial effusion. Severe cases may have behaviour disturbances, lapse into coma and die.

Investigations

The diagnosis is confirmed by a low blood P.B.I., and low radioactive iodine uptake by the thyroid, and there may be thyroid antibodies in the blood. The serum cholesterol is high, for unknown reason.

Treatment

The treatment is thyroxine, initially in small doses so as not to over-stimulate the heart, then a maintenance dose of 0·3 mg daily for life. Patients tend to stop their tablets when they feel better, so it must be explained that life long therapy is required to remedy their thyroid deficiency. Severe cases presenting in coma require hydrocortisone injection, followed by tri-odothyronine and thyroxine.

CARCINOMA OF THE THYROID

This is rare, but should be suspected in middle-aged patients presenting with a hard lump in the thyroid. They are not usually thyrotoxic, indeed the nodule will often be found to be a 'cold' one, which does not take up radio-active iodine, and may be delineated on a radio-scanning with a counter over the neck. Occasionally, the first presentation is as metastases in lungs or bones. Treatment is surgical where possible. The few cases causing thyrotoxicosis may be helped by thyroidectomy followed by radio-active iodine in a dose sufficient to destroy the functioning metastases.

Parathyroid disorders

These four little glands, situated behind the thyroid, control calcium and phosphorus metabolism, preserving the normal blood calcium level. Excess parathyroid hormone raises the blood calcium by action on kidneys and bones.

There is, however, also a recently discovered hormone, *calcitonin*, produced mainly in the thyroid gland. It tends to lower the blood calcium.

HYPOPARATHYROIDISM

This may occur spontaneously or following inadvertent removal of the parathyroids at thyroid operation. The blood calcium falls, causing increased irritability of nerves with painful muscle cramps and spasm—tetany. There is painful flexion of the wrists with metacarpo-phalangeal joints, with extension of the fingers. There may also be spasm of the larynx. Tapping over the facial nerve produces twitching of the facial muscles. Tetany may be provoked by over-breathing, leading to loss of carbon dioxide and tendency to alkalosis with lowered effective blood calcium (see page 242).

Treatment

Calcium gluconate, 10 ml 10 per cent solution by intramuscular or slow intravenous injection relieves the acute symptoms of tetany. Hypoparathyroidism could theoretically be treated by parathyroid hormone, but a satisfactory preparation is not available. Vitamin D (calciferol) however, has a similar effect in doses of 500 micrograms —2 milligrams (20,000–80,000 units) daily orally. (It should be noted that this is a high, 'pharmacological' dose, as distinct from the small doses of 10–100 micrograms (400–4,000 units) sufficient to treat rickets). The blood calcium level should be frequently checked to avoid overdosage, which causes calcium deposition in the kidney.

HYPERPARATHYROIDISM

Over-activity is usually due to a benign tumour of one parathyroid gland. It is rarely palpable. Radio-isotope scan (using labelled methionine) may aid in its location. This is *primary* hyperparathyroidism.

Symptoms and signs

In severe cases, calcium is dissolved from the bones, producing osteitis fibrosa cystica, and fractures—von Recklinghausen's disease of bone.

Calcium is high in the blood and urine, and may be deposited in the kidneys and cause renal calculi. There is often polyuria. Hyperparathyroidism may also be associated with duodenal ulceration.

Mild cases are easily missed, but a raised serum calcium gives the clue to diagnosis.

Treatment

The treatment is surgical removal of the offending parathyroid gland.

'*Secondary*' hyperparathyroidism may complicate renal failure, where there may be complex disturbances of calcium metabolism.

Thymus gland

This gland is situated behind the breast-bone in front of the great vessels, and is large in infancy. The thymus influences the production of the type of lymphocytes responsible for the 'cell-mediated' part of immunity but its continued presence does not seem to be essential. Thus the thymus is often atrophic in adult life. In the rare disease myasthenia gravis (a disorder causing muscle weakness) there may be enlargement or tumour of the thymus, and patients not responding to neostigmine may benefit from thymectomy

Adrenal glands

The adrenal or suprarenal glands are situated one on top of each kidney. The adrenal gland has a *cortex*, essential to life, and a *medulla* which functions independently producing adrenaline-like hormones, but is not essential.

Disorders of the Adrenal Cortex

The cortex produces three groups of hormones—the three S's.

1. *S*tress—hydrocortisone (cortisol)—a gluco corticoid—so called because it increases protein breakdown resulting in increased production of glucose; essential for normal response to stress and injury; also has sodium retaining action.

2. *S*alt—aldosterone, concerned in sodium and water balance through its action on the renal tubule. Causes sodium retention. A mineralo corticoid.

3. *S*ex hormones, which are dominantly masculinizing (androgenic) even in women.

Overaction

1. CUSHING'S SYNDROME—*Overproduction of cortisol*

This is usually due to pituitary overactivity, with excessive production of A.C.T.H. which causes bilateral adrenal enlargement and over-production of cortisol. Some cases are, however, due to a primary tumour of the adrenal, benign or malignant.

Symptoms and signs

The effects are the same as in cortisone over-treatment, when patients become 'Cushingoid'.

There is 'mooning' of the face which is often high-coloured, obesity of the trunk with thinning of arms and legs (like a lemon on sticks), muscular weakness, thinning of the skin with easy bruising, thinning of the bones causing osteoporosis and sometimes fractures, hypertension and diabetes mellitus.

Similar effects may be produced by certain tumours, e.g. carcinoma of bronchus, which may produce an A.C.T.H.-like substance.

Investigations

The diagnosis is confirmed by high urinary and blood cortisol levels estimated as 11-hydroxycorticosteroids, and raised A.C.T.H. (estimated by a technique called radio-immunoassay) if there is a primary pituitary overactivity. In cases due to adrenal tumour, the blood cortisol fails to be suppressed by dexamethasone (dexamethasone suppression test).

Treatment:

surgical removal of affected gland if due to tumour.

removal of both glands, bilateral adrenalectomy, in the more usual type secondary to pituitary overactivity. This gives better results than operations on the pituitary itself. Subsequent replacement therapy with cortisol and fluorohydrocortisone (as for Addison's disease) is necessary.

2. ALDOSTERONISM

Primary aldosteronism (Conn's syndrome) is due to a tumour, usually benign, producing excess aldosterone, causing hypertension, weakness and polyuria. The serum potassium is low, and the blood shows a tendency to alkalosis. The condition is rare but important as surgery offers cure.

Secondary aldosteronism occurs when there is a threat of a lowered plasma volume, as in nephrotic syndrome and cirrhosis of the liver; it may also occur, for unknown reasons, in congestive cardiac failure. It results in salt and water retention with increased *oedema*. Treatment is that of the cause, where possible, plus diuretics which promote sodium loss directly (e.g. bendrofluazide) or indirectly by antagonizing the action of aldosterone on the renal tubule (e.g. spironolactone).

3. ADRENAL VIRILISM

This is due to inappropriate production of masculinizing sex hormone by the adrenal cortex. It may cause precocious puberty, or difficulties in sexual designation of infants who are really female but appear male. Cases in adults are usually due to malignant tumours of the adrenal; surgical cure is sometimes possible.

The urine contains an excess of hormone breakdown products, measured as 17-ketosteroids (oxosteroids). These may also be raised in Cushing's syndrome, and used to be the only hormone test available, but cortisol can now be more precisely estimated, for example as 11-hydroxycorticosteroids.

Underaction of the adrenal cortex

Causes

1. Destruction following tuber-
   culosis (now rare).   } Primary adreno-cortical
2. An 'auto-immune' destruction.   } failure—*Addison's disease*.
3. Secondary to A.C.T.H. lack, from pituitary disease, or as the result of long continued administration of steroids, causing suppression.

ADDISON'S DISEASE

This is a result of deficiency of cortisol and aldosterone.

Symptoms and signs

Loss of appetite and of weight, vomiting, and low blood pressure. There is a brown pigmentation of the skin, well seen in flexures (e.g. axilla) and scars and in the forehead at the hair line. Dark bluish spots occur inside the lips and mouth. The cortisol deficiency causes an increased secretion of A.C.T.H. by the pituitary and this is associated with increased secretion of M.S.H., a hormone which stimulates the production of the melanin pigment.

There is progressive weakness, with poor resistance to stress and infection. If treatment is neglected, the patient becomes dehydrated from vomiting and may lapse into coma and succumb.

Investigations

1. Serum sodium—usually low.
2. *Water-load test:* Patient drinks 20 ml of water per kg body weight over $\frac{1}{2}$ hour. All urine is collected for the next 4 hours. Normal patients excrete over 80 per cent of the load in this period—reduced in Addison's disease, correctable by cortisol. Not a specific test, and there is danger of causing water intoxication.
3. *Plasma cortisol and tetracosactrin (Synacthen) test.*

Patients with underactivity of the adrenal cortex have a low plasma cortisol level and in cases due to primary adrenal disease, i.e. Addison's disease, it fails to rise after A.C.T.H., most easily given as tetracosactrin (Synacthen) 0·25 mg intramuscularly—the blood is taken for test before, and $\frac{1}{2}$ hour after injection.

Treatment

Replace the deficient hormones—hydrocortisone, or as cortisone, usually 25 mg in the morning and 12·5 afternoon. The natural salt-retaining hormone aldosterone is not available in satisfactory form, and the best substitute is fluorohydrocortisone, 0·1 mg daily. Androgenic hormones are not usually necessary.

Increased dosage of cortisone is necessary to cover stress such as injury, operation or infection.

SIDE EFFECTS OF CORTISONE-LIKE (CORTICOSTEROID OR STEROID) DRUGS

Cortisol (hydrocortisone) is essential to life, and the adrenal cortex secretes about 30–40 mg daily, the replacement dose in Addison's disease. More is required to cover the stress of injury or infection. Apart from its replacement role, cortisol (or cortisone, which is changed to cortisol in the body) can be used *pharmacologically* in much bigger dosage to treat conditions such as severe asthma and status asthmaticus, overhwleming septicaemias, haemolytic anaemia, and disturbances of immunity. But, inseparable from such beneficial action are undesirable actions which would ultimately result in a Cushingoid state with moon face, muscle weakness, thinning of the bones, hypertension, tendency to diabetes and possible worsening of peptic ulceration.

In an attempt to avoid such effects, synthetic steroids similar to cortisol have been produced. These include prednisone and prednisolone, 5 mg equalling 25 mg cortisone in potency. These drugs may have less of the salt-retaining, hypertensive properties of cortisone, but Cushingoid effects will still be seen in long-continued dosage.

Moreover, such steroids will inhibit production of pituitary A.C.T.H., so that the body's own adrenal cortex becomes atrophic, and if the administered steroid is then withdrawn, the patient will pass into a state of adrenal cortical insufficiency with hypotension and collapse.

Steroid drugs such as prednisone are thus a valuable contribution to therapy in many otherwise intractable conditions, but their misuse can be disastrous.

Side effects of oral contraceptives ('the pill')

These contain hormones of oestrogen and progesterone type, similar to the naturally-occurring ovarian hormones. Part of their action may be due to suppression of pituitary function and inhibition of ovulation, but they also affect the secretions of the cervix of the uterus. They are, chemically, steroids, but in clinical practice the word steroid is generally used to mean cortisone-like drugs. Side effects of oral contraceptives include alteration in blood co-agulation factors with an increased tendency to venous thrombosis, and to cerebral arterial thrombosis. The drugs may also affect the liver causing jaundice, and sometimes cause deterioration of diabetic control. Thus, history-taking in young women must now include enquiry as to whether they are taking an oral contraceptive 'pill'.

The adrenal medulla

Phaeochromocytoma is a simple or, rarely, malignant tumour which secretes excess adrenaline or nor-adrenaline—the hormones released at sympathetic nerve endings.

There is hypertension, often paroxysmal, severe sweating and pallor. The tumour may be palpable, or detectable at I.V.P. or on x-ray after retroperitoneal injection of gas. Adrenaline breakdown products (catecholamines) are detected in a 24 hour urine collection as excess vanillyl-mandelic acid (V.M.A., H.M.M.A.).

Though rare, the condition in important as a treatable cause of hypertension, so that '24 hour urine for V.M.A.' is a useful screening test.

Treatment is surgical removal, using adrenergic blocking drugs during the operation, and nor-adrenaline infusions post-operatively until normal blood pressure is maintained.

Pituitary gland

This is a small gland, about the size of a pea, situated in the pituitary fossa of the skull. Above it is the optic chiasma, and the pituitary stalk is connected with the part of the brain called the hypothalamus. This is concerned with emotional response, sleep, appetite and salt regulation. Pituitary secretion is in turn influenced by such factors. The pituitary gland has two parts, anterior and posterior.

Hormones of the anterior pituitary (*'the leader of the endocrine orchestra'*)

Human growth hormone (H.G.H.).
Thyroid stimulating hormone (T.S.H.).

Adrenocorticotrophic hormone (A.C.T.H.) and melanocyte-stimulating hormone (M.S.H.).

Gonadotrophins

follicle-stimulating hormone (F.S.H.)—acts on ovary—oestrogens.

luteinizing hormone (L.H.)—acts on ovary—progestogens.
or on testis—testosterone.

Prolactin—affects milk production from breast of nursing mother.

Hormones released by the posterior pituitary

Vasopressin (antidiuretic hormone).

Oxytocin (contracts smooth muscle of uterus and blood vessels, and causes milk ejection from lactating breast? releases prolactin).

Obesity in children used to be ascribed to pituitary upset (the 'fat boy' of Frohlich's Syndrome) but the few cases originally described were probably due to tumours of the hypothalamic region. Such tumours are rare and usually associated with visual upset from involvement of the optic chiasma and evidence of a space-occupying lesion. In the vast majority of cases of obesity there is no demonstable pituitary endocrine disturbance or obvious hypothalamic lesion. There may, however, be some disturbance of appetite control causing overeating, the usual reason for obesity.

Disorders of anterior pituitary

Growth hormone deficiency my arise from tumour or spontaneously and causes shortness of stature in children. Other causes of dwarfism, such as cyanotic congenital heart disease, coeliac disease, and chronic renal disease should be excluded. The diagnosis is confirmed by finding a low H.G.H. level in the blood, and it fails to rise normally after the stimulus produced by a drink of Bovril. H.G.H. is now available for treatment.

ACROMEGALY

Excessive production of growth hormone causes *gigantism* if it occurs before the epiphyses of the bones have united. In adults, it results in *acromegaly*. This literally means enlargement of distal tissues—hands and feet, and also the lower jaw which becomes prominent, with coarsening of the facial features. Some cases are due to tumour, and the optic chiasma may also be involved, causing visual field defects. Diabetes may also be associated, as H.G.H. is diabetogenic. Active cases require surgery or pituitary ablation with radio-active yttrium seeds, which can be implanted through a nasal route. There are varying degrees of deficiency of other pituitary hormones, which may require replacement therapy.

Excess production of A.C.T.H. causes Cushing's syndrome, already described—see Overactivity of the adrenal cortex. If bilateral adrenalectomy is carried out as treatment, there may be a subsequent exacerbation of an A.C.T.H. producing pituitary tumour, and M.S.H. is also produced in excess, with increasing pigmentation. Direct therapy to the pituitary may be necessary in such cases.

Lack of pituitary gonadotrophins causes amenorrhoea and infertility. Lack of the gonadal hormones secondary to gonadotrophin deficiency causes loss of sexual characteristics, and the skin becomes fine and excessively wrinkled.

PANHYPOPITUITARISM (SIMMOND'S DISEASE)—UNDERACTIVITY OF THE ANTERIOR PITUITARY

Causes

This may occur after *post-partum haemorrhage*, when it is called *Sheehan's syndrome*, but may also arise *spontaneously*, or as a result of *tumour* or infiltration of the anterior pituitary gland.

Effects

There is a failure of production of the trophic hormones, which normally stimulate the distal endocrine glands, and as a result, their secretion fails. Thus the effect of panhypopituitarism is to cause deficiency of the hormones of the ovary (or testis in a man), adrenal cortex and thyroid, in varying degree.

Symptoms and signs

There is commonly a history of failure to lactate after pregnancy, and the periods do not return and sexual hair disappears from lack of gonadotrophin effect. The skin is pale yet the patient is not anaemic. There need not be weight loss. The patient is weak and hypotensive from lack of cortisol, and there is varying degree of hypothyroidism.

Investigations

The diagnosis is confirmed by finding low blood levels of cortisol and thyroxine (measured as P.B.I.), produced respectively in the adrenal cortex and thyroid, two of the important target organs for the trophic hormones. Tests of the 'pituitary—adrenal axis' help to localize the fault in the anterior pituitary. These include response to A.C.T.H., insulin hypoglycaemia and the substance metyrapone.

Treatment

Treatment is by replacing the deficient hormones—cortisone 37·5 mg in the day, as in Addison's disease. There is seldom need for salt-retaining hormones such as fluorohydrocortisone. Thyroxine 0·3 mg daily remedies thyroid deficiency.

The only pituitary trophic hormone available is human gonadotrophin, which is now being used for infertility in females. The dose is uncertain, and multiple pregnancies have tended to follow its use.

Disorder of the posterior pituitary

The posterior pituitary releases the antidiuretic hormone (A.D.H., vasopressin) in response to a signal from an area of the hypothalamus sensitive to increased tonicity (osmolality) of the blood. A.D.H. acts on the renal tubules, causing reabsorption of water into the circulation and correcting the tonicity of the blood—and less urine is formed, i.e. there is an anti-diuresis.

DIABETES INSIPIDUS

This is due to lack of A.D.H., which may follow destruction of the posterior pituitary by tumour, trauma, or infection (such as encephalitis), but in about a third of patients there is no apparent cause.

Symptoms and signs

The patient passes large quantities of extremely dilute urine—specific gravity around 1·000—just like water. There is great thirst and if fluid is withheld the patient will go to any extreme to obtain water. This is helpful in diagnosis, which can be confirmed by measurement of the osmolality (tonicity) of the plasma, and by the response to treatment.

Treatment

Treatment is by replacing the deficient hormone—pitressin tannate in oil given by injection intramusculary daily or alternate days, or vasopressin nasal spray. Strangely, the thiazide diuretics such as bendrofluazide have an antidiuretic effect in diabetes insipidus, and chlorpropamide, as used in diabetes mellitus, is also effective in the treatment of diabetes insipidus—the reasons are obscure.

Inappropriate secretion of antidiuretic hormone may occur with certain tumours (e.g. brochogenic carcinoma) and be associated with weakness and a low blood sodium.

Hormones and cancer

Certain cancers are hormone-dependent. Improvement, especially of metastases, may occur if the hormonal balance is influenced by giving another hormone—thus cancer of the prostate can often be controlled by oestrogens such as stilboestrol. Side-effects include an increased thrombotic tendency.

Cancer of the breast in young women can be influenced by male sex-hormone, and in older women by female sex hormone such as an oestrogen. Adrenal and pituitary hormones (e.g. growth hormone) have been suggested as exacerbating factors in disseminated breast carcinoma, and adrenalectomy and pituitary ablation have been tried as palliative measures, but the long term results are disappointing.

Some disorders of sexual differentiation

Each body cell has 46 chromosomes, which carry the genetic, inherited characteristics of the cell. There are twenty-two pairs of chromosomes, plus two X chromosomes in females or an X and a Y chromosome in males—the sex chromosomes. One is contributed from the father's side in the sperm, the other from the mother's side in the ovum. There may be faults at fertilization, so that the ovum and foetus ends up with lack, or excess of sex chromosomes.

Lack of an X chromosome is found in *Turner's syndrome*—which presents as failure to menstruate in an apparent 'girl', usually of small stature and sometimes with webbing of the neck. The uterus is small or absent and secondary sexual development, such as breast enlargement at puberty, does not occur.

An extra X chromosome on top of an existing XY inheritance constitutes Klinefelter's syndrome, and apparent 'males' with this condition fail to develop normal male characteristics at puberty, and may have breast enlargement.

Recently the XYY syndrome has been discovered in tall 'males' of delinquent propensity in criminal institutions. The XXX 'super female' is in fact tall and spindly and lacks secondary sexual characteristics.

(In mongolism, Down's syndrome, there is an extra non-sex chromosome.)

Such chromosome abnormalities may be detected by examining cells from scrapings of the mucosa of the cheeks (buccal smear) or by culture of white blood cells.

Apart from such genetic troubles, there may be disturbances of sexual development from pituitary gonadotrophin failure, or from primary disease of the gonads. A not uncommon primary ovarian cause of infertility and hirsutism (excessive body hair) is called the Stein-Levinthal Syndrome.

Most people reported as undergoing change of sex are in fact transvestists, who are physically normal, but desire to adopt the opposite sex, and seek hormonal and surgical treatment to accomplish this. Again, homosexuals seldom have physical abnormality, but appear to be psychologically deviated towards each other—there is, however, some recent evidence that their hormone levels may be different from those in normal people.

15

Diseases of the joints, connective tissue, bones and muscles

Structure of joints

Fibrous joints, such as those uniting the tibia and fibula are composed of tough ligaments which allow only slight twisting movement. Cartilaginous joints are found only in the mid-line and include those of the vertebral column. Here the bone surfaces are covered with cartilage and united by a disc of fibro-cartilage surrounded by a ring of fibrous tissue attached to the periosteum of the bones; again, movements are limited but the column provides strong support. The synovial joints, found in the limbs, are free to move. The bones are united by a joint capsule which is lined by synovial membrane, the parts of the bones in contact with each other are coated with smooth articular cartilage lubricated by a layer of synovial fluid.

Arthritis and rheumatism—the meaning of terms

Arthritis means inflammation of a joint. Acute infective (septic) arthritis, with swelling and pus formation, occurs from direct bacterial invasion from neighbouring bone sepsis (osteomyelitis) or via the bloodstream from a distant septic focus. Causative organisms include the staphylococcus, the tubercle bacillus, and brucella. The management is with antibacterial drugs, though surgical drainage may be necessary. It should be noted that a damaged joint is more liable to infection, and an infective arthritis may complicate rheumatoid arthritis.

Post-infective arthritis occurs in rheumatic fever as a *reaction* to a preceding streptococcal throat infection; several joints in succession are involved, but they are not invaded by the organisms, the reaction is an allergic or hypersensitivity one, and there is usually no residual damage.

Arthritis may also be *traumatic*, or follow haemarthrosis in *haemophilia*.

Chronic arthritis includes the group of conditions called the *Chronic Rheumatic Diseases:*

rheumatoid arthritis, an inflammation of many joints, with systemic upset

osteoarthritis or osteoarthrosis, a degenerative disease of weight-bearing joints

gout, a disturbance of metabolism with deposition of uric acid in joints

ankylosing spondylitis, an inflammation of spinal joints.

These are definable rheumatic disorders, conforming to a pattern and considered in detail below.

The unqualified word 'rheumatism' (from the Greek, a flow) is a lay term to describe any ache or pain, usually associated with stiffness, and attributed to trouble in or around joints. Terms such as 'muscular rheumatism' and 'fibrositis' are equally unsatisfactory, as discussed later. However, although sometimes difficult to define, the rheumatic disorders are important, ranking second only to upper respiratory infections as a cause of sickness absence.

Connective tissue (collagen-vascular) diseases—definition

In this group of diseases, degenerative changes occur in connective tissues. These contain fibres of a protein material called collagen, but it is now uncertain whether the primary change is in it. The degeneration may be due to an inflammation in the small blood vessels and probably represents a disturbance of the immunity mechanism. The group includes rheumatic fever, where streptococcal allergy is involved, and rheumatoid arthritis, where there is no known antigen, hence the term 'auto-immune' disease, destructive of 'self'. The term 'connective tissue disease' is, however, customarily restricted to rarer members of the group such as systemic lupus erythematosus, described below. The inflammatory element in these diseases is suppressible with corticosteroids.

Bone diseases and pain

Bone diseases may be associated with aches and pains, from direct involvement of the bone in Paget's disease and in secondary carcinoma, or through bone collapse affecting surrounding joints and nerves. (Thus a complaint of 'rheumatism', meaning pain, may in fact be due to such disease.)

Rheumatoid arthritis

Rheumatoid arthritis is a chronic arthritis of small joints. It may cause only slight disability, or result in crippling deformities. It affects over 3 per cent of the population and is three times commoner in females. It usually presents in young adults in their thirties and forties, a group which includes housewives with young children and wage-earners, so the condition is of considerable social and economic importance. A rare form called Still's disease occurs in children. Rheumatoid arthritis does not usually shorten life, so its results are very commonly seen in the elderly. Despite previous statements to the contrary, its occurrence is not confined to cold, damp climates, but they may exacerbate symptoms. There is a slight familial tendency.

Pathology

There is an inflammation and proliferation of the synovial lining membrane of many joints, which may proceed to cause their destruction. In addition, there is constitutional upset and the term rheumatoid *disease* makes it clear that the condition is not simply an arthritis but a systemic disorder in which the main brunt falls on the joints.

The cause is unknown. The current theory is that rheumatoid arthritis is a disturbance of immunity, possibly a type of delayed hypersensitivity reaction to an unknown micro-organism, or an autoimmune reaction, causing enzyme release and joint inflammation. In most cases the blood contains an abnormal globulin called *rheumatoid factor*, an antibody, but its role in the inflammatory process is uncertain.

Symptoms and signs

The condition presents as aching pain, stiffness and often swelling of the joints, especially the smaller joints such as the metacarpophalangeal and proximal interphalangeal joints of the hands and fingers, and the wrist joints. The elbows, knees and feet may become affected and even the mandibular joints and the upper cervical spine. The shoulders may be involved, but rarely the hips (in adults) or the ankle joints.

Symptoms are often worst in the morning, when there is pain and stiffness in the fingers passing off in an hour or two but recurring the next day, or subsiding completely for weeks or months. Alternatively, the onset may be acute with severe pain and swelling of joints and tendon sheaths, and the forming of rheumatoid nodules near the elbows. Constitutional upset includes fever, fatigue, loss of appetite, loss of weight and anaemia.

Course

The condition may burn itself out over a year or so (and there is some evidence that the cases which are most acute initially are more likely to do this) or persist with remissions and relapses over many years. Apart from joint inflammation there is an associated arteritis, leading to circulatory disturbance and cold fingers and feet. There is muscle weakness and wasting, the hands tending to drop towards the ulnar side, ulnar deviation, and destruction of tendons causes further disability. Ultimately there may be severe crippling deformity with contractures, or sometimes a curious atrophy and floppiness of the fingers.

A milder form of arthritis of rheumatoid type may be associated with the skin disorder psoriasis.

Complications

These include an atrophy of the lacrimal (tear) and salivary glands (Sjogren's syndrome) leading to dry eye and tendency to corneal and scleral inflammation, and a dry mouth. There may be splenic enlargement associated with decreased white cells (Felty's syndrome) —usually there is a mild leucocytosis.

Dislocation of the upper cervical joints may cause spinal cord compression, so injudicious manipulation or handling (e.g. at operations) must be avoided.

Other complications include peripheral neuritis, fibrosis of the lungs, and amyloid disease.

Further investigations

R.A. (rheumatoid arthritis) Latex test—detects rheumatoid factor in the blood. Blood count shows anaemia (normochromic, but can be hypochromic from disturbed iron absorption, or occasionally macrocytic from relative folic acid deficiency), raised white cell count, and *high E.S.R.*—which is a guide to the activity of the disease. X-rays show joint deformity and adjacent bone rarefaction (osteoporosis).

Treatment

There is no known cure. The aims of treatment are to relieve pain and suppress inflammation, to prevent deformity, and to maintain the general well-being of the patient in the community. There are four aspects of treatment:

1. *General measures.*
2. *Local measures.*
3. *Drugs.*
4. *Long-term care.*

1. General measures

Bed rest. In the active stages of the disease, and with fever or constitutional upset, the patient should be admitted to hospital for a period of bed rest. Early admission induces remission most quickly and improves prognosis. Bed rest should be complete, apart from toilet purposes. The mattress should be firm, a backrest can be used by day and a low pillow at night. A bed cage and foot rest are provided, but pillows must not be placed behind painful knees, or contractures may develop.

Diet. No special dietary measures are indicated, but the diet should be adequate in protein, calcium, iron and vitamins, and include meat, milk, eggs and fresh fruit.

2. Local measures

Splinting. Splinting has two main purposes—to rest an inflamed joint, and to prevent deformity. In the acute stages plaster of Paris or plastic splints are applied to the wrists, and a plaster back-slab to the knees to keep them extended. Later, continued use of splints at night may be helpful. A plastic collar may be indicated for cervical arthritis. Sometimes 'serial' splinting is tried to correct existing deformities.

Exercise. An inflamed joint should be rested and short-term splinting does not cause contractures. Thus passive or active movements should not be carried out when there is pain. Once acute symptoms subside, the physiotherapist instructs the patient on static exercises (muscle tensing) and passive joint movements to maintain their range. Later graduated active exercises are practised to build up the muscles, with gradual weight-bearing and ambulation.

Heat in the form of wax baths to the hands is often comforting. Local heat from hot-water bottles or an infra-red lamp may also be used, but such measures are not required if the joints are pain-free at rest.

Steroid injections. This may be helpful if only one or two joints are involved. Hydrocortisone is injected intra-articularly, having ascertained that there is no infection present. Inflammation is suppressed, but repeated injections may increase joint destruction.

Surgical synovectomy. This is sometimes carried out in acute rheumatoid arthritis of the knees and finger joints, removal of the inflamed and proliferating synovial membrane decreasing pressure in the joint and preventing cartilage destruction.

3. *Drugs*

Aspirin remains the drug of choice and in doses of 600 mg 3 or 4 times daily relieves pain and suppresses inflammation. Both plain and soluble aspirin can cause gastric irritation, and aspirin-glycine (Paynocil) or enteric-coated preparations may be tried instead. Aspirin-induced gastro-intestinal bleeding is usually occult, and may contribute to the anaemia.

Phenylbutazone (Butazolidin) 100 mg tablets and indomethacin (Indocid) 25 mg capsules are also effective in treatment, but again are gastric irritants; phenylbutazone may also depress the bone marrow, and cause fluid retention. Indomethacin can be given as a suppository, effective for some hours.

Newer drugs include ibuprofen (Brufen) and the fenamates (Arlef, Ponstan). Chloroquine is little used now because of toxic effects on cornea and retina. Gold injections are helpful if other measures fail, but toxic effects include skin rashes, marrow depression, and kidney damage with albuminuria.

Steroids such as prednisone have a remarkable suppressive effect and may allow return of mobility, but their side-effects preclude their use in all but the most severe cases. It may occasionally be justified to continue a small dose of prednisone (7·5 mg daily or less) where it is the only measure allowing a patient to pursue his occupation.

Immuno-suppressive drugs such as azathioprine have been tried in treatment, but preliminary results are disappointing.

The anaemia of rheumatoid arthritis is partly due to toxic marrow depression, and partly to aspirin-induced blood loss. Iron supplements by mouth (ferrous sulphate) may help, but this is one of the few conditions where intramuscular iron may be more effective. Occasionally the anaemia is due to folic acid deficiency, when supplements are appropriate.

4. *Long-term care*

Wherever possible the patient should resume his or her normal daily duties. Activity is to be encouraged provided there is no pain. Exercises should be continued to maintain muscle power. If splints are worn they should be checked to ensure a correct fit. Out-patient surveillance is usually indicated.

Surgical measures such as tendon reconstructions and transplants, and arthrodesis (joint fixation) may prevent disability. Thus in the hand a patient may be enabled to grip with two fingers with a fixed, but painless wrist. Flexion deformity of the knees may be corrected into fixed but straight knees, thus avoiding a chair-bound existence.

Domestic and social adjustments. There are many gadgets available which assist a disabled patient—thus appliances with long handles and wire controls enable patients with stiff elbow and shoulder joints to feed and dress themselves. Elbow crutches may improve mobility and a 'half-step' fixed to a walking stick assists stair climbing. Hand-rails and ramps should be provided in public buildings.

Employment. Often the trouble is in getting to work—it is difficult for the arthritic to climb into a bus. Suitably adapted motor cars are available, or even a motorized wheel chair permits independence. Where a patient is unable to follow his usual occupation, industrial retraining and rehabilitation may be helpful—it is desirable for the patient to be able to earn his own living.

PROGNOSIS

The individual prognosis is difficult—the outlook is better for cases with onset before the age of forty, especially if early treatment is given. Probably about 20 per cent of patients become symptom free, about 60–70 per cent have slight or moderate disability and only 10 per cent become severely crippled and dependent on others. Elderly and severely crippled patients may require permanent hospital care. In them, care of the skin is important as they are especially liable to pressure sores, so that frequent turning in bed is essential, and some measure of ambulation should be encouraged.

Reiter's syndrome

This is a triad of urethritis, arthritis (affecting joints in feet, legs or lumbo-sacral spine) and conjunctivitis. It occurs mainly in men and may follow a venereal infection with organisms of the group Bedsonia, which are intermediate between viruses and bacteria. The urethritis may respond to tetracycline or possibly to trimethoprim-sulphamethoxazole (Septrin, Bactrim) but only symptomatic treatment can be given for the arthritis. The condition tends to burn itself out in months or a year or two.

Osteoarthritis

Osteoarthritis or osteoarthrosis is best regarded as a degenerative disorder of the larger, weight-bearing joints. It results from a wearing-away of the cartilage on the opposing bone surfaces. Trauma and obesity contribute to it, and it is very common in the hips and knees of fat, middle-aged and elderly people. There is no systemic upset, but there may be an associated slight degenerative joint change in the terminal interphalangeal joints of the fingers. Little nodular swellings called Heberden's nodes are often seen here, and the patient can be reassured that they do not have the serious significance of the proximal interphalangeal joint swellings of rheumatoid arthritis—crippling hand deformity does not occur in osteoarthritis. The type with Heberden's nodes is called primary osteoarthrosis and is seen especially in post-menopausal women.

Symptoms and signs

(a) *Limb joints.*

There is pain and stiffness with creaking and grating of the large joints, especially after a period of immobility. The pain is sometimes episodic, possibly due to the irritation of little pieces of cartilage or osteophyte which break off into the joint. Cold and damp may precipitate an attack, but psychological factors such as depression also play a part—it is often difficult to relate the symptoms to the clinical and x-ray appearances, those with obvious damage may have few complaints while others with minor changes may complain bitterly.

In severe cases, there is joint deformity and destruction, and in the hips and knees this can result in serious disability and crippling. This is a common reason for hospitalization in the elderly.

(b) Arthritis of the spine.

Similar degenerative disease of the spinal joints has been described in Chapter 13 (page 347). Arthritic changes are especially liable to occur in the cervical spine in association with disc degeneration, causing the condition called *cervical spondylosis*. This is present in many people after middle age and may cause no symptoms. When symptoms occur, they include aches at the neck and restricted movement, often with tenderness and spasm in the surrounding muscles. Nerve root pressure may cause discomfort in the arms. It should be noted that osteoarthritis rarely affects the shoulder joint and symptoms here may be due to an inflammation of the joint capsule causing 'frozen shoulder' or to polymyalgia rheumatica, described below.

In the lumbar region arthritis may be associated with the low backache called lumbago and disc degeneration and prolapse may cause 'sciatica'—pain in the distribution of the sciatic nerve at the back of the leg from pressure on the roots contributing to the nerve.

TREATMENT

General measures

These include weight reduction, avoidance of trauma, and analgesics as necessary to relieve pain. Aspirin or paracetamol often suffice, but indomethacin, by capsule or suppository is useful. Phyenylbutazone is effective, but in view of its side effects the other drugs should be tried first. Oral steroids should not be used.

Heat and physiotherapy

The purposes of these are:

1. to relieve pain and relax muscles in spasm and thus allow mobilization of stiff joints,

2. to build up the muscles which guard and stabilize the joints.

Local heat is comforting and can be applied by wax baths, hot water bottles, warm flannel, or an electric pad. Heat from an *infra-red lamp* has only little penetration, but is safe, the only risk being of burning the skin. An ordinary electric fire is a reasonable source of infra-red heat.

Short wave diathermy produces heat in deeper tissues by the passage of a high frequency electric current. The affected part is placed between two electrodes situated a short distance from the skin. Short wave diathermy should be given only by a skilled physiotherapist, for there is no warning of overheating the tissues.

Ultrasound is a newer method of creating heat at a depth and is at present being evaluated.

Massage has fallen from favour in deference to active exercises, but it can be helpful in relaxing muscles in spasm. It may have greater application in non-articular or 'muscular' rheumatism—see below. As deep penetration of drugs through the skin does not occur, it makes little difference what substance is used in massage. Many popular remedies produce a feeling of warmth by slight skin irritation—oil of Wintergreen, methyl salicylate, actus thus and smells impressive though massage with olive oil is probably equally effective.

Exercises:

static and active quadriceps exercises build up the knee muscles;
sling and pulley exercises for the hips;
active exercises for spinal muscles.

These are practised in the physiotherapy department and continued at home.

Hydrotherapy—exercises in a deep warm pool may help to improve the range of movements as the effect of gravity is removed and the warmth is soothing. Regarding spa therapy, there is no evidence that 'taking the waters' internally has any special virtue. However, the relaxed atmosphere of spa resorts may contribute to a feeling of well-being and increased mobility may result.

Manipulation of joints is a way of increasing their mobility by force, but this must be gentle or further damage will result.

Local injection therapy

Hydrocortisone injection into an affected joint may relieve pain, but repeated injections cause joint destruction.

Infiltration of a painful area of soft tissue or muscle with a local anaesthetic such as lignocaine or procaine may alleviate symptoms temporarily, but has more application in 'muscular' rheumatism.

Supports and appliances

A cervical collar of felt or polysterene is useful in cervical spondylosis with nerve-root pressure. Lumbo-sacral supports tend to be worn for a few weeks then discarded. Calipers are of little value in supporting arthritic knees. Raising of a shoe may help if there is deformity and leg shortening.

Surgical measures

These include replacement of the hip joint with a metal or plastic prosthesis. The results are often gratifying.

Arthrodesis of a joint such as the knee may also be helpful.

Change of climate

Chilling and dampness should be avoided, but it is uncertain what influence, if any, barometric pressure and atmospheric humidity have in causing symptoms. Thus, while moving to a new district carries no guarantee of benefit, wintering in a warm climate may be helpful, if circumstances allow.

Gout

Gout is a metabolic disease associated with a high blood uric acid, crystals of which are deposited in joints causing recurrent attacks of arthritis.

The high blood uric acid is usually due to an over-production in the body, but there may be a defect in renal tubular excretion in addition. The over-production is a result of abnormal purine metabolism—purines are proteins present in many body cells, especially those of the pancreas and liver. Excessive consumption of foods such as sweetbreads (pancreas) and liver, and of alcohol, does not cause gout, as used to be thought, but may precipitate an attack. The gouty tendency or diathesis is inherited as a dominant, but gout is 95 per cent a male disease, and usually presents after the age of 50. There are racial predispositions, a high uric acid being common in Pacific islanders.

Apart from primary gout, the blood uric acid may be raised in blood diseases such as polycythaemia and following the use of oral diuretics, and gouty attacks may occur.

Symptoms and signs

There are recurrent attacks of pain and inflammation in one or more joints, probably due to uric acid crystal deposition at the time. The metatarso-phalangeal joint of the big toe is commonly affected and symptoms characteristically come on during the night, but may be precipitated by a heavy meal or alcohol, or by an infection or operation. The pain may be excruciating, the joint is swollen, and the part is red and shiny and exquisitely tender. The finger joints may also be affected. Recurrent attacks may be followed by a degenerative arthritis.

Deposits of uric acid may also be seen as white 'tophi' under the skin especially at the cartilage of the ears. These give the disease its name—gutta means 'a drop'. Deposition also occurs around the tubules of the kidney, predisposing to pyelonephritis and to renal failure. The 'gouty diathesis' may also be associated with arteriosclerosis and hypertension, and there may even be a gouty pericarditis with effusion. However, with treatment, the prognosis of gout is generally good.

Treatment

Excessive intake of purine-containing foods should be avoided.

Acute attacks respond to phenylbutazone (200 mg 6 hourly till pain relieved) or indomethacin (25 mg 4–6 hourly) which have tended to replace the older drug colchicine.

Long term treatment has as its object, the removal of the excess uric acid pool. Probenecid (Benemid), ethebenecid (Urelim) and sulphinpyrazone (Anturan) do this by increasing renal excretion and are called uricosuric drugs. The dose of probenecid is 0·5–1·0 G twice daily. Allopurinol (Zyloric) acts by lowering uric acid production, and is used if there is renal impairment, dose 100 mg 3 times daily. All these drugs may initially precipitate attacks of gout, so that the 'acute' drugs should be to hand. Aspirin antagonizes the action of the uricosuric drugs.

A high fluid intake helps to prevent uric acid deposition in the urinary tract. Treatment with uricosuric drugs must usually be lifelong to keep the blood uric acid normal.

Ankylosing spondylitis

This is an inflammatory disease of the joints of the spine, of unknown cause, affecting young men. The condition is *not* a form of rheumatoid arthritis, for rheumatoid factor is not found in the blood.

Symptoms and signs

The first symptoms usually occur before the age of thirty and the condition should be suspected in a previous healthy man complaining of back-ache or pains in the thighs. The sacro-iliac joints are first affected, changes are seen on x-ray, and the E.S.R. is raised. There is pain and stiffness of movement of the lumbar spine, spreading up to involve dorsal and even cervical spine, and in later stages bony fixation (ankylosis) of the joints occurs and the patient has a rigid 'poker-back' or 'bamboo spine'. The rib articulations may be involved, but respiration is seldom seriously impaired. In neglected cases the cervico-dorsal junction may become fixed in flexion with chin-on-chest deformity as a result. There may be minor involvement of hip joints and knees.

Iritis (inflammation of the iris of the eye) and rarely aortitis causing aortic incompetence are complications.

Occasionally the course is rapidly progressive, but usually pain settles as the spine becomes increasingly rigid over a period of years, and many patients can continue at work despite their disability.

Treatment

Symptoms are often worse after a period of rest, and ankylosing spondylitis is a type of arthritis in which immobilization is undesirable. Patients should be encouraged to keep on the move during the day, and at night should sleep on a firm mattress with a low pillow.

Aspirin, indomethacin or phenylbutazone afford symptomatic relief. Where they fail, x-ray therapy may be effective and may arrest the disease in some cases, but there is a raised incidence of leukaemia as a result of its use, and some consider this risk unjustifiable.

Muscular rheumatism—'fibrositis'

As noted, the term rheumatism is popularly used to mean aches, pains and stiffness attributed to disorders in joints, ligaments or muscles—if the latter, the term is qualified to 'muscular' rheumatism. Inflammatory disease of muscles is not, however, a common cause of recurrent symptoms—the only common inflammation or infection is epidemic myalgia or Bornholm disease, caused by a Coxsackie virus, presenting as chest wall pain and tenderness, and settling within a week or ten days. Abscesses of muscle may occur in the tropics. Myositis may occur in the rare connective tissue diseases described below.

The word fibrositis came into being in the 1930's when it was believed that little tender nodules, sometimes palpable in the neck and back muscles in those with aches and pains, were the cause of the symptoms. These nodules were ascribed to an inflammation in fibrous tissue, 'fibrositis', and were suggested as 'trigger spots' causing rheumaticky pains, possibly by nerve irritation—the word 'neuritis' may also be used by the lay person to describe his symptoms. There is now doubt as to whether there is such an entity as fibrositis, and any apparent nodulation may simply be a normal finding. However, infiltration of tender spots in the soft tissues or muscles with a local anaesthetic does sometimes relieve symptoms.

When a patient complains of rheumatism or fibrositis, it is important to exclude definable conditions such as the chronic rheumatic disorders described, local post-traumatic conditions such as frozen shoulder (inflammation of the tendons and capsule of the shoulder joint), polymyalgia rheumatica (see below) and bone disorders. Osteoarthritis of the spine is probably a common cause of many rheumaticky pains. Muscle spasm, from nerve irritation or in an attempt to protect the joint from undue movement, may explain some of the aches and tenderness around the part, and the symptoms are ascribed to the muscles instead of to the causative disease.

In many cases however, the cause of rheumaticky pains remains uncertain. Such troubles form a large proportion of sickness certifications and absence from work. The occurrence of symptoms is often ascribed to undue strain, or exposure to draughts, cold and dampness, and a warm climate may improve them. Again, symptoms are worse in those who are depressed—depressive illness may present with rheumatic pains.

As spontaneous improvement tends to occur simply with the passage of time, the results of many 'treatments' are difficult to evaluate, and placebo measures (i.e. the use of inert drugs which satisfy the patient) often help, as may the therapies of nature cure specialists and quacks—provided the patient is not suffering from serious disease.

Treatment

This follows the lines of that described for osteoarthritis. Measures include the correction of obesity and the avoidance of strains such as heavy lifting, but reasonable activity should be encouraged. Analgesics, heat, possibly massage, exercises as practised in the physiotherapy department, local anaesthetic infiltration—any or all of these may be helpful. In some cases, anti-depressive drugs may be indicated. The place of spa therapy and the possible benefit of a change to a warm climate have already been discussed.

Connective tissue ('collagen vascular') diseases

As noted this is a group of diseases in which there is degeneration of connective tissue in association with inflammation of small blood vessels. They may be disturbances of the immune mechanism of the body, and abnormal globulins and antibodies may be detectable in the blood, with a raised E.S.R. While rheumatoid arthritis (and rheumatic fever) could be included in the group, the term connective tissue diseases is customarily restricted to those described below.

SYSTEMIC (DISSEMINATED) LUPUS ERYTHEMATOSUS

This relatively rare condition occurs in young women. The cause is unknown, but many tissues are involved, possibly from deposition of immune complexes in the small arteries supplying them, with resultant inflammation and degeneration. The condition gets its name from an erythematous (erythema means redness of the skin) rash across the nose and cheeks, a 'butterfly' distribution. However, this rash is not always present and can occur as a local skin condition in the absence of any systemic disease. A lupus erythematosus-like syndrome may follow the use of drugs, including hydrallazine (occasionally used in hypertension) and procainamide, used in cardiac (ventricular) arrhythmias.

Symptoms and signs

Any system may be involved, and general symptoms include fever and malaise.

Joints. Patients often present with polyarthritis, similar in distribution to rheumatoid arthritis, but more transient, and constitutional disturbance is more marked than joint changes.

Skin. The 'butterfly' erythema at nose and cheeks may be present, often mild but worsened by exposure to sunlight. Erythema at the nail bases, due to dilated small vessels (telangiectasis), is characteristic. Purpura may occur. Thrombosis in small arteries may cause cold, pale finger tips with gangrenous patches.

Kidneys. Lesions may cause acute glomerulonephritis and risk of renal failure, or the more chronic picture of nephrotic syndrome with albuminuria and oedema.

The pleura may be involved with pleurisy and effusion, occasionally there are heart valve lesions, there is a tendency to haemolytic anaemia, and there is increased drug sensitivity with rashes.

Investigations

Systematic lupus erythematosus should be borne in mind as a cause of an obscure illness with fever, joint aches and blood changes in a young woman. The white cell count is low. Diagnosis is confirmed by a positive L.E. Latex test, which detects the abnormal antibody in the blood. This antibody affects the white cells, some of which engulf others and appear as the typical 'L.E. cells' on a blood smear. Various anti-nuclear factors are present. The E.S.R. is high. The blood urea may be raised.

Treatment

Rest is essential in acute phases. Analgesics such as aspirin may relieve symptoms but all severe cases should be treated with steroids —prednisone, initially 10 mg four or six hourly, reducing the dose as symptoms are controlled.

The prognosis is poor if there is renal involvement with high blood urea, but early cases now seem to do well over several years with appropriate steroid therapy.

POLYARTERITIS NODOSA AND CRANIAL ARTERITIS

Polyarteritis nodosa is a rare disturbance of small arteries throughout the body, commoner in middle-aged men. There is fever, tendency to arterial thrombosis with nodulation related to arteries, peripheral neuritis, raised white cell count with many eosinophilic cells, and high E.S.R. There may be a patchy recurrent pneumonia.

The diagnosis may be confirmed by muscle biopsy, the blood vessels in the muscle showing characteristic changes.

The condition known as *cranial (or giant cell or temporal) arteritis* is best regarded as a localized form of the same condition. It occurs in the elderly, presents with severe headache and there may be tenderness over the affected temporal artery, biopsy of which confirms the diagnosis. Its importance is its association with involvement of the retinal artery with the threat of blindness.

Treatment

Prednisone is a useful suppressive drug, and should be used without delay in cranial arteritis to prevent the risk of blindness. Maintenance doses are required for some months, when the disease may be found to have gone into remission.

POLYMYALGIA RHEUMATICA

This condition is given many different names and its exact nature is uncertain, but the clinical picture is clear cut. It presents in people over sixty as severe pain and stiffness at the muscles of the shoulder girdles (sometimes at the hips), especially in the early morning so that there may be difficulty moving from bed and dressing. Abduction of the shoulders is difficult and there is muscle tenderness, but slow passive movement can be carried out (unlike 'frozen shoulder'). The E.S.R. is raised and the condition may be related to polyarteritis or cranial arteritis. Its importance is, like the latter, that the retinal arteries may become involved. Patients are therefore best treated with prednisone, and usually a small dose suffices. If the E.S.R. remains normal, the drug can be discontinued after some months when the disease will commonly be found to have burnt itself out.

Other rare members of the 'Connective Tissue diseases' are:

DERMATO MYOSITIS—fever, skin-rash and painful tender muscles —sometimes associated with a carcinoma elsewhere which may not be clinically manifest.

SCLERODERMA and SYSTEMIC SCLEROSIS—here there are painful stiff fingers, the skin becoming hard and bound down to underlying structures. The face may be affected, so that the patient has difficulty in opening his mouth. Oesophageal involvement causes dysphagia. Sometimes the condition is preceded by Raynaud's phenomenon—episodic coldness and blueness of the fingers—usually an innocent condition due to vasospasm from sympathetic overactivity, but here actually due to disease of the small vessels.

Steroids are sometimes of value, and the drug d-penicillamine is being tried, but the condition is usually a progressive and disabling one.

Structure of bone

Bone contains living cells, in a protein matrix in which calcium salts are deposited. Flat bones such as the sternum, vertebrae and pelvis contain active marrow concerned in blood formation. However, even the long bones are not simply supporting structures, they are metabolically active, calcium deposition and resorption occurring all the time.

Rarefaction of bones occurs in osteoporosis, osteomalacia, hyperparathyroidism, myelomatosis and in metastatic bone disease.

Osteoporosis

Osteoporosis is a thinning of the bones, a loss of bone density, Normal stresses and strains protect against it, and if a limb is immobilized, osteoporosis occurs. Thus it may be seen locally in the bones round splinted joints, but occurs more generally if a patient is confined to bed. Rarely, osteoporosis has a known endocrine causes, such as Cushing's syndrome. Post-menopausally, it may be due to urinary calcium losses from hormonal deficiency.

Osteoporosis is very common in the elderly. The cause is uncertain. Though it has been regarded as a normal ageing change, current opinion relates it to calcium deficiency. There seems to be a fall in calcium absorption after the age of 70 (possibly due to mild vitamin D deficiency not amounting to that producing osteomalacia). The discovery of the hormone calcitonin (secreted mainly in the thyroid and concerned in maintaining the calcium content of the bones) has been followed by the suggestion that deficiency of it may play a part in osteoporosis.

Symptoms and signs

Osteoporosis especially affects the spine, the vertebrae becoming smaller, so that elderly people do become shorter in stature and may have prominent transverse skin-creases across the abdomen. Much bone has to be lost before x-ray changes of rarefaction are seen. There are aches and pains in the back. Some crush fractures of the vertebrae may occur but acute symptoms with nerve root involvement are rare—the old person seems to adapt to the gradual nature of the process.

Fracture of the neck of the femur, a common result of a fall in the elderly, may be more liable to occur if there is osteoporosis.

In osteoporosis alone, the blood calcium is normal.

Treatment

Calcium supplements have been given by mouth and claims made that bone pain decreases over some weeks, but no improvement has been proven on x-rays. More recently, calcium infusions have been tried. Hormones with an 'anabolic' effect—i.e. increasing protein deposition, have been given, with doubtful benefit. The hormone calcitonin is currently being evaluated.

Osteomalacia

This is the adult equivalent of rickets in childhood; it is defective mineralization of bone due to lack of calcium deposition, which in turn is due to deficiency of vitamin D. In rickety children, bones became soft, bent and deformed, changes being especially noticeable in the legs. In severe adult osteomalacia, there is gross deformity of the pelvis and spontaneous bone fractures. The blood calcium is low. Osteomalacia can occur in the elderly, but is less common than osteoporosis. See page 239, vitamin D deficiency.

Hyperparathyroidism—osteitis fibrosa cystica (von Recklinghausen's Disease of Bone)*

Hyperparathyroidism may cause generalized demineralization or local cyst formation with risk of fractures. The blood calcium is high, and there is excessive urinary calcium loss. The condition is described under Endocrine Disorders, page 363.

Myelomatosis (multiple myeloma) and amyloid disease

Myelomatosis is described under Diseases of the Blood. There are osteolytic (bone destructive) lesions in the vertebrae, pelvis skull and other flat bones due to deposits of plasma or myeloma cells. These lesions have a punched-out appearance on x-ray, and there may be a general bone rarefaction. Bone pains, fractures and spinal cord compression may all occur. The myeloma cells produce abnormal globulins which are found in the blood and are associated with raised E.S.R. and sometimes with Bence Jones protein in the urine. X-ray therapy may be used locally in treatment, and the cytotoxic drug melphalan (or cyclophosphamide) is given by mouth.

Amyloid disease may be appropriately referred to here. It may complicate chronic infections such as bronchiectasis, or destructive processes such as rheumatoid arthritis, and it also occurs in association with myelomatosis. Amyloid is a waxy substance, a degenerative product of collagen, and is formed when there is disturbance of globulin production. It is deposited in the spleen, liver and kidneys, causing enlargement of these organs, and may be associated with nephrotic syndrome with albuminuria and oedema. In myelomatosis

---

* von Recklinghausen's name is also given to Neurofibromatosis, an entirely different condition.

(and in a rare primary type of amyloidosis of unknown cause) deposits in the tongue cause macroglossia, there may be cardiac involvement, and deposits in the small intestinal wall result in malabsorption. However, the alimentary tract seems to be affected in any presentation of amyloid disease, for the diagnosis can be confirmed by biopsy of the gum or rectum, which contain the amyloid tissue. Amyloidosis is rare (though the primary form has been claimed to be a cause of heart failure in the elderly) and there is no effective treatment.

Metastatic bone disease

Malignant secondary deposits (metastases) are a common cause of bone disease. Bone arches and pains occur—symptoms may precede those of the primary tumour. X-ray changes are late, but bone scanning using radio-active strontium may allow earlier detection. Spontaneous 'pathological' fractures may occur, and in the spine these may cause cord compression and paraplegia.

The primary site may be in the prostate, breast, thyroid or lung. Oestrogenic hormones are of value in prostatic cases, otherwise only palliative treatment can be offered though such measures as pituitary ablation have been tried for disseminated breast carcinoma.

Paget's disease of bone* (osteitis deformans)

This is a disorder of the elderly, rather commoner in men. There is a thickening and deformity of the bones, the skull, tibia, femur and pelvis being especially affected. The cause is unknown. Characteristically, the skull enlarges, the patient complains of headaches and requires increasing sizes of hats. The legs become bowed, and with spine involvement, the afflicted patient shuffles along with the help of sticks and can be a most distressing sight. Bone pains occur. The circulation to the bones is increased, and murmurs may be heard with the stethoscope. In severe cases, heart strain and failure results. There is a risk, too, of development of malignant tumours called sarcomas in the affected bones.

There are typical changes on x-ray, and the blood alkaline phosphatase is extremely high, confirming the diagnosis.

Up till recently analgesics were all that could be offered in treatment but calcitonin and the drug mithramycin appear to be helpful.

* Paget's disease of the nipple is an entirely separate disease—an inflammation of the nipple associated with a carcinoma of a duct of the breast

Diseases of muscle—myopathy

The word myopathy can be applied to any disorder of muscle, inflammatory or metabolic, but is customarily used to describe diseases presenting with muscle weakness.

THE MUSCULAR DYSTROPHY GROUP (INHERITED MYOPATHIES)

This is a group of rare, hereditary disorders affecting mainly young people, and causing muscular weakness.

Types

Duchenne type—pseudo-hypertrophic muscular dystrophy. Presents in infancy, occurs only in boys—it is a sex-linked recessive disorder (as is haemophilia). Waddling gait, weakness and tendency to contractures, muscles appear bulky (pseudo-hypertrophic) but become progressively paralysed—child rises from the floor by 'climbing up his legs'. Prone to infection, heart complications and early death.

Limb-girdle type—adolescents affected, both sexes, autosomal recessive, weakness of shoulders and in raising arms, difficulty climbing stairs—progressively weaker over 10–20 years.

Facio-scapulo-humeral type—less severe and may present in adults —autosomal dominant inheritance so that affected individuals pass it on to half their children, so family planning advice is necessary. Weakness of facial muscles and difficulty in closing the eyes and puffing the cheeks, winging of scapulae, some weakness in arms and legs again with tendency to waddling gait. Often remains in this mild form over many years.

Dystrophia myotonica may also be classified in this group, but presents in adults—dominant inheritance. Weakness and wasting of facial muscles and sterno mastoids, and *myotonia*, which means continued active contraction of a muscle after voluntary stimulus is over—stiffness and inability to 'let go' after shaking hands. Associated frontal baldness, cataracts, gonadal atrophy and progressive mental deterioration.

Investigations

Serum enzymes—creatine kinase raised in Duchenne type.

Electromyography—investigation of electrical activity of the muscles, which is disturbed. There is a recent suggestion that the abnormality may be in the motor nerve supply in some cases rather than in the muscles themselves.

Muscle biopsy.

Treatment

There is no known cure. Drugs such as quinine, procainamide and phenytoin may help myotonia. Patients should keep active as far as possible, helped by courses of physiotherapy. The diseases are worsened by bed rest, with added risk of complications such as pneumonia. Surgical correction of deformities may be required.

Genetic considerations and prevention

Female carriers of the gene causing the severe Duchenne type may now be identified with the aid of serum enzyme and other tests, and family planning advice given to prevent the birth of boys who would be affected by the disease.

ENDOCRINE, METABOLIC AND CARCINOMATOUS MYOPATHIES

Proximal myopathy, weakness of the muscles of the shoulder-gridle and thigh, may complicate thyroid disorders (thyrotoxicosis, myxoedema) and is common in Cushing's syndrome. The patient has difficulty in raising the arms above the head, and in stair climbing. There may be wasting of the affected muscles. A similar picture may occur in osteomalacia, causing a waddling gait, and may be related to low serum calcium.

A low serum potassium level (*hypokalaemia*) causes muscular weakness, and occurs in aldosteronism, but the excessive use of diuretics is by far the commonest reason. In the treatment of heart failure and oedematous states, potassium supplements should be given.

Familial periodic paralysis is a rare disease causing episodes of muscle weakness usually associated with a low serum potassium and occurring after a period of rest (unlike myasthenia gravis, where weakness occurs in tired muscles).

Rare defects of muscle sugars and enzyme abnormalities are associated with muscle weakness.

Carcinoma, especially *bronchogenic carcinoma*, may be associated with myasthenia-like (see below) muscle weakness and should be considered in obscure cases in the middle-aged and elderly.

Myasthenia gravis

Myasthenia gravis is an uncommon disease with onset in adult life or late childhood. It is due to a defect in the transmission of the nerve impulse at the neuromuscular junction so that the muscle fails to contract and remains flaccid. This flaccidity and paralysis resemble that caused by the arrow-poison curare, derivatives of which are used by anaesthetists to cause muscle relaxation during operations. However rather than being due to a curare-like effect, it is now believed that the disturbance in myasthenia is an impaired synthesis or release of acetylcholine, the neuromuscular transmitter substance. This disturbance may be due to a factor produced by the thymus gland which may be enlarged (or contain a tumour), in some cases of myasthenia. The disorder may result from some disturbance of immunity (an auto-immune disease).

Symptoms and signs

The patient experiences muscle weakness, especially of muscles of the face, so that he may have difficulty in keeping his eyes open, in chewing, and even in swallowing. The arms may also be affected. Symptoms are worse towards the end of the day when the muscles are tired. Cases have been described where an affected child was unable to keep his eyes open or hold his head up in the classroom, and a policeman was unable to apprehend a criminal due to muscular weakness as he was about to make the arrest. Thus, though rare, the diagnosis should be considered in such patients who might otherwise be labelled 'neurotic'.

Diagnosis and treatment

The diagnosis is confirmed by the slow intravenous injection of edrophonium (Tensilon) 10 mg, a cholinergic drug which produces an immediate return of muscular power. The longer acting drug neo-stigmine (Prostigmine), tablets of 15 mg and the even longer acting pyridostigmine (Mestinon) are used in treatment. In cases showing a poor response, thymectomy (removal of the thymus) may be helpful.

16

Diseases of the skin

Structure of the skin

The outer layer, or *epidermis*, consists of stratified epithelial cells which are continually replaced from below, losing their nuclei and becoming progressively worn as they reach the surface where their remains form the scaly or horny surface layer.

The deeper *dermis* or true skin has projections into the epidermis, making their junction serrated, as seen under the microscope. The dermis consists of loose connective tissue and contains the nerves, blood vessels, hair follicles with their sebaceous (oil-secreting) glands, and the sweat glands.

Functions

1. Protective, and also a sense organ for pain, temperature and touch.

2. Temperature regulation.

3. Concerned in fluid and mineral metabolism, excessive losses in insensible evaporation or visible sweating causing water and salt depletion.

4. Production of vitamin D by action of ultra-violet light.

Infections

(*a*) *Bacterial*

Boils are due to staphylococcal infection in a hair follicle and may go on to abscess or carbuncle formation, when systemic antibacterial therapy is indicated—pencillin if the organism is sensitive.

Impetigo is an infection caused by staphylococci and streptococci together, and consists of blisters, tending to become pustular and crusted, on inflamed skin. It may follow neglect, scratching and lack of cleanliness after abrasions or septic spots, and is seen mainly in children. Treatment is local cleansing with cetrimide and pencillin locally or systemically.

Erysipelas is a spreading inflammation in the superficial layers of the skin near a muco-cutaneous junction such as the lips or nose. It is a streptococcal infection which responds to systemic penicillin.

Cellulitis is a spreading inflammation in the subcutaneous tissues from a septic area or ulcer. The cause is usually a staphylococcal or streptococcal infection, and treatment is appropriate antibacterial drugs.

It should be noted that the mild redness of the skin around a varicose ulcer, and the slightly purulent base of the ulcer are not indications for systemic antibacterial drugs. The organism cultured is usually one of low virulence, or an extension of the normal skin flora. Local cleansing and wound toilet are usually all that is necessary.

Tuberculosis of the skin of the face, lupus vulgaris, is now rarely seen.

Leprosy should be remembered as a cause of skin disease in under-developed countries.

(b) Fungus

Infection of the mouth with the fungus *Candida* (*Monilia*) results in the white patches called *thrush*, which is found in debilitated patients or those receiving broad-spectrum antibiotics. A similar infection may occur in the vagina, causing *pruritus vulvae*, and is especially likely to occur in *diabetics*.

Intertrigo is a moist red rash occurring where two surfaces rub together and cleanliness is lacking, and may be due to an eczema reaction (see below) complicated by a low grade infection with a fungus of the Candida group. It is common under the breasts of obese women—there is an offensive oozing patch with a red edge containing pin-point vesicles. The condition responds to cleansing and application of amphotericin (Fungilin) lotion, nystatin ointment, or simple dusting powders.

Tinea is a term applied to other human fungus infections of the skin, conditions sometimes called *Ringworm*. In children, ringworm may affect the hair but in adults the condition is seen in moist areas—between the toes (*Athlete's Foot*) and at the groins (dhobi itch—from its occurrence in India and the tropics). Between the toes the skin becomes soggy and macerated. At the groins there is a spreading red ring (which gives the disease its name) of inflammation, with healing tending to occur in the centre of the patch—the same appearance as intertrigo, with considerable irritation and some odour. Tinea responds to cleansing and the application of paints and fungicides such as Whitfield's ointment (contains salicylate) or the more modern tolnaftate creams (e.g. Tinaderm). Tinea can also affect the nails. Severe cases are treated with the oral drug griseofulvin. Other forms of ringworm are acquired from contact with infected animals.

Fungal infections may be complicated by a more chronic inflammatory skin reaction, and by bacterial infection if treatment is neglected.

(c) *Virus*

Herpes simplex is a virus infection, causing 'cold sores' around the lips and nose, sometimes in association with lobar pneumonia. Though a mild infection when confined to the skin, the virus is highly dangerous in newborn infants, where it may invade the nervous system causing encephalitis—thus sufferers should keep away from the nursery.

Herpes zoster (shingles) is a vesicular eruption along the line of a a nerve—seen usually on the trunk, sometimes in the face from involvement of the ophthalmic division of the fifth cranial (trigeminal) nerve. Pain may be severe, with tendency to secondary infection. The virus responsible also causes chicken pox, yet contact spread is rare.

Molluscum contagiosum is a virus infection causing little watery blisters—it may be acquired at swimming pools. Touching the blisters with phenol is an effective treatment.

Common warts are induced by virus infection, though the reasons for their appearances and disappearances are obscure. They may be removed with carbon dioxide snow. *Senile warts* are larger warty outgrowths in the skin of the elderly, and are of no serious significance.

Infestations

LOUSE INFESTATION (PEDICULOSIS)

Lice are small flat insects which feed on blood. Head lice may infest the scalp of children, young women and youths with long hair, the eggs or nits being attached to the shaft of the hair. The nits are greyish-white specks which can be cracked between the finger nails and in severe infestation the hair may be covered with them. The irritation of the adult lice causes scratching and minor skin infection, with enlargement of the occipital and cervical lymph glands as a result. Infestation spreads easily in schools.

Body lice affect people who are dirty—vagrants, and those living huddled together in squalid conditions in refugee camps. Lice transmit typhus, which was the scourge of armies and beleaguered cities. The principal effect of lice is, however, the irritation caused by their bites—the bites appear as small red spots, and there is much scratching and slight secondary infection. The louse lives in the seams of clothing, where it lays its eggs.

Crab lice affect the pubic region and are spread by sexual intercourse.

Louse infestation is treated with insecticides such as D.D.T. (dicophane) or gamma benzene hydrochloride (gamma B.H.C.). Two applications a week apart are necessary for head lice, to kill the parasites hatching from the nits. The whole family should be treated.

SCABIES

Scabies is an infestation with a small mite called the acarus. The female acarus is just visible to the naked eye and burrows into the epidermis, causing severe itching. Favourite sites are the clefts of the fingers, the front of the wrists and elbows, axillary fold and pectoral region—areas which can be scratched, the parasite being spread by the finger nails. The burrows are visible as greyish lines up to a centimetre in length and there may be a raised red eruption which tends to secondary infection. Minor epidemics of scabies occur in school children and in the elderly in hospital, the condition being very contagious in institutions. It should be remembered in any patient with intractable itch. The acarus can be picked out with a pin and identified under the microscope.

Affected patients are given a hot bath, then painted from chin to toes with benzyl benzoate application, or gamma B.H.C. Application is repeated the next day, and the following day the preparation can be washed off by bathing. All contacts should be treated at the same time. Elaborate disinfestation of bedding is not required.

FLEAS

Fleas have become uncommon, but flea bites should be borne in mind as a cause of itchy, raised red spots with a central bite-mark even in people who pride themselves on their cleanliness.

Dermatitis and eczema

Dermatitis means inflammation of the skin and includes the *'eczema reaction'* which typically starts with erythema (reddening) followed by the formation of tiny fluid-containing vesicles and 'weeping', followed by a more chronic scaling stage when the skin may become thickened or 'lichenified'. Eczematous lesions are usually extremely itchy. The terms dermatitis and eczema are sometimes used interchangeably.

Eczema may be present in infancy and be followed by flexural eczema (Besnier's prurigo) in childhood. There is an association with asthma, and such patients are said to manifest atopy, an inherited tendency to show hypersensitivity or allergic reactions. The eczema and asthma may improve in adolescence, but the skin seems to remain very sensitive. People with no previous allergic history may also have skins which are prone to show the eczema reaction. The primula plant produces a reaction on contact with the skin in many normal people, but in those with the eczema tendency, many substances innocuous to others also result in dermatitis. Thus chemicals and drugs cause contact dermatitis in susceptible subjects—nickel-plated suspender and brassiere clips produce an eruption where they rub the skin, and reaction may develop to eye-shadow and lipstick. Soaps and detergents, and substances met with at work (occupational or industrial dermatitis) may cause contact dermatitis, the handling of pencillin and streptomycin. Sunlight sometimes makes such reactions worse—photosensitivity.

A skin reaction may also be provoked by the ingestion of a substance to which the person is hypersensitive, and this occurs in many drug reactions considered below.

Some patients are prone to a form of eczema, sometimes called seborrhoeic eczema or seborrhoeic dermatitis, occurring especially in flexures, e.g. behind the ears causing fissuring, in the axillae, groins or under the breasts. Seborrhoea means increased sebum and there is an association with dandruff and dermatitis near the hair follicles, but these are not necessarily present in this adult flexural eczema. Eczema may follow any infection of the skin, though it is not in itself contagious. Flexural eczema may be associated with a low-grade fungus or bacterial infection and is the basis for the *intertrigo* under the breasts already referred to.

Varicose (gravitational) eczema is a result of low-grade infection and irritation following venous stasis.

Pompholyx is a vesicular eczema of the hands, with tiny pin-point water blisters on thickened skin, and may be a reaction to skin irritation or infection elsewhere, e.g. tinea of the feet.

A note on treatment

In any dermatitis, it is a good principle to use only simple local applications such as calamine lotion until the condition either disappears or is diagnosed by a dermatologist. This is especially true in the eczema reaction, where the application of preparations containing antibiotics may only make matters worse.

Corticosteroid lotions, creams and ointments often produce a rapid improvement. There are many preparations available, the simplest being hydrocortisone 1 per cent. Their indiscriminate use may, however, allow spread of infection, repeated applications can cause atrophy of the skin, and with some preparations systemic absorption may lead to steroid side-effects and depression of adrenal cortical function.

Drug rashes

These are very common in hospital practice, and while the eruption may follow local application or contact, usually it is due to a drug that has been taken by mouth. Drug eruptions are a result of a delayed hypersensitivity, cell-mediated allergic reaction.

Barbiturates especially phenobarbitone may provoke a diffuse blotchy-red itchy rash, or many red spots tending to coalesce rather like measles.

Aspirin, sulphonamides, antibiotics especially ampicillin, and oral anticoagulants such as phenindione may cause a skin eruption in sensitive subjects—it may be of any pattern, but tends to be repeated if the drug is inadvertently given again, and here there may be a more severe general reaction.

However, any drug may cause a rash, and in doubtful cases it is wise to stop all but essential medication to see if the rash clears.

Anti-histamine drugs such as chlorpheniramine (Piriton) are often given in treatment, but probably only ease the itching, the rash subsiding spontaneously when the offending drug is stopped. Anti-histamine drugs should not be used as ointments or creams for they are liable to provoke rashes themselves in this form.

Iodine-containing substances, used in x-ray contrast media and in proprietary cough bottles, may cause a characteristic vesicular rash.

Heavy metals such as gold, used in the treatment of rheumatoid arthritis, may cause a severe *Exfoliative Dermatitis* (*Erythroderma*) with generalized reddening of the skin and there may be extensive peeling. This is a serious condition demanding fluid replacement, steroids, and antibiotics to treat secondary infection.

Urticaria

This is the appearance of itchy red lumps in the skin, from oedema and inflammation in the deeper layer (dermis). In some cases, the patient using his finger nail or a match stick may be able to write his name on his skin.

Some individuals have this heightened reactivity when exposed to nervous stress, such as examinations, to a hot or cold bath or to contact with or ingestion of substances ranging from tomatoes to drugs, or following insect bites.

Urticaria is due to the 'immediate' type of allergic reaction in which *histamine* is released, and the reaction can be suppressed by anti-histamine drugs.

Severe cases go on to '*angio-neurotic oedema*' when there is a puffy oedematous swelling of the eyes and face, and the larynx may also become swollen from oedema. Treatment is the immediate injection of adrenaline 0·5–1·0 ml of 1 in 1000 solution subcutaneously, followed by hydrocortisone 100 mg and an antihistamine drug intravenously.

Acne

Acne occurs in adolescence, especially in males, and is an effect of male sex hormone on the hair follicles, stimulating their secretion of sebum (the natural hair oil). The hair follicles become blocked with secretion and scales, forming blackheads (comedones) with some swelling and redness causing little raised papules in the affected area, often the chin and neck. Removal of blackheads, cleansing with cetrimide, and a small dose of tetracycline by mouth are often helpful.

Rosacea

This is sometimes mis-called acne rosacea, but the condition has no relation to acne. Rosacea is an erythema of the cheeks affecting middle-aged women due to dilated skin vessels, and may be worsened by stress and possibly by hot or spicy foods. However, tetracycline orally may again be helpful. Topical steroids should not be used as they may cause further dilatation of facial capillaries, making the flushing worse.

Lupus erythematosus

This is an erythematous rash on the nose and face which may be patchy or conform to the 'butterfly' distribution across nose and cheeks. The skin may become thickened and there may be scarring with disfigurement. It occurs in young and middle-aged women either alone or in association with systemic lupus erythematosus, and is worsened by exposure to sunlight. Thus patients may be helped by wearing a wide-brimmed hat, and sun-screening creams such as Uvistat can be tried. Severe cases respond to local application of steroid creams. Chloroquine orally may help, but used long-term may affect the cornea and retina.

Psoriasis

This is a common chronic skin disease, often presenting in adolescence, but it may occur at any age. It is characterized by scaly patches on the skin. The cause is unknown but there is a familial tendency, and although the lesions appear discrete, there is a disturbance of function throughout the epidermis.

The scaly patches often occur over extensor surfaces such as elbows and knees, but in severe cases may be much more diffuse. The patches are disc-sized or larger, reddish and slightly raised, the scales producing a silvery appearance with a white line on scraping. The condition is unsightly, with much flaking of the scales, but there need be no itch. In more severe cases the patches are at times red and weepy, and here there is more irritation. Psoriasis may be associated with an arthritis rather like rheumatoid arthritis, though the terminal joints of the fingers are more liable to be involved and psoriasis of the nails may be associated.

Treatment includes the application of steroid creams under occlusive polythene dressings, or the preparation dithranol, but recurrence is common.

Pityriasis rosea

This is a rash of slightly itchy pink spots with scaly edges, occurring on the trunk, in young adults. The rash may be preceded by a single 'herald patch', and disappears in 4–6 weeks. The cause is unknown. Calamine lotion is usually all that is necessary.

Erythema multiforme

This is a red or heliotrope patchy rash of the trunk, and may be a sensitivity reaction to sulphonamides. Severe cases are associated with conjunctivitis and inflammation around the genitals, the Stevens-Johnson syndrome.

Lichen planus

Here reddish-violet raised areas, papules, appear especially at the flexor surfaces of the wrists and elbows, but lesions can occur in the mouth. The cause is unknown. Itching may be severe. Local steroids (such as hydrocortisone or the more powerful fluorinated compounds) may be used under occlusive polythene dressings, but in severe cases oral treatment may be justified.

Dermatitis herpetiformis

This is a recurrent vesicular eruption of unknown cause. The lesions have some resemblance to those of herpes zoster. Adults are affected the vesicles tend to occur in groups on the elbows, knees, upper part of the back and where there is pressure from clothing, and they have a raised red base. There is intense itching. The condition is sometimes associated with intestinal mucosal atrophy similar to that in coeliac disease, resulting in a malabsorption syndrome. The eruption responds to the drug dapsone (also used in the treatment of leprosy) and to sulphapyridine.

Pemphigus

This is a serious skin disease of the elderly and may be a disturbance of immunity. Fluid-containing *bullae* form in the epidermis and appear as blisters or larger blebs, the thin roof of which gives way leaving an oozing inflamed surface—parts of the epidermis may be shed. Lesions also appear in the mouth. Treatment is oral steroids in large doses, but the prognosis is often poor.

Pemphigoid is a less dangerous condition of unknown cause—bullae form at the basal layer of the epidermis; they are rather thicker-walled and more tense than those of pemphigus. Steroid treatment is often effective. Similar bullous lesions are sometimes seen in barbiturate poisoning.

Tumours of the skin

PRIMARY TUMOURS

The rodent ulcer or basal cell carcinoma is a slow-growing tumour occurring on the face near the nose, eye or ear of an elderly person. It responds well to x-ray therapy.

A squamous cell carcinoma is a more rapidly growing malignancy which spreads to lymph nodes, so that therapy has to be more extensive and is less satisfactory.

The common mole or naevus rarely becomes malignant, but the malignant melanoma is a pigmented spot of high malignancy which spreads locally, and metastasises commonly to the liver; there is no satisfactory treatment.

Mycosis fungoides is not a fungus infection as the name suggests, but a type of skin malignancy presenting as almost any type of rash followed by nodulation and ulceration. Treatment is unsatisfactory and the prognosis is poor.

SECONDARY TUMOURS

Secondary deposits present as little lumps in the skin, which may ulcerate. The primary is commonly a carcinoma of the lung or stomach. Skin involvement means that the spread is extensive and the outlook poor, with only palliative treatment being possible.

Skin deposits may also occur in leukaemia and the reticuloses.

Acanthosis nigricans is a dark scaly eruption which is a reaction to carcinoma in the alimentary tract. The latter may not be clinically manifest, but the appearance of the characteristic skin eruption should lead to a search for its presence.

Alopecia

Alopecia means loss of hair, and may be partial, or total, causing baldness. Systemic causes include myxoedema. Patchy loss may

result from any lesion causing scarring. It also occurs in the condition
alopecia areata, where one or more hairless patches appear; the
cause is unknown and there is no satisfactory treatment. In young
people regrowth usually occurs spontaneously, but in older age
groups the loss may be permanent and a wig may be required. Loss
of hair is a possible complication of therapy with the cytotoxic drug
cyclophosphamide.

The skin in systemic diseases

Purpura should not be confused with Campbell de Morgan's spots—
little red vascular spots common in the skin of those over forty and
of no significance. The spider naevi of cirrhosis should also be distinguished. Multiple telangiectases, little dilated capillaries, may
occur in association with a generalized telangiectasia, where there
may be bleeding from lesions in the alimentary tract. Often the
telangiectases are well seen at the lips and under the tongue. The
Peutz-Jegher's syndrome is the association of pigmented spots at
the lips with haemangiomatous lesions in the gut.

Xanthomas are little raised yellow spots at the elbows, buttocks
and sometimes over the Achilles tendon at the heel. There may be
an associated yellow pigmentation in the 'lines of life' in the palms.
Xanthomas occur in disturbances of lipid metabolism, usually with
raised serum cholesterol and increased risk of atherosclerosis from
deposits in the arteries.

Erythema nodosum consists of dusky red, coin-sized, slightly
raised, itchy lesions over the shins and lower legs. It occurs as a reaction to several conditions, tuberculosis, sarcoidosis and streptococcal infection being likely causes in Britain. In the United States the
fungal infection coccidiodomycosis, and in underdeveloped countries
leprosy, may precipitate the reaction. It may occur in ulcerative
colitis and Crohn's disease, or be due to drugs, but sometimes no
cause can be found. There may be associated joint aches and swelling. In idiopathic cases rest and analgesics suffice, the condition
settling in a week or two.

Sarcoidosis may also present as a scattered papular rash, or as a
chilblain-like redness at the tip of the nose and at the finger joints.
Chilblains themselves are due to poor circulation in the skin capillaries on exposure to cold, but do not signify deficiency or serious
disease, and protection from cold is all that is required. Cold
exposure may also precipitate Raynaud's syndrome (cold blue or

white fingers) due to vasospasm, but where similar skin changes occur in warm surroundings, one should suspect small-vessel disease as in systemic lupus erythematosus, scleroderma or other 'collagen-vascular' disorder.

Exposure to sunlight may cause rashes and vesicular eruptions in certain types of porphyria, rare disorders of haemoglobin metabolism associated with abnormal urinary pigments, and sometimes worsened by barbiturates.

PIGMENTATION OF THE SKIN

The normal pigmentation is largely due to melanin formed by special cells, melanocytes, in the basal region of the epidermis. In the *albino* there is a recessively inherited defect in the melanocytes, which fail to produce melanin. In hypopituitarism, there is a lack of melanocyte-stimulating hormone (M.S.H.) and patients are pale as a result.

Pallor of the skin is, of course, much more commonly due to anaemia.

Vitiligo, patchy loss of pigmentation, is due to lack of melanocytes in the affected areas of skin (often in the arms, face and neck) and may occur in auto-immune diseases such as pernicious anaemia and thyroiditis.

Pigmentation is increased in sun-tanning. Addison's disease (pituitary M.S.H. being produced along with A.C.T.H. which attempts to stimulate the atrophic adrenals), and haemochromatosis —in the latter, there is increased melanin as well as iron deposition in the skin. Poisoning with the heavy metals arsenic and silver (argyria) also causes abnormal pigmentation.

Patches of increased pigmentation called café-au-lait spots occur in neurofibromatosis, von Recklinghausen's disease (not to be confused with von Recklinghausen's disease of bone, which is due to hyperparathyroidism). This is a disease of dominant inheritance. The neurofibromas may be visible or palpable as little swellings in the skin or subcutaneous tissues, and associated with similar lesions in the central nervous system, causing root and cord compression, or the 'acoustic neuroma' at the cerebello-pontine angle.

Jaundice is yellow discoloration due to deposition of bile pigment (bilirubin) in the skin.

PRURITUS (ITCHING)

Local irritation in scabies, insect bites, eczema, urticaria, lichen planus and dermatitis herpetiformis has already been described. It

14—EM * *

also occurs in prickly heat in the tropics, possibly a result of sweat gland obstruction.

Pruritus ani, itching around the anus, may be due to threadworms, or fungus infection and lack of cleanliness, but may be associated with anxiety and depressive states. Pruritus vulvae may occur in an atrophic inflammation in middle-aged women, or from trichomonas vaginalis infection, but candida (thrush) infection is a common cause, in association with diabetes mellitus, and the urine must always be tested for sugar.

Other systemic diseases causing a more generalized itch include obstructive jaundice, Hodgkin's disease, leukaemia, carcinoma, and chronic renal failure with uraemia. Old people often scratch themselves for no apparent reason, and psychogenic factors sometimes play a part in younger age groups.

Pruritus may occur with cocaine or morphine, and in hypersensitivity to many other drugs.

EFFECTS OF SKIN DISEASE ON OTHER SYSTEMS

Extensive inflammatory skin lesions impose a considerable demand on the circulation and may contribute to cardiac failure in those with existing heart disease. The effects of fluid losses and disturbance of temperature regulation have also to be borne in mind.

Dermatitis herpetiformis and some other diseases may be associated with flattening of the intestinal mucosa as in coeliac disease, and malabsorption, which improves with treatment of the skin condition.

Absorption of steroids from topically applied creams may result in systemic steroid side-effects and depression of adrenal cortical function.

Though the skin is often 'the mirror of the mind', skin diseases can be disfiguring, causing embarrassment and distress and resulting in depressive illness—treatment directed to the latter may improve the skin condition.

17

Mental disorders

Psychiatry is the branch of medicine devoted to the diagnosis and treatment of mental disorder. Mental disorder is divided into two groups—*mental subnormality*, and *mental illness.*

Mental subnormality (mental retardation)

Here there is a failure of normal brain development.

Known causes include:

(i) *chromosome abnormality*—mongolism (Down's syndrome)—extra chromosome. Other defects becoming recognized.

(ii) *gene abnormality*—phenylketonuria, an enzyme defect, excess amino-acid (phenylalanine) damages brain, but detection at birth (Guthrie test) and special diet prevent this.

(iii) *damage to embryo*—rubella (German measles) and toxoplasmosis in early pregnancy.

(iv) *injury at birth.*

(v) *post natal*—infections (e.g. meningitis); hypothyroidism if untreated (cretinism).

In many cases the cause is unknown.

Mentally subnormal persons may be grouped according to Intelligence Quotient (I.Q.). Normal I.Q. is taken as 100. Those with I.Q. over 80 may be educable normally, I.Q. 50–80 are subnormal require special schooling, I.Q. under 50 are severely subnormal. However, personality and emotional adjustment, and family and social background influence management, as does the type of society—the mentally handicapped may be better accepted in a rural community than in an industrial city. Mentally handicapped children should be managed at home or within the community as far as possible—confinement to institutions results in social isolation, worsening their plight. Admission to special hospitals is unfortunately still required for a proportion of the mentally subnormal.

Mental illness

Types
    (*a*) *Due to an organic lesion.*
    (*b*) *Non-organic—Psychiatric.*
    (*c*) *Personality disorders.*

(*a*) ORGANIC

Here a known physical disease affects the brain, e.g. neurosyphilis, cerebral tumour, or arteriosclerosis. *Dementia*, deterioration of intellect and memory, may result and is considered below.

(*b*) NON-ORGANIC—PSYCHIATRIC

1. *Anxiety and depressive states*—often called the neuroses or affective neuroses, there being a disturbance of the emotions or 'affect'. The patient retains his insight—he realizes he is suffering from such a state. Anxiety neuroses include obsessive-compulsive states, and phobias (irrational fears). Depressive illness is extremely common in all societies.

2. *Psychosis*—a severe disorder in which the patient fails to realize he is mentally ill. Schizophrenia (literally 'splitting of the mind') is the classical example, and the patient may be completely detached from reality.

3. *Psychosomatic and hysterical disorders*—here the patient has symptoms for which there is no physical basis.

(*c*) PERSONALITY DISORDERS

1. *Psychopathic disorder.* A psychopath is a person who fails to conform to accepted social standards or conduct without being aware that he may be doing wrong. Psychopaths may be aggressive, creative, or inadequate, dependent on charity and often guilty of petty crime.

2. *Alcoholism and drug dependence.* Dependence exists when a person is compelled to take a drug for its psychic effects. Withdrawal may result in feelings so unpleasant that the habit is resumed.

GENERAL MANAGEMENT OF MENTAL ILLNESS
It will be seen from the above classification that there is often no firm distinction between physical illness and mental illness—indeed as the workings of the mind are unravelled, it is becoming clear that many so-called mental disorders have a physical cause. Thus depression may be due to disturbed function of the emotional system connected with the hypothalamus, some schizophrenics have an abnormality of amine production, and an extra Y chromosome may be found in some criminal psychopaths. These considerations apart, physical illness may present as a mental illness such as depression. Again, the mental state of the patient affects his reaction to systemic disease—'there are no diseases, only sick people'—one cannot separate psyche (the mind) from soma (the body).

Thus the division of mentally ill patients into a group to be kept apart in a special institution is no longer justified. The disturbed behaviour associated with mental disorders was often due to lack of understanding by relatives or doctors, leading to resentment and agitation in the patients who were quite unjustifiably confined behind locked doors. Some of the symptoms attributed to mental illness were in fact due to such institutionalization and social isolation. Modern psychiatric units are therefore part of the general hospital service.

Most patients who are mentally ill can be handled through normal channels, by referral to the psychiatric out-patient department and admission if required, the patient usually being willing to accept hospital care if so advised. In cases of urgent necessity, when the patient's behaviour is a danger to himself or others, in Britain Section 29 of the Mental Health Act allows one doctor to order detention in hospital for seventy-two hours. This period permits psychiatric assessment and advice on further care.

Organic mental illness

TOXIC-CONFUSIONAL STATES (DELIRIUM)
A toxic confusional state or delirium results from disordered function of the brain—there is clouding of consciousness, disorientation, confusion and restlessness, often accompanied by hallucinations (false perceptions). A toxic confusional state has an organic cause—fever, infection, toxaemia, electrolyte depletion, hepatic failure (portal systemic encephalopathy) poisoning with alcohol or drugs, and, most important, any condition causing cerebral anoxia. A slight

decrease in the oxygen supply to the brain cells is especially important where there is pre-existing brain damage or degeneration (as in dementia). Thus respiratory infection or heart failure are common causes in the elderly. A toxic confusional state is reversible if the cause can be treated.

The differentiation from an acute behaviour disturbance accompanying psychiatric illness such as schizophrenia or hysteria is not usually difficult, for in these there is no background of physical illness.

A restless or agitated patient may require sedation with chlorpromazine (Largactil) 100 mg intramuscularly, or diazepam (Valium) 5–10 mg slowly intravenously. Haloperidol (Serenace) 5–10 mg, or paraldehyde may be required in the severely disturbed.

DEMENTIA

Dementia is a deterioration of mental function following brain damage or disease—such damage is usually severe and extensive.

There is impairment of intellect, associated with impairment of memory—the patient has a loss of memory for recent events but may be able to recall happenings of many years ago. The memory disturbance causes disorientation in time and place. There is a deterioration and coarsening of personality, and emotions may be shallow or disturbed. Thus social behaviour disintegrates, personal appearance and hygiene are neglected, and the patient may become filthy in his toilet habits. Conversation with the patient, enquiries as to his name, address, age, and family ties, day of the month, current events, simple arithmetic (subtracting 7 from 100), giving him numbers to remember—these usually suffice to confirm the diagnosis. Dementia is usually a permanent state, but symptoms may be worsened by intercurrent infection or anoxia, especially in the elderly.

Causes

Dementia is usually a result of slowly progressive cerebral disease and is commonest in old age. Senile dementia is seen especially in women and may be an ageing change—the brain undergoes shrinkage and plaques of degenerate tissue resembling amyloid may be found. Arteriosclerotic dementia also occurs in the elderly, especially in men, but can usually be differentiated by its association with previous strokes and pyramidal tract signs or other evidence of cerebral arterial disease, with or without hypertension; the deterioration of personality may not be so complete.

The pre-senile dementias are a group of conditions presenting in patients below the age of sixty—Alzheimer's disease (probably an early form of senile dementia), Pick's disease, Huntington's chorea, and Creutzfeldt-Jakob disease (? slow virus infection)—all relatively rare.

Neurosyphilis (G.P.I.), rarely other infections, cerebral tumour, and chronic alcoholism are other causes. Deficiency of thyroxine in myxoedema, or of vitamin B_{12} in pernicious anaemia are unusual causes, but they should be borne in mind, for the dementia is unusual in that it will improve if the deficiency is remedied—dementia is otherwise an irreversible condition. Acute injury is a rare cause, but the repeated brain trauma sustained by boxers may lead to dementia.

Management

With the exceptions noted (thyroxine and B_{12} deficiency), there can be no cure. Patients may deteriorate during infection or other illness, and early treatment will improve this. Attention should therefore be directed to maintaining normality in other systems as far as possible. Drugs of vitamin B group are only of value if there is a deficiency—no drug can reverse brain destruction.

Patients are generally best managed at home for as long as possible, for they are better in familiar surroundings with relatives. Patients with senile and arteriosclerotic dementia form the largest group, and their management at home and in hospital is further considered in Chapter 18, Care of the Elderly.

Anxiety and depressive states

Anxiety and depression are extremely common. They may not be complained of, but will be admitted to, in many patients attending hospitals ostensibly with other complaints. They may be regarded as exaggerations of normal response to stressful situations, grief and bereavement. While they may exist in 'pure' form as *anxiety state* and *depressive state*, they are commonly inseparable. Moreover, a severe depressive state may present as anxiety. There may be many concomitants including strange fears and feelings of unworthiness and guilt. Patients complain of sleeplessness and of feeling 'always tired'. Depression may be classified as 'reactive' (i.e. reaction to an existing stressful situation such as financial trouble or a broken love affair) or 'endogenous' (in which the personality may basically be a depressive one and there may be a family history). The reactive depressives have difficulty in getting-off to sleep, whilst the endogenous depressives wake up in the small hours feeling extremely low in spirits and unable to get back to sleep. Such classification is not rigid, though response to drugs does tend to justify it. Enquiry into sleep disturbance, and the direct question 'Are you depressed?' help to confirm the diagnosis.

Severe cases become extremely miserable and withdrawn, and unable to pursue their normal activities. Concentration at book work becomes impossible. The lay-term 'nervous breakdown' usually applies to this condition.

Such patients may attempt suicide as the only relief from their misery.

Treatment

Sympathetic understanding is most important. The mere fact that the patient can talk about his troubles to the physician or nurse is helpful to him. The patient often cannot or will not confide in his relatives, and their well-meaning suggestions may only distress him further. Exhortations to the patient to 'pull himself together' are useless and harmful.

Most anxiety-depressive illness gets better with the passage of time—weeks or months—and it is a question of tiding the patient over until spontaneous recovery ensues. During that time, in severe cases, it may be necessary to admit the patient to hospital. Here, the disciplined environment often produces marked improvement within a few days.

Drug therapy

Modern drugs, which are specific, have transformed management, which can usually continue on an outpatient basis. Only rarely is recourse to electro-convulsive therapy (E.C.T.) now necessary. It must be remembered however, that there is always the risk of suicide in such patients, so close surveillance is necessary.

Anxiety relieving drugs. Barbiturates, e.g. sodium amylobarbitone (Sodium Amytal) are very effective in calming the patient in the acute situation. Because of the danger of overdose with barbiturates however, drugs of benzodiazepine group such as diazepam (Valium) and chlordiazepoxide (Librium), which are safe even in high dosage, have become increasingly used instead.

Anti-depressants. These are of two main groups, the mono-amine-oxidase inhibitors (M.A.O.I. group) which are especially effective in reactive depression with strange fears (phobias), and the tricyclic compounds, for endogenous depression. Because of severe effects such as hypertension and headache when a patient on a M.A.O.I. drug eats amine-rich foods such as cheese (or is given a drug such as pethidine) there is a tendency to prefer drugs of the tricyclic group initially for all forms of depression—imipramine (Tofranil) which tends to be stimulant, and amitriptyline (Tryptizol) which is sedative and therefore used in agitated depressive states.

These drugs produce great benefit in most cases within a matter of weeks. Maintenance doses are usually necessary for months or longer, under the supervision of the psychiatrist.

The psychoses

A psychosis or psychotic state is a severe mental illness, in which the patient has no insight, and is often detached from reality. Very severe depressive illness may merge into this category and there may be swings of mood from melancholia to acute excitement and violence amounting to mania. This is manic–depressive psychosis. In mania, the patient appears uncontrollably excited with flights of ideas, delusions (false beliefs) and hallucinations (false perceptions, the patient hearing or more rarely seeing things that are not there).

The term schizophrenia or schizophrenic psychosis is used to describe mental illness characterized by deterioration of emotional stability and personality, disordered judgement, and failure to act in accord with reality. The cause is unknown, but there may be a genetic predisposition and a biochemical abnormality in cerebral amine metabolism.

Schizophrenia presents in young people who, having been apparently normal, become withdrawn, decline to mix with others, and develop disorders of thought and of emotion. Abstract thinking is impaired, the thought process may suddenly become 'blocked' and the patient may believe that his thoughts are being influenced by outside sources—he may hear voices (auditory hallucinations), and there may be delusions of persecution, the paranoid state. There is emotional flattening with swings from apathy to inappropriate laughter or outbursts of rage with aggression and destructiveness. In advanced cases, there is an incongruity or 'splitting' of affect (emotional display) and thought, which gives the disorder its name.

Mild cases often go unrecognized, the patient presenting himself repeatedly at hospital with many complaints, for which multiple investigations may have been carried out. The clue to such a state is the difficulty the doctor experiences in attempting to get a lucid history—after an hour's interview, he feels no further forward in the consultation.

Severe cases are very distressing to parents, who witness rapid deterioration in personality and behaviour in a son or daughter who becomes quite incapable of living in normal society without treatment.

Treatment of schizophrenia

Early recognition and treatment is vital. Treatment has been revolutionized by the phenothiazine drugs, which do not cure the illness but usually halt its progress. Chlorpromazine (Largactil) in large doses may be used initially, or depot injections of long-acting phenothiazines. A drug of different type, haloperidol (Serenace) is also effective. After initial hospital treatment, therapy is maintained on an out-patient basis as far as possible, for it is most important to keep the patient in contact with his environment, relatives and friends. Many patients are now able to return to work—a far cry from the results of the former methods of institutional care.

Psychosomatic and hysterical disorders

The mind, psyche, has a powerful influence on the body, soma. Where there appears to be no physical basis for complaints, they are often labelled 'psychosomatic' or 'functional' or 'psychoneurotic'. Terms such as 'neurotic' or 'low-pain threshold' can however, too easily be applied to patients. They also tend to prevent the application of the proper sympathy and understanding that all patients merit. (Malingering—pretence of sickness to avoid work—is in fact rare.)

Hysteria literally means a 'wandering of the womb' (having the same derivation as the term 'hysterectomy'). It is classically a disorder of young women, and this mechanism was believed responsible! The term has been used for an emotional upset, in which the patient complains loudly in an attempt to draw attention to herself, the symptoms multiplying and exhibitionism increasing in front of an appropriate audience. This was the picture of the Victorian 'vapours' —the modern generation tends rather to use 'self-poisoning' (see below) as a means of gaining medical attention. The hysterical emotional outburst usually responds to firm handling.

Hysteria is used in a different sense to describe a mental state in which part of normal consciousness is missing or 'detached'. Thus there may be a hysterical paralysis of a limb, or the patient may fail to appreciate painful stimuli such as pin-prick, the sensory loss not conforming to a recognized pathological pattern. Severe complaints may be described by a patient whose smiling appearance is incompatible with them—the attitude called 'la belle indifference'. Occasionally there may be memory loss or a 'fugue' in which the patient apparently does not know his or her identity and may be found wandering by the police. Hysterical fits, not of the pattern of true epilepsy, also occur. The cause of such hysterical symptoms is uncertain, but personal gain may be the motive, albeit at subconscious level.

Hysteria is not a diagnosis to be made lightly—the symptoms may in fact have a serious physical or psychiatric basis even in those whose behaviour or history suggests a hysterical personality.

In the treatment of hysteria, it is often necessary to treat and remove the symptom before one can deal with the underlying condition. Patients are often very suggestible at consultation, or under hypnosis in suitable cases.

'Mass hysteria' is a well-known term to describe the reactions of crowds to political agitators. A form of mass hysteria may be responsible for 'epidemics' of sickness and drop-attacks in school children, and an epidemic of an encephalitis-like illness which affected members of staff of the Royal Free Hospital in London in 1953 may have had a similar basis.

Anorexia nervosa

This is a condition found in young women. They stop eating, with marked loss of body weight, presenting as extreme emaciation in severe cases. The cause may be related to emotional disturbance or to an obsession that they are too fat and they proceed to put themselves on a starvation diet. They then develop a curious lack of insight into the fact that their physical appearance has become less, instead of more attractive. Amenorrhoea is usually present, but the secondary sexual characteristics such as pubic and axillary hair, are retained, unlike hypopituitarism, with which anorexia nervosa has been confused. Severe cases may go on to extreme weakness and collapse.

Treatment includes an attempt to resolve any underlying emotional conflict. Temporary removal from home environment may be necessary, and large doses of chlopromazine (Largactil), 100 mg 3 or 4 times daily, sometimes allow the patient's attitude to food to be more reasonable—once meals are accepted, improvement occurs. In this condition, chlorpromazine does not produce the marked sedation that might be expected. In severe cases, forced feeding by nasogastric tube or even intravenously (using fructose, sorbitol, fat emulsions and protein hydrolysates such as Aminosol, is required.

The outcome is not always satisfactory, and follow-up is required as the condition may recur. Sometimes patients swing to the opposite extreme, over eat, and become obese. Thus disorder of the appetite regulating centre in the hypothalamus at the base of the brain, which is concerned also with emotional response, has been suggested as a cause.

Alcoholism

ACUTE ALCOHOLIC INTOXICATION

The effects are well known—disturbance of balance, dysarthria, emotional and intellectual changes. Alcohol is a cerebral depressant, and while inhibitions may be released, judgement is impaired. There is a high association with road traffic accidents. In Britain it is illegal to be in charge of a motor vehicle with a blood alcohol level of 80 mg per 100 ml or over. Alcohol is also a gastric irritant, and a diuretic.

The management of alcoholic coma is that of any state of coma, ensuring patency of the airway, maintaining respiration, and considering the use of gastric lavage. In the conscious subject, the drinking of water speeds the urinary excretion of alcohol and helps to prevent hangover, which is largely a dehydration effect.

CHRONIC ALCOHOLISM

The alcoholic, or alcohol-dependent person is one who has lost control of his drinking and cannot stop. He should be distinguished from the regular heavy drinker, who can still stop if advised to do so—signs of alcoholic poisoning such as peripheral neuropathy, cirrhosis, or alcoholic heart disease and failure are good reasons for this advice.

It is estimated that 1 per cent of the population in Britain are alcholics, but many conceal their addiction. They do not usually display signs of acute drunkenness, but their lives revolve around their need for alcohol. Alcoholism may follow excessive social drinking in those of previously good personality, or the habit may have followed a drinking bout after depression or stress, an escape from the cares of the world. Some alcoholics have underlying psychotic disorders, many are psychopaths and the history often includes a broken home and family alcoholism.

Symptoms and signs

Morning drinking or solitary drinking may be the first signs. 'The shakes' occurs on rising, following the withdrawal of alcohol during the period of sleep—there is tremor and irritability, and the subject reaches for another drink. At this stage insight is retained. Gradually there is deterioration of personality and concentration at work, and all money is diverted to procuring alcohol—cheap wines (and sometimes methylated spirits) replacing the previous whiskies or gins. A respectable business man may become a pathological liar, and will go to great pains to conceal his supplies and his addiction; much distress may be caused to his wife and family.

Delirium tremens (D.T.'s) is caused by intercurrent infection or sudden withdrawal of alcohol. Delirium is a state of clouding of consciousness, with restlessness and hallucinations—here they frequently take the form of small animals running over the body (seldom are they 'pink elephants'). There is fear, confusion, and a tremor. Wernicke's encephalopathy is due to the vitamin B_1 deficiency so common in the alcoholic from his poor diet. There are haemorrhages at the base of the brain, causing confusion, paralysis of eye muscles with visual upset such as diplopia, nystagmus and ataxia. This may proceed to loss of memory for recent events, and *confabulation*, the patient giving a fictitious account of his movements— the picture called *Korsakov's psychosis*. In the late stages of alcoholism there is progressive degeneration of cells in the cortex of the brain, with memory loss, intellectual deterioration and complete disintegration of standards of personal hygiene and behaviour.

Treatment

Complete abstention from alcohol is imperative—where insight is retained the patient will be able to co-operate. The help of wife or relatives should be enlisted. Withdrawal symptoms can be treated with chlordiazepoxide (Librium), chlormethiazole (Heminevrin) or possibly chlorpromazine (Largactil). In delirious states and psychosis large doses of vitamin B complex should be given by injection— Parentrovite is a useful preparation. It may be wise to give vitamin B supplements in all cases of alcoholism. Treatment of cirrhosis and heart failure may also be required.

Disulfiram (Antabuse) is a drug which produces unpleasant symptoms such as severe headache if alcohol is taken, but its place in therapy has proved limited. Some alcoholics may be helped to stop drinking by joining Alcoholics Anonymous. Though the results of treatment of chronic alcoholism are often disappointing and many patients default, a determined attempt to help the patient and his family should always be made.

Drug dependence (addiction)

Dependence may be defined as a compulsion to take a drug on a continuous or periodic basis in order to experience its psychic effects and sometimes to avoid the discomfort of its absence. Thus withdrawal of some drugs of dependence results in symptoms such as agitation and anxiety—the brain has adapted to the drug and its absence may cause such symptoms, which may be related to a rebound excess activity of dream (R.E.M.) sleep. Tolerance to the drug, that is the need to take increasing doses to produce an effect, may or may not be present. Tolerance may be due to the production of increased enzymes by the liver, speeding destruction of the drug.

Opium-smoking is as acceptable in the Far East as social drinking is in the West. However, the introduction of opiates (morphine and heroin) to the West has been followed by misuse and dependence. In Britain, addiction to *morphine* occurred in a small group who had received the drug for medicinal purposes. *Heroin* addiction became a problem after a quantity had been stolen, and following lax prescribing by a few doctors. Heroin mixed with cocaine (H and C) and injected intravenously ('mainlining') has euphoriant effects. These are powerful drugs of dependence and tolerance, so that subjects had to procure further supplies, generally illegally. Tight control has resulted in some improvement in heroin abuse in Britain, and addicts can only be supplied at special clinics. In the United States, however, heroin addiction remains a major problem.

Cannabis (marihuana, hashish, hemp, pot) is commonly smoked in Mexico. In Britain, according to some sources, it was introduced by jazz musicians and spread by pop groups and their followers, influencing young people. It is said to remove inhibitions and improve the mood, giving a feeling of peace, but its effects are partly dependent on the subject's existing frame of mind and his social surroundings. Cannabis also causes dilatation of the conjunctival vessels. The smoke has a characteristic smell. Although there is no proof that its use has resulted in serious harm or dependence, those who smoke cannabis are at risk from their social associations with others who may use more dangerous drugs.

LSD (lysergic acid diethylamide) is a dangerous drug which produces hallucinations and may cause brain damage.

Almost any sedative or stimulant drug can be misused. Thus amphetamines cause stimulation but also psychotic episodes. Apart from such effects, intravenous use and sharing of syringes may result in sepsis and hepatitis. Amphetamines have little medical application, and curtailment of prescribing has resulted in less misuse. Thus drug-takers have turned to barbiturates and non-barbiturate hypnotics, often mixed with alcohol, in their search for psychic effects.

The management of drug dependence is as much a social as a medical problem. Young people should be discouraged from experimenting with drugs, and their elders can reconsider their own tobacco and alcohol-drinking habits. Doctors and nurses may in fact have contributed to the dependence of many middle-aged women on barbiturates and other hypnotics—their routine issue in hospital is to be deprecated and their long-term use has no rational basis.

Self-poisoning—attempted suicide

The vast majority of persons who take an overdose of drugs do so as an impulsive gesture, as a 'cry for help'. They will generally be admitted to hospital and they realize that their action affords an opportunity for their misery to be attended to. Only a small proportion intend to kill themselves and they make a planned attempt away from the public gaze, and if foiled, try again. The term 'self-poisoning' is now therefore preferred to cover all cases with or without serious suicidal intent. Self-poisoning accounts for over 10 per cent of acute admissions to British hospitals. There are some 6,000 deaths annually from poisoning, but most patients admitted to hospital now recover.

Corrosive acids and coal gas used to be the common methods, but the former is now regarded as unpleasant, and as natural gas contains no carbon monoxide, attempts with the gas oven are ineffective. Car engine (petrol, not diesel) exhausts are, however, a source of carbon monoxide (and inadequate combustion or ventilation using any fuel can result in its production).

CARBON MONOXIDE POISONING

The gas fixes to haemoglobin, forming carboxyhaemoglobin and preventing oxygen carriage by the blood. Although carboxyhaemoglobin is pink, patients suffering from poisoning appear pink only if moribund. Earlier they are cyanosed and pale, confused or unconscious; breathing is maintained to a late stage. Treatment is in a hyperbaric (pressurized) oxygen chamber if available, or by giving pure oxygen by face mask. Apparent recovery may be followed by intellectual deterioration or Parkinsonism, from cerebral or basal ganglia damage.

The establishment of Poisons Information centres has helped to define the problem of self-poisoning. The lay-public thinks in terms of an 'antidote', but only in a very few cases is such available—an alkali such as bicarbonate of soda is the obvious antidote to an acid and generally a stomach tube should not be used for such corrosive poisoning. Again, the small boy who has eaten 'berries' may be helped if these can be identified and their dangers defined by the Poisons Information Centre. In the vast majority of cases, however, the patient has taken a quantity of commonly available or prescribed drugs such as aspirin, barbiturates, other hypnotic, anxiety-relieving or anti-depressant drugs, or a mixture of these. It is important to seek information as to drugs taken, and to preserve any tablets, as well as specimens of vomitus and urine.

ASPIRIN (SALICYLATE) POISONING

It should first be made clear that acute aspirin poisoning does not cause unconsciousness in adults—even drowsiness is unusual though it does occur in children. If an adult patient with aspirin poisoning is unconscious, he is either at death's door, or another drug has been taken in addition.

Aspirin stimulates the respiratory centre causing rapid deep breathing. Though normal doses are antipyretic, overdosage causes metabolic stimulation, restlessness, *pyrexia* and sweating. There is tinnitus (noises in the ears). Gastric irritation causes vomiting and patient becomes dehydrated. An initial respiratory alkalosis (due to over-breathing washing out CO_2) is followed by metabolic acidosis. There is potassium upset and hypokalaemia. Aspirin competes with vitamin K, resulting in lowered prothrombin level and bleeding tendency.

Treatment

1. Pass a wide-bore stomach tube, aspirate and preserve the gastric contents, and carry out lavage with warm water. (Aspirin is re-excreted into the stomach).

2. Blood is taken for serum salicylate and potassium estimation.

3. In severe cases (serum salicylate over 40 mg %), *forced alkaline diuresis* is carried out—intravenous fluids, initially 1–2 litres hourly (500 ml normal saline, 500–1000 ml 5% dextrose or laevulose, plus 500 ml 1·26% sodium bicarbonate)—excretion of salicylate is speeded by an alkaline urine, pH 8 on indicator paper. Urine volume must be charted and noted to be adequate.

It is essential to have frequent checks of the patient's blood, for the potassium level may fall (leading to weakness, cardiac irregularity and arrest if untreated) and there is disturbance of acid-base balance as noted.

4. In very severe cases, haemodialysis with the artificial kidney.

5. Vitamin K_1 to counteract bleeding tendency—10 mg intramuscularly.

6. Prochlorperazine (Stemetil) may allay vomiting and the discomfort of tinnitus.

Aspirin poisoning often appears mild initially, but the biochemical effects are complex and often delayed, so it is important to admit, and carefully observe and treat all but the most trivial cases.

PRINCIPLES OF MANAGEMENT OF THE UNCONSCIOUS POISONED PATIENT

Management is largely the same as that of coma—note the level of consciousness, clear the airway, confirm that respiration is occurring and the heart is beating, chart pulse and blood pressure. Seek information from relatives as to drugs taken. Consider gastric lavage —it is not indicated if more than 4 hours since drug taken (except in aspirin poisoning, when always indicated). Keep specimens. Bear in mind that the most important principle is to maintain vital functions, such as respiration and the heart, until the poison is naturally eliminated. See also below.

BARBITURATE POISONING

All barbiturates depress the level of consciousness and respiration. Only in very severe cases does the heart stop. The important principle therefore is to make sure that the patient's respiration is adequate.

Treatment

1. Gastric lavage is of value only if the drug has been taken within four hours. It should be performed only if the patient is conscious enough to cough. If deeply unconscious, a cuffed endotracheal tube should be passed first to prevent aspiration into the lungs.

2. Insert an airway, and if the ventilatory movements and air entry (heard with the stethoscope over the lung) are still poor, the doctor may pass an endotracheal tube so that mechanical ventilation with a respirator can be carried out. He will be guided by measurements with a portable spirometer and blood gas analysis. Respiratory stimulants such as nikethamide are of only temporary value. (Circulatory depression with systolic blood pressure below 90 mm Hg may be helped by elevating the foot of the bed and giving injections of metaraminol (Aramine) or intravenous fluids. These measures are seldom necessary if ventilation is maintained). Oxygen may be helpful, but again it does not replace the need to maintain respiration.

3. Blood may be taken for barbiturate estimation.

4. If the blood barbiturate is high and a long acting barbiturate such as phenobarbitone (which is not broken down, but excreted unchanged in the urine) has been taken, forced alkaline diuresis (as for aspirin poisoning) is helpful. Its value is less certain for barbiturates that are metabolized—the shorter acting ones such as pentobarbitone (Nembutal) and cyclobarbitone.

5. In very severe cases, peritoneal dialysis or, preferably, haemodialysis with artificial kidney.

Most patients admitted with barbiturate poisoning recover with the simple supportive measures described.

POISONING WITH NON-BARBITURATE SLEEPING DRUGS

Properly used, barbiturates are remarkably free from serious side effects. Because of the danger of overdosage, however, a series of drugs thought to be safer have come into use. They include glutethimide (Doriden), methaqualone compounds such as Mandrax, and nitrazepam (Mogadon). Glutethimide and Mandrax have in fact turned out to be very dangerous if taken in excess. There is no anti-dote, forced diuresis may actually be harmful, and again it is a question of maintaining respiration. Nitrazepam so far appears safe.

ANXIETY RELIEVING DRUGS AND ANTIDEPRESSANTS

The benzodiazepines such as Valium and Librium appear safe, overdosage producing drowsiness but seldom deep unconsciousness.

Antidepressants such as amitryptyline and imipramine cause atropine-like effects, with dry mouth, blurring of vision and varying degrees of restlessness with possible disturbance of consciousness. Cardiac arrhythmias may occur.

Monoamineoxidase inhibitors such as phenelzine (Nardil) or tranylcypromine (Parnate) may produce dangerous states of excite-ment followed by coma.

Supportive therapy, the maintenance of respiration and use of fluids intravenously to combat dehydration, are all that can usually be offered in such poisoning.

IRON POISONING (e.g. FERROUS SULPHATE, FERROUS GLUCONATE)

This occurs mainly in children, who are attracted by the brightly coloured tablets—hence manufacturers have changed the sugar coat-ing from green to brown to make them less appealing, and special press-through packets may foil little fingers.

Iron is irritant to the stomach, producing vomiting, and extremely toxic when absorbed causing convulsions, coma and death.

Gastric lavage is performed and 5–15 G of desferrioxamine (Desferal) in 200 ml normal saline is instilled into the stomach. This substance 'chelates' or binds the iron. It should also be given by intravenous drip.

SELF-POISONING—FOLLOW-UP

After they have recovered from the overdose, all patients should be seen by the psychiatrist so that the precipitating depressive or other illness can be assessed and treated.

18

Care of the elderly

Principles of geriatric care

The medical care of the elderly is called geriatric medicine. There is no difference in the approach to, and application of medical principles in the elderly—cause, symptoms and signs, diagnosis and management must be carried out in just the same way as in the young. Geriatrics should not therefore be considered apart from medicine as a whole, but the concept of geriatric care has produced an improvement of standards towards those who were so often neglected in the past.

There are several accompaniments of old age—a decrease in strength, a loss of body height due to osteoporosis, and a difficulty in retaining new information. Intellectual function may, however, be well preserved until advanced years. The secrets of longevity are not known, but a good family history is a favourable omen. While degenerative disease such as arteriosclerosis might be expected, it is by no means invariable. Indeed, arterial disease strikes down people in their fifties and sixties, and those who live to eighty and ninety seem to be constitutionally destined to do so. Some elderly people do gradually fade away and one might be justified in ascribing this simply to senility, but many an elderly person succumbs to treatable disease such as anaemia, chest or urinary infection, or to the effects of neglect, loneliness and depression.

For unknown reasons, women live longer than men. Perhaps the stimulus of keeping house and caring for their husbands keeps women going. Perhaps too, the compulsory retirement of so many men at age sixty-five is not a good thing—people are healthiest when they are busily engaged in some occupation. Preparation for retirement and ability to pursue hobbies such as golf, and gardening are important aspects of preventive medicine in the elderly.

Indeed, preventive medicine assumes much more importance in the elderly than in any other group. It is wrong that an old person should put off calling for the doctor until he or she is sick. Overt illness is only the 'tip of the iceberg'. Large numbers of elderly people put up with disabilities which are remediable. It should be the duty of social and medical services to ensure that home visiting of the elderly is carried out. Cataract, causing visual impairment, and anaemia can be cured, heart failure treated, and dietary inadequacies corrected. Loneliness should not occur if relatives, friends, Ministers of the Church, doctors—and also postmen, milkmen and tradesmen—are aware of an old person's predicament, and can call on the help of community and welfare services.

Thus there should be no need for acute hospital admission simply because a person is old. On the other hand, the elderly person may fall victim to any of the disorders of younger people and is entitled to the same medical attention.

So long as they are able, elderly people should be encouraged to continue to live in their own homes. Many cherish their independence and refuse to move to a new home, which may be easier to run, but different from their established ways. When they become very frail, it may be wise for old people to accept offers of hospitality from their relatives, even for short periods, which at least ensure one or two square meals daily—the meals-on-wheels service is of course a boon to the elderly.

Social customs have changed and younger women who might previously have devoted their lives to looking after elderly relatives, are now out at work. Nevertheless, many families go to great pains to take turns in looking after their old folks. It is often said that the younger generation cares nothing for the elderly. This is not true. It must be remembered that the number of persons over sixty-five has more than doubled in the last fifty years. The successful fight against illness and disease has enabled a rising proportion of the population to realize their potential life span. However, there has not been much progress in increasing this span, the degenerative diseases, especially vascular disease, continuing to be the major cause of death.

There is no special pathology of the aged but disease has a greater effect on the aged body. In young people, it is an important principle to try to establish one diagnosis for multiple symptoms. In the elderly, multiple disorders are much more likely to be present.

GERIATRIC ASSESSMENT

1. Daily activities

walking ⎤ can the old person   (a) unaided
dressing ⎬ do these   (b) with help
eating   ⎦   or (c) is he incapable of doing
                                     them at all?

2. Is he continent of urine, occasionally incontinent, or frequently incontinent?

3. Mental condition

(a) normal ⎤
(b) mildly confused ⎬ Psycho-geriatric assessment.
(c) demented ⎦

4. Faculties

(a) sight
(b) hearing
(c) speech

In addition full physical examination, urine testing, blood count and chest x-ray are carried out.

THE GERIATRIC DAY HOSPITAL

A day hospital is attached to a general hospital, and shares facilities such as physiotherapy, occupational therapy, social workers, x-ray and laboratory services. Old people attend one day a week in a group of 20–30, being brought from their homes. Some may have recently been discharged from the ward.

The day hospital bridges the gap between home and hospital, and allows assessment, rehabilitation (especially after a stroke) social care (meals, baths, chiropody), medical surveillance, and nursing care—dressings, injections, catheter changing. It enables old people to remain in the community, and this is much preferable to long-term hospital admission. (Often admission on a month-in, month-out basis can be arranged, with the help of the social worker, in cases where an elderly patient is periodically staying with relatives.)

Disorders common in the elderly

1. *Cardiovascular disease*

Myocardial infarction, which may be relatively silent.

Arterial insufficiency in the legs, with tendency to ulcers and gangrene of the feet if neglected.

Congestive cardiac failure—usually amenable to diuretics and digoxin, though the elderly are often *very sensitive* to this drug.

Venous insufficiency in the legs, with tendency to oedema and ulceration, with poor healing.

2. *Cerebrovascular disease*

Tendency to 'strokes'.

3. *Parkinson's disease.*

4. *Degenerative arthritis*

Osteoarthrosis—especially affecting hips and knees, with risk of immobilization.

5. *Rarefaction of bones*

Osteoporosis is very common, may be associated with low backache; immobilization worsens it—no drugs are of proven value in treatment.

Osteomalacia though rarer, does occur, especially if there is slight malabsorption (as may follow stomach operations) or inadequate intake of vitamin D. There may be spontaneous fractures, abnormal calcium and other levels in the blood. Treatment is with vitamin D.

Fractured neck of femur may follow trivial falls, and it is always wise to x-ray the part. Surgical pinning allows early mobilization.

6. *Disturbances of nutrition*

Though gross malnutrition is rare, living on 'tea and toast' causes vitamin and mineral deficiencies. Thus scurvy may be seen, and may actually occur in institutions as vitamin C tends to be lacking in bulk-prepared meals. Anaemia may rarely result from dietary iron or folic acid deficiency.

The appetite of the elderly in hospital, is however, surprisingly good—they eat well.

7. *Constipation and spurious diarrhoea. Diverticular disease of the colon*

Neglect of the call to stool, and previous purgation habits may predispose to constipation; faeces impacted in the rectum cause spurious diarrhoea. Regularity can usually be re-established by occasional oral laxatives after initial use of suppositories or gentle enemas.

8. *Cancer*

This accounts for one-sixth of the deaths over sixty-five, not really a very high proportion. Cancers in the elderly are often slow growing, and may be an incidental finding. The cancers that do kill, include those of lung, stomach, pancreas, colon, breast and prostrate. Many can be alleviated, the patient often dying from intercurrent illness. The problem of cancer management is not a major one in geriatric wards.

9. *Incontinence of urine.* ⎫
10. *Dementia.*   ⎬ See below.
11. *Hypothermia.*   ⎭

URINARY INCONTINENCE IN THE ELDERLY
Causes:

   (i) *urinary tract infection*;
  (ii) *diminished bladder size* or muscle function—sometimes due to faecal impaction;
 (iii) *pelvic floor muscle weakness*—stress incontinence;
 (iv) *neurogenic*—following a stroke, or associated with dementia.

Urinary infection may be associated with frequency, dysuria, rigors and pyrexia, but quite often the infection is 'silent', the patient presenting with vague malaise or disorientation. Bacteriological examination of a fresh specimen of urine is indicated, and the appropriate therapy, usually a sulphonamide, is curative.

During any illness in the elderly, especially if there is brain involvement, there may be transient incontinence, presumably related to disturbance of bladder motility or innervation. Temporary catheterization may be required. Improvement occurs when the patient is ambulant.

After a stroke, bladder function may be disturbed but may return to normal in time. There is no way of predicting this, but in general if the patient recovers full consciousness and mental acuity, regained control of bladder function is to be expected.

Diminished bladder capacity, often associated with neurogenic upset, may be improved by the anticholinergic drug emepronium (Cetiprin) 100–200 mg at bedtime or during the day—this drug is worth a trial in incontinent elderly patients. Electrical stimulation of the external bladder sphincter, using battery-powered electrodes or pessary is being tried, but this muscle often remains weak and lax in the elderly.

With general mental deterioration, incontinence is common. It is sometimes of the 'infant' type before toilet training, the patient apparently being indifferent to wetting himself. This can be managed by ensuring that he or she is taken to the toilet (or provided with a urinal) at frequent intervals. An occasional lapse can be allowed for by using easily laundered pants or trousers. Permanent transurethral catheterization in men should be avoided—sometimes a condom drainage device is feasible. Plastic disposable catheters of Foley self-retaining type are especially useful in females. They must be changed weekly, with full aseptic precautions, and connected to a plastic bag allowing continuous drainage, while at the same time permitting the patient to be ambulant. Even over a period of years, such a measure need not be associated with serious urinary infections, though fever should be an indication for urine culture, with appropriate chemotherapy if positive. A high fluid intake helps to prevent such infections.

DEMENTIA AND PERSONALITY DISORDERS (PSYCHO-
GERIATRIC MEDICINE)

A mild degree of deterioration in mental acuity, forgetfulness (leaving the kettle on, for example) and obstinacy are common in the elderly. There tends to be an exaggeration of previous personality traits— the tolerant and gracious may become increasingly likeable, while the querrulous and demanding become unreasonable and awkward. The former tend to have willing relatives. The latter are not popular in society, and when they become old, relatives will not have them—there tends, therefore to be a somewhat higher proportion of such patients in hospital.

It is surprising how many mildly demented elderly people manage their day-to-day lives, if they are helped at home and served by understanding shopkeepers. When they become neglectful of personal hygiene and a danger to themselves and others (e.g. fire hazards) then hospitalization is required. Transfer to unfamiliar surroundings may, however, cause an old person to become noisy and aggressive initially.

Senile dementia is seen mainly in women, possibly because it is an ageing change and they live longer than men. Dementia may also be due to arteriosclerotic disease, especially if there has been a history of strokes, and signs of pyramidal tract disorder.

There are, however, some factors which worsen the symptoms in those already predisposed by their age. These include:

1. infections—pneumonia, urinary infection
2. cardiovascular disease such as myocardial infarction or congestive heart failure leading to cerebral anoxia
3. anaemia
4. occasionally vitamin B_{12} deficiency in the absence of anaemia.

It is vital to bear such conditions in mind for treatment may allow improvement in the patient's mental state.

Chronic cases are a test for the forbearance and skill of nursing staff. It is often surprising how well patients adapt to hospital routine. As far as possible, however, they should not be allowed to become institutionalized as occurred in the old mental hospitals, and transfer to purely psychiatric hospital care may still, unfortunately have such connotation. In fact mental hospitals have been utilized to such an extent that more than half their occupants are over sixty-five.

The object is to keep patients out of bed except for sleeping purposes—which should be during the night. Diversional or occupational therapy such as knitting, playing simple games, making baskets and pottery, watching television, and pursuit of any hobbies, should be encouraged. Free visiting in hospital is desirable.

Surprisingly few drugs are needed. Chlorpromazine may be useful in initial management and can be given in larger dose as a sedative at night. Barbiturates cause disorientation in some elderly patients, and chloral hydrate or nitrazepam (Mogadon) are preferable if a hypnotic is required. Some phasic behaviour disturbances may have an epileptic basis from brain scarring in the elderly, and phenobarbitone of phenytoin may be indicated here.

HYPOTHERMIA IN THE ELDERLY

Hypothermia means low body temperature. It exists if the rectal temperature reading is less than 95°F (35°C). The rectal temperature is used as it measures the heat in the body core, and as the ordinary clinical thermometer may not read below 95°F, a special low-reading instrument should be used.

Hypothermia occurs in the elderly due to failure of the temperature-regulating mechanism in the hypothalamus at the base of the brain and is usually, but not always, associated with a cold environment—the homes of elderly people are often inadequately heated in winter. Precipitating factors include loss of mobility due to arthritis or after a stroke (the old person perhaps lying undiscovered for hours), coronary thrombosis, infection or simply forgetfulness and exhaustion, but sometimes there is no obvious cause.

Mild degrees of hypothermia, with a temperature of 90–95°F (32·2–35°C) may not be serious, but temperatures below 90°F (32·2°C) are associated with deterioration of vital functions and below 85°F (29·4°C) there is a danger of ventricular fibrillation or asystole.

Clinical features

Characteristically, the old person is found lying on the floor by neighbours or the police. There is mental slowing, confusion or apathy which may have progressed into a state of *semi-consciousness* or *coma*, and respiration is shallow. There may be a curious puffiness of the face, simulating myxoedema, a rare cause of hypothermia.

The skin feels *cold*—like touching marble, and this is the clue to the diagnosis. There is no shivering, the mechanism for this has failed. The pulse is slow, but sometimes there is atrial fibrillation. The blood pressure is low.

Signs of a precipitating cause may be obscured, but injury, stroke, chest or urinary infection should be borne in mind.

The diagnosis is confirmed by taking the rectal temperature. There may be characteristic E.C.G. changes, and sometimes the serum amylase is raised, from effects on the pancreas.

Treatment

The best measures are preventive ones—such as a warm house and adequate visiting of the elderly in their homes.

Hypothermia is a medical emergency and hospital admission is essential.

The principle is to nurse the patient in warm surroundings but avoid direct heating, which would take blood away from the vital centres.

Thus the patient is placed flat in bed with a normal covering of blankets. The room temperature should be raised, and maintained at 85°F (29·4°C).

Generally, the patient should be disturbed as little as possible—if there is doubt about his breathing, an airway may be inserted. E.C.G. should be monitored to detect dangerous arrhythmias, but atrial fibrillation need not cause concern. Intravenous fluids are not advised unless there is a clear indication for their use, but patients are seldom dehydrated.

Drugs. Hydrocortisone 100 mg four hourly by intravenous injection is customarily given, but there is no proof of its value. Thyroxine or tri-iodothyronine should only be used if the patient is known to have myxoedema. Antibacterial drugs are indicated if there is evidence of an infection, and other precipitating causes should be appropriately treated.

Improvement may take several hours and in the recovery stages metabolic upset such as acidosis may become manifest; blood tests including sodium, potassium, urea, pH or bicarbonate level, and blood sugar should be taken so that therapy can be given if necessary.

The prognosis is very variable, some patients recovering completely despite a very low initial temperature, but severe hypothermia generally carries a high mortality.

Care of the dying

It is in the diseases for which there is no cure that the needs of the patient are often greatest. The patient who is dying continues to merit the care and attention accorded any other patient, plus a compassion and understanding that comes only with experience.

We do not know how many patients realize they are dying for, unlike Victorian times, death is not a usual topic of conversation, but one authority put the figure as high as 80 per cent. Nor do we know how many patients wish to talk about death, but most welcome the opportunity to participate in some form of conversation. The important thing is to allow time to listen, no matter the subject. The patient may welcome the chance to express his feelings, but it is unusual to be asked 'Am I going to die?'. It is generally unwise to tell a lie but the whole truth need not be disclosed and most important of all, one must never take away hope. The patient may be entitled to more precise information if he insists on knowing and has business affairs to put in order.

Many patients fear not so much death, rather the process of dying. They are worried that they may have pain, that their courage may fail, or that they may be neglected at a time of need. Some become depressed, a few may react with anger. With increasing weakness and the necessity for complete nursing care, a patient may feel remorse at having become so dependent. His great need is for reassurance, and comfort comes from the fact that people still care for him. He may seek spiritual help, and this should be available, a minister of the Church being a valuable member of the hospital team.

The place of drugs

Patients with incurable disease, in whom deterioration is obvious, sometimes have a curious detachment from reality, rendering them oblivious to it, and making their management easier when the end is near. They slip quietly into a coma and pass away. The most distressing conditions are those in which mental acuity is retained till a late stage, such as motor neurone disease and bulbar palsy. A patient with advanced malignancy rarely dies in agony—indeed, it is never necessary for any patient to suffer pain. The drug chlorpromazine (Largactil) is useful in emulating nature's sense of tranquillity and simple analgesics may suffice in the early stages. It is, however, important to anticipate pain or suffering, when a mixture of diamorphine and cocaine such as the Brompton mixture should be given and continued regularly, with opiates by injection if necessary. Prochlorperazine (Stemetil) is useful if there is vomiting.

The patient's relatives

It is important that time be spent with relatives, who must be kept fully informed of the position from day to day. Generally, unless the patient finds it trying, free-visiting should be encouraged— the patient will appreciate the fact that his relatives still care, and that he will not be left alone. The relatives themselves require understanding and support, and if they have a brave attitude it is a great help in management. The good nurse can offer much comfort not only to the patient, but also to his family.

19

Man, his environment and occupation

Hazards of smoking

King James I in 1604 described smoking as 'a custom loathsome to the eye, hateful to the nose, harmful to the brain, and dangerous to the lungs'. Tobacco smoke has a complex composition, including nicotine (which affects the autonomic nervous system), carbon monoxide (which impairs the blood's capacity to carry oxygen) and hydrocarbons proven to be carcinogenic to animals. Cigarette smoking appears to be especially dangerous, having the following effects:—

1. causes lung cancer
2. predisposes to chronic bronchitis and emphysema
3. increases the risk of coronary heart disease, arterial disease of the legs and cerebral arterial disease causing strokes
4. delays the healing of gastric (and possibly of duodenal) ulcers
5. is associated with increased incidence of cancer of mouth, larynx, oesophagus and bladder
6. during pregnancy may be followed by the birth of babies of lower than average birth weight and increased neonatal mortality
7. raises the risk of tobacco amblyopia, a rare form of blindness.

Doctors and nurses who are foolish enough to ignore these risks have at least a duty not to smoke in front of patients. Cigarettes should not be sold in wards, with the possible exception of geriatric wards. Governments have a responsibility to introduce legislation to curb cigarette smoking, a bad habit and a costly and unnecessary hazard to a nation's health.

Environmental hazards—ecology

Ecology is the study of man in relationship to his environment. Civilization has brought with it atmospheric pollution, contaminating the air we breathe, food production methods which carry risks, and waste disposal methods which threaten our water supply.

ATMOSPHERIC POLLUTION

The pollutants include smoke (carbon particles) and sulphur dioxide, derived from the burning of coal and fuel oil. These are lung irritants, especially when combined with fog (water vapour) as in the British form of 'smog'. They are used as indices of atmospheric pollution. Atmospheric pollution is especially liable to occur in large industrial cities and is associated with a high incidence of chronic lung disease—chronic bronchitis and emphysema. In cold winter fogs, those with chronic lung disease are prone to infection causing acute exacerbations and pneumonia. Smoke control legislation has recently resulted in an improvement in atmospheric pollution in Britain.

In the United States, the motor vehicle is responsible for 60 per cent of the total weight of atmospheric pollutants. Pollution is especially important in a city such as Los Angeles, where geographical factors result in 'temperature inversion', where the hot air is at a height instead of at ground level, as is usual. Pollutants are therefore not dispersed by an upward flow of air, but tend to be carried downwards to form a 'smog'. Motor exhaust contains oxides of nitrogen and hydrocarbons, and sunlight acts on these to produce substances extremely irritant to the eyes and respiratory tract. In addition, the petrol engine emits carbon monoxide, and lead (added to motor fuel to increase its octane, anti-knock ratio). Legislation will limit such emissions.

Radio-active strontium is discharged into the atmosphere following the testing of nuclear explosive devices, and is deposited in the bones. International cooperation in nuclear disarmament should eliminate this hazard.

FOOD PRODUCTION

'Natural' foods may themselves be hazardous—lathyrism occurs in India from eating large quantities of a pea-like vegetable which at times contains a chemical causing a form of spastic paraplegia. Fungal contamination of ground nuts causes production of aflatoxin, which causes liver damage and cancer in animals.

Effects of pesticides

The most widely used pesticide is D.D.T. (dicophane), which has made a major contribution to the elimination of insect-borne diseases such as malaria in large parts of the world. Serious toxic effects in man are rare. However, bird life may be affected, with thinning of egg shells. D.D.T. is not broken down, but stored in fat, and in view of long-term uncertainties, its use has now been restricted. Insecticides of the 'nerve gas' type, exemplified by parathion, act by interfering with the enzyme that destroys acetylcholine. Poisoning causes 'cholinergic' symptoms including headache, vomiting, diarrhoea and pin-point pupils, the antidote being atropine. Parathion becomes broken down in nature, and poisoning is liable to occur only at the time of crop spraying if precautions are neglected. However, in 1967 sixty-three people in Colombia died after eating bread baked from flour on which parathion had spilled. Paraquat is a soil contact weedkiller. If swallowed, it causes lung necrosis and death, the fate of a Scots youth who drank paraquat stored in a lemonade bottle.

Intensive farming methods

The modern practice of keeping birds or animals in close quarters increases the risk of spread of infection. Thus battery-reared chickens may carry salmonella infection and food poisoning results if cooking does not raise the temperature sufficiently to kill the organisms. Antibiotics fed to cattle to promote their growth result in the emergence of resistant strains of bacteria which could be passed to man—such use of antibiotics is now restricted.

Food additives

Preservatives include sodium nitrite, excess of which causes methaemoglobinaemia, a discoloration of the haemoglobin pigment. Excessive monosodium glutamate, a flavouring agent favoured in Chinese cooking, causes neck pains and malaise, Kwok's quease or the Chinese restaurant syndrome.

DISPOSAL OF WASTE—WATER POLLUTION

Instead of being used as manure on the fields, animal excreta is now often hosed away to form a 'slurry' reaching streams or drains. In addition to carrying bacteria, streams and rivers may also contain nitrogenous fertilizers washed from fields. The excess nitrate may be converted to nitrite and poisoning has occurred in children from drinking contaminated water. Moreover, the natural balance of river life is upset, and if industry adds a quota of effluent, rivers and lakes become lifeless, heavily polluted and unpleasant. Even the sea has become a dumping ground, and mercury poisoning followed eating fish from Scandinavian waters contaminated with effluent from wood pulp mills. High mercury levels have recently been reported in tuna fish.

Oil slicks appear to be another hazard of twentieth century life. Nature does not take kindly to upset in her established order. Ecology is now an important aspect of the public health.

Personal hazards

DISORDERS DUE TO HEAT

Sunburn is due to excessive exposure to ultra-violet rays, and is an erythema followed by blistering if severe. Exposure to the sun should be gradual in those visiting the tropics or the ski-slopes. There is no evidence that the desired bronze tanning conveys any special medical benefit, but of course a tan offers protection against the sun's rays.

Salt-deficiency heat exhaustion follows hard work in hot atmospheres with sweating and salt-loss. Symptoms include weakness, muscular cramps and vomiting, and the treatment is to take extra salt.

Prickly heat is a prickly rash of tiny vesicles from blockage of sweat ducts, occurring in hot climates and usually diminishing on acclimatization.

Anhidrotic heat exhaustion may follow prickly heat and is associated with patchy lack of sweating, weakness, irritability and collapse. Unless the subject is removed to a cool environment, there is danger of the condition going on to Heat Stroke.

Heat stroke—heat hyperpyrexia. This is due to an overloading and breakdown of the temperature regulating mechanism and occurs in hot climates on severe exposure or complicating an infection such as malaria. The temperature may be 106°F (41°C) or higher with headache, confusion, extreme thrist and sometimes polyuria. Sweating may continue, or the mechanism may fail. The condition is a medical emergency demanding rapid cooling by sponging and encouraging evaporation by the use of fans. Any coexisting infection should be treated.

DISORDERS DUE TO COLD

Hypothermia in the elderly is described above. Serious hypothermia exists if the rectal temperature is below 90°F (32·2°C).

15—EM * *

Prevention is better than cure. Treatment is by nursing in a warm room, avoiding direct heating.

Cold air exposure in hikers can be prevented by taking shelter before fatigue occurs. Simple measures such as covering with a plastic bag (a useful item of equipment) afford some protection. Hypothermia here is treated by slow rewarming. Frostbite, freezing of tissues may have affected exposed parts. If tissues are still frozen when the patient is seen, they should be immersed in warm water, dried and exposed to the air. If gangrene follows, surgery is required.

Immersion in near-freezing waters following shipwreck causes a rapid and dangerous loss of heat from the body core to the cold skin. Heavy outer garments are protective, and frantic swimming about is to be avoided. Treatment is to reverse the heat loss as quickly as possible by rapid rewarming in a hot bath.

DROWNING

Immersion causes either (*a*) spasm of the glottis and death from asphyxia without water entering the lungs—dry drowning, or (*b*) inhalation of water into the lungs; fresh water is then absorbed into the circulation causing haemolysis; salt water by its osmotic effect attracts water from the circulation causing haemoconcentration. In both cases there is lung irritation and risk of delayed pneumonia in those that survive.

Immediate treatment includes clearing the airway, mouth-to-mouth respiration, cardiac massage and attention to arrhythmias. Intubation, aspiration of air passages and oxygen may be required. Resuscitative measures should be continued even in apparently hopeless cases for recovery may follow.

Intravenous fluids are often required to maintain the circulation, and while hypertonic fluids are in theory indicated for fresh water cases, in practice plasma or dextran should be used in any case of drowning pending blood analysis. Careful watch for lung infection is required, and antibacterial drugs may be necessary.

LIGHTNING AND ELECTRIC SHOCK

Apart from the current and voltage, the effects of electricity depend on its route of passage through the body, and there is a further hazard of burning.

Lightning may cause damage to the central nervous system similar to severe head injury with haemorrhage of the brain, or there may be coma or temporary paralysis. A man touching an overhead cable may be jerked off a pylon, but seizing a live domestic wire may cause tetanic muscle spasm, and 'holding-on' to the wire. If the current traverses the respiratory centre in its passage through the body, then breathing may stop, but it is more common for the route of passage to be through the limbs and chest, and ventricular fibrillation and cardiac arrest is in fact the usual cause of death.

Thus treatment may necessitate not only mouth-to-mouth respiration, but cardiac massage or defibrillation. It should be noted that breathing may restart although the heart is not yet beating. While bizarre burning and weakness or sensory loss may follow electrical injuries, these are not common and if a victim survives the first few hours after electric shock he can be expected to recover completely.

BEE AND WASP STINGS

The barb left behind by the insect should be scraped off rather than pulled, for squeezing may express further venom from the terminal sac. The venom contains a mixture of chemicals including histamine. Local applications are of little value. Stings in the mouth or neck may however be followed by swelling and laryngeal obstruction, and some individuals may develop an anaphylactic reaction to a single sting at any part. Treatment is immediate injection of 0·5 ml of 1 in 1000 adrenaline intramuscularly, followed by intravenous hydrocortisone. Antihistamine drugs are of little value in this acute situation, but may relieve irritation in the more usual cases.

SNAKE BITE

In Britain, the only poisonous snake is the adder, a shy creature unless disturbed. A venous tourniquet can be applied above the bite for a few minutes to cause bleeding and wash away the venom, but generally rest to the part is sufficient. If there is a severe reaction with swelling and pain, steroids can be used. Antivenom is rarely needed. In other countries, snake bite can be more dangerous, the venoms including powerful neurotoxins, haemolysins, coagulant and anti-coagulant substances and antivenoms appropriate to the local species of snakes should be available.

HAZARDS OF AIR TRAVEL

Travel sickness. This may be due to unusual sensitivity of the vestibule and semicircular canals of the inner ear in certain individuals, may be worsened by fatigue and anxiety, and presents as faintness, malaise and vomiting. Hyoscine 0·6 mg, or an antihistamine drug half an hour before the journey may be helpful.

Effects of altitude. Modern aircraft cabins are pressurized to be equivalent to an altitude of 5,000–7,000 feet. The reduced oxygen pressure is only a hazard to those with chronic respiratory disease, heart failure, or recent myocardial infarction. Pressure changes may cause discomfort or ear damage in those with head colds and blocked eustachian tubes.

Rapid crossing of time-zones. Long journeys involving crossing of several time-zones may be followed by upset in the body's normal rhythms, including that of sleep, and the cyclical variation in cortisol secretion. It is said that concentration and judgment may be impaired professional and business men should postpone important decisions until normality is restored in a day or two.

Occupational hazards

A case history must include details of the patient's present and past occupation. Enquiry must be made as to exposure to toxic chemicals —many of these enter the body by inhalation. It should be ascertained whether dust suppression, or removal by methods such as exhaust ventilation is carried out, and whether recommended procedures are observed. If doubt remains, the employer should be contacted and he will usually be found to be most helpful.

LEAD POISONING

Lead has been used since ancient times. The Romans may have invaded Britain to obtain supplies; absorption from cooking pots, water pipes and wine vessels may have caused lead poisoning which is said to have contributed to the decline of the Roman Empire.

Lead is used in pigments and paints, for lead sheeting, water pipes, plates for electric accumulators, in solder and ceramic glazes. Tetra-ethyl lead is an organic compound added to petrol to raise its octane value—foliage near main roads may be contaminated by deposits of lead.

Causes of poisoning

Lead smelting, car battery manufacture or burning of old batteries for scrap, ship-breaking—inhalation of fumes or ingestion of lead can occur in these processes. Prevention includes exhaust ventilation, hand washing and prohibition of eating or drinking in work-rooms.

High concentrations may occur in the domestic water supply if very soft water dissolves lead from pipes. Young children are liable to poisoning from 'pica'—ingestion of substance which is not a food— they tend to put things in their mouths, and may lick or nibble paint—lead paint should not be used indoors or on toys. Poisoning has occurred from paint nibbling in old property.

Symptoms and signs

Lead affects enzyme systems and haemoglobin synthesis.

In adults there is pallor from anaemia, lassitude, constipation and severe colicky pains which may simulate an abdominal emergency. There are muscular cramps and lead palsy, due to a peripheral neuropathy or toxic effect on muscle, and wrist drop. A blue line (from lead sulphide) may be seen at the gums if the patient has teeth, and round the anus. Long-term effects include renal damage and liability to cerebro-vascular disease.

In children the picture is different—pallor, headache and vomiting from raised intracranial pressure, and the signs can be confused with those of meningitis—this is called lead encephalopathy, and is a serious condition.

Further investigations

Blood shows hypochromic anaemia, and 'stippling' of the red cells on the stained film is characteristic. Blood and urinary lead levels are high, and haemoglobin metabolites (including porphyrins) are detectable. In children x-rays may show lead lines in the bones, where lead is deposited.

Treatment entails:
  (i) removal from exposure.
  (ii) removal of the excess lead by chelating agents which bind with it and allow its excretion in the urine—calcium E.D.T.A. (edetate, Calcium Disodium Versenate) intramuscularly or intravenously, or oral penicillamine.

MERCURY POISONING

Though it can be absorbed through the skin, poisoning occurs mainly by inhalation, and results in salivation, stomatitis, tremor, aggressive behaviour, and nephrotic syndrome. Mercury salts are used in the felt industry, and these symptoms in workers have resulted in the terms 'hatter's shakes' and 'mad as a hatter'.

Organic mercury compounds are used as fungicides in seed dressings and poisoning causes a unique neurological syndrome of ataxia, dysarthria and constriction of the visual fields.

ARSENIC POISONING

Arsenic compounds are used in the refining of ores and manufacture of glass, as preservatives of hides, and as insecticides. Poisoning can follow inhalation or ingestion, or contact with the organic compounds. Acute arsenical poisoning is a gastro-enteritis with severe abdominal pain, vomiting, diarrhoea, collapse and possibly coma and death. Chronic poisoning follows exposure to small amounts over a long period. The arsenic is deposited in the skin, causing 'rain-drop' pigmentation and thickening with risk of carcinoma. There is also liver dysfunction with jaundice, and a peripheral neuropathy with paralysis and muscle wasting. Arsine gas (arseniuretted hydrogen) is liberated in some industrial processes—inhalation is followed by haemolysis with jaundice, haemoglobinuria and renal damage.

CHROMIUM POISONING

Chromium attacks the skin causing an ulcer known as 'chrome hole', and perforation of the nasal septum is common in chrome workers.

BERYLLIUM POISONING

Beryllium, used in fluorescent lamp tubes causes acute lung irritation, and chronic exposure causes lung fibrosis, general weakness and loss of weight.

OCCUPATIONAL DISEASES OF THE LUNG

Coal-workers' pneumoconiosis
Silicosis
Asbestosis   See page 104.
Byssinosis
Farmer's lung, bird-breeders' lung

Vapours produced in the manufacture of polyurethane, the basis of many plastics and paints, may cause lung irritation with cough and asthmatic symptoms. However, awareness of the older industrial risks and the enlightened approach of most manufacturers have resulted in safer working conditions in modern industries.

INDUSTRIAL CANCER

Cancer of the scrotum formerly occurred in chimney sweeps from contact with coal tar derivatives. Workers in the aniline dye industry were found to have a high incidence of papilloma and carcinoma of the bladder, from excretion of a carcinogenic product in the urine. Substances related to aniline used in the manufacture of electric cables, and benzidine-like substances (formerly used to test stool specimens for occult blood) carry a similar hazard, and have been withdrawn. Exposure to 'blue' asbestos causes tumours in lung, pleura and peritoneum—sometimes years later. Nickel dust causes cancer of the nasal sinuses, and the wood dust to which cabinet makers are exposed can carry a similar hazard. Girls who licked the point of the brush used to paint the dials of luminous watches with a radio-active substance later developed bone tumours.

DECOMPRESSION SICKNESS—CAISSON DISEASE

A caisson is a chamber in which a number of men work in compressed air. It is used in bridge construction to lay foundations on the bed of a river. Compressed air is also used in tunnel construction and in diving bells or suits. It balances the hydrostatic pressure of the water, preventing the ingress of mud or sand to an area under construction. When a man is exposed to compressed air, oxygen is used in the normal way but nitrogen becomes dissolved in tissues, especially in fat. Decompression sickness is thought to result from the formation of nitrogen bubbles in the tissues or circulation, the gas expanding as the pressure is lowered. This is less likely to happen if the decompression process is carried out slowly.

Symptoms include 'the bends'—pains in the limbs near major joints, and more serious symptoms possibly due to bubbles in the blood and central nervous system (which is rich in fat in the myelin) —vomiting, 'the staggers' with vertigo, weakness and paralysis and hypotensive collapse. These symptoms occur a few hours after too-rapid decompression, but there is an additional late hazard not necessarily preceded by them—this is a bone necrosis developing in compressed air workers months after exposure. It rarely occurs in divers.

Treatment of decompression sickness is immediate recompression in a compressed air chamber, which, by law, must be available on the construction site. Very gradual decompression is then carried out. No known treatment affects bone necrosis. It is hoped that the incidence of decompression sickness may be lowered by detecting bubbles in the circulation before they cause symptoms, using an ultrasonic detector clipped on the ear.

RADIATION HAZARDS

Man has always been exposed to natural sources of radiation but this 'background level' carries no hazard—risk only occurs with exposure to radium or to man-made radio-active isotopes or x-rays. Atomic radiation includes alpha particles, beta particles or electrons, and gamma radiation. The latter is similar in its penetrating effect to x-rays, so that these two forms of radiation constitute the main practical hazard.

Gamma rays and x-rays affect rapidly growing tissues, such as the bone marrow and mucosal cells lining the intestine. Massive exposure causes acute radiation sickness from death of many cells, with vomiting, diarrhoea and death from circulatory collapse. Smaller doses of radiation result in destruction of the actively dividing cells of the bone marrow, resulting in thrombocytopenia, leucopenia and infections, and aplastic anaemia. There is also a delayed hazard of skin cancer.

Such risks occur in industry—x-rays being used to detect flaws in metal, and isotopes being used as flow indicators—and the danger is greater where inexperienced operators are unaware of the nature of substances they may be using. In atomic power-stations and isotope laboratories, meticulous precautions assure greater safety.

In hospital, risks occur from radium, isotopes, and x-rays and those exposed must wear badges of radio-sensitive paper which measure radiation levels and indicate any undue exposure. There is no absolutely 'safe' level, and all exposure is to be avoided unless there is a clear diagnostic or therapeutic indication. Tomograms (multiple films to localize a lesion) and x-ray screening (e.g. barium meals) cause high radiation exposure, though for the radiologist this can be minimized by the use of television (image-intensifier) techniques as well as use of lead lined gloves and aprons.

20

Hazards of therapy. The dangers of hospital care. Iatrogenic illness

The importance of keeping patients out of hospital

This has been emphasized in many parts of the text. Conditions should be recognized and treated early, on an out-patient basis as far as possible, the object being to have as little disruption as possible of the patients normal way of life. Attendance at hospital need not be a reason for a prolonged spell off work.

It is especially important that the elderly be kept out of the hospital environment, for they tend to become 'institutionalized' and apathetic if removed from their simple interests at home. A day-care centre will often allow such old people to manage at home for most of the time, or admission on a month in/out basis may be possible with the help of the social worker.

In the eighteenth and early nineteenth centuries patients were terrified of being admitted to hospital, for infection rates were so high that many died—only the poorest people would go into hospital, those who could afford medical attention realizing they had a better chance if they were nursed at home. Following the control of infection and better understanding of disease hospitals are now relatively safe places. No longer does the patient risk streptococcal septicaemia, the miseries of excessive purgation, or chloroform poisoning from crude rag-and-bottle anaesthesia when he comes into hospital. He does, however continue to risk the dangers of rest in bed and the ill health which may be provoked as well as prevented by some modern therapy. Disorders caused by doctors and their drugs are called iatrogenic disorders.

Causes of iatrogenic illness

1. *Improper diagnosis and handling*—e.g. making a cardiac neurotic of someone by diagnosing non-existent cardiac disease.

2. *Rest in bed*—venous thrombosis and pulmonary embolism;
   stiffening of joints;
   osteoporosis;
   urinary incontinence; constipation;
   impaired respiration, pneumonia;
   demoralization, depression and sleeplessness.

3. *Imposed diets*—old fashioned 'gastric' diets deficient in vitamin C;
   low residue diet makes diverticular disease worse not better;
   'diabetic diets' should be applied only if existing diet is unbalanced—timing of meals often more important than content;
   'no protein diet' unwise in renal failure, as body protein breakdown goes on—low protein, high carbohydrate better;
   'crash diets' (no calories') dangerous—some calories plus protein essential.

4. *Fluid restriction*—dangerous after haematemesis, patient needs fluid. Provided a patient is passing urine, it is generally safe to let him have fluids, and the oral route should be used unless severity of dehydration necessitates intravenous route as well.

5. *Hazards of blood transfusion*—wrong grouping or clerical error and resultant haemolysis;
   danger of transmission of hepatitis;
   formation of antibodies and subsequent transfusion reaction;
   circulatory overload;
   acidosis and calcium upset after massive transfusion.

6. *Misuse of oxygen*—high concentration dangerous in those with chronic respiratory disease.

7. *Drug induced disease*—see below.

8. *Investigations*—x-rays may be hazardous to reproductive system and bone marrow.

Further risks may be incurred from the misinterpretation of

laboratory data—the increasing help that is obtained from laboratory investigations should not blind one to its limitations, especially in three fields: (i) sputum examination—purulent sputum means infection even if the laboratory report says 'normal flora only'.

(ii) antibiotic sensitivities in the laboratory do not always correspond with effects of the drugs in the patient.

(iii) blood samples may apply only to the relatively small and accessible part of the body fluids, and may not reflect the intracellular state.

Drugs and disease

Before 1930 drug therapy did not greatly alter the natural history of disease, though potent drugs such as digitalis, thyroid and insulin were available. The past forty years has witnessed a therapeutic explosion and many modern drugs are potent for evil as well as for good. Disorders may be caused as well as cured by antibiotics, tranquillisers and steroids.

Some of the applications, and hazards, of drugs mentioned in the text will now be reconsidered.

DIGOXIN AND DIURETICS

Oral diuretics are so potent in clearing oedema that they are tending to displace digoxin from its traditional place in the therapy of cardiac failure. Digoxin's good effects (depression of rate of conduction in A.V. bundle, stimulation of the ventricle) become toxic effects if the dose is pushed, causing bradycardia and coupling, but sometimes an irregular tachycardia. These effects occur more easily if the patient is depleted of potassium, which is a side effect of diuretic therapy. In severe cases the patient becomes weak with low blood pressure and may develop paralytic ileus. Cirrhotic patients are prone to potassium deficiency. Potassium should be replaced in the form of potassium chloride, a rather irritant substance, some preparations of which (now withdrawn) caused ulceration of the bowel.

ADRENALINE AND ISOPRENALINE

These are useful in relieving broncho-spasm in asthma, but may cause dangerous tachycardia if used to excess.

ASPIRIN AND ANALGESICS

Aspirin may precipitate haematemesis from gastric erosion.

Phenacetin-containing drugs may cause 'analgesic nephropathy'—
kidney damage. Paracetamol is a related substance, and liver
damage has been reported. Indomethacin and phenylbutazone
are gastric irritants and the latter also causes sodium retention and
agranulocytosis.

STEROIDS

Steroids such as prednisone mimic cortisol (hydrocortisone). They
are useful in severe asthma, some forms of leukaemia and haemolytic anaemia, nephrotic syndrome and auto-immune diseases such
as rheumatoid arthritis. Side effects—mooning of the face, thinning
of arms and legs and of the skin with bruising tendency, osteoporosis
muscular weakness, sodium retention and oedema, exacerbation of
diabetes and of peptic ulcers. In addition steroids suppress cortisol
production and if suddenly withdrawn the patient becomes hypotensive and may pass into coma.

Hormone preparations containing oestrogen-like substances are
used as oral contraceptives and in the management of cancer of the
prostate. They increase the risk of venous and cerebral thrombosis,
and may cause liver cell dysfunction.

DRUGS USED IN HYPERTENSION

Methyldopa (Aldomet) causes a 'safe' lowering of the blood pressure,
but 10 per cent of patients develop a disturbance of immunity causing
a positive Coombs' test in the blood, and may proceed to haemolytic
anaemia.

Reserpine is a 'mild' hypotensive, but may cause depression, and
fluid retention.

Guanethidine (Ismelin) and bethanidine (Esbatal) are sym-
pathetic-blocking drugs, producing marked postural hypotension,
especially in the morning, so dosage should be adjusted depending
on the blood pressure after standing and after exertion. They may
cause impotence. The older ganglion-blocking drugs also cause
parasympathetic blockade, with disturbance of visual accommodation, dryness of the mouth and sometimes urinary retention.

ANTICOAGULANTS

Heparin and drugs such as phenindione (Dindevon) nicoumalone
(Sinthrome) and warfarin prevent venous thrombosis. Overdosage
results in haematuria and bleeding. Heparin is short-acting and
can be neutralized by protamine sulphate. The other drugs deplete

clotting factors formed in the liver and can be antagonized by vitamin K.

DRUGS ACTING ON THE NERVOUS SYSTEM

Morphine and diamorphine—still the best pain relieving and sedative drugs in myocardial infarction, relieve breathlessness in left ventricular failure. Side effects include vomiting and depression of respiration, so they must not be used in respiratory disease. Pethidine is less potent. All are drugs of addiction, but this should not preclude their proper use in the right circumstances.

Pentazocine (Fortral) has been claimed to be as effective, yet nonaddictive, but a rise in pulmonary artery pressure has been reported after its use.

Barbiturates produce sedation and sleep (but it is not a natural sleep); their only severe effect is that of overdosage, causing respiratory depression and coma; folic acid deficiency anaemia occurs in epileptics on long continued phenytoin and sometimes with phenobarbitone.

Benzodiazepines—such as chlordiazepoxide (Librium) and diazepam (Valium) produce sedation. Intravenous diazepam produces a dreamy state with some analgesic action, allowing the carrying out of procedures such as intubation and electrical conversion of arrhythmias.

Anti-depressants such as amitriptyline may provoke cardiac irregularity. Mono-amine oxidase inhibitors such as phenelzine (Nardil) cause raised blood pressure and headaches if the patient eats cheese, and pethidine and anaesthetics may provoke hypotension in patients on M.A.O.-inhibitor drugs.

Chlorpromazine and other phenothiazine tranquillizers are most useful drugs, but may cause jaundice and Parkinsonism.

ANTIBIOTICS

Penicillin remains the best drug for sensitive Gram positive infections, such as streptococcal throat and pneumonia due to pneumococcus. The related drugs cloxacillin and flucloxacillin (Orbenin and Floxapen) and methicillin (Celbenin) are often effective against penicillin-resistant staphylococci, and ampicillin (Penbritin) against Gram-negative organisms, except pyocyanea, where carbenicillin (Pyopen) may be used. Skin reactions and fever may occur with any of these penicillin-related antibiotics.

Tetracyclines are broad spectrum antibiotics, but indiscriminately destroy gut organisms, some of which may be good ones to have. Other resistant organisms, such as certain staphylococci may take over, causing severe enterocolitis; monilial infection of the mouth is also a complication. Tetracyclines are deposited in growing bones and teeth, causing an irreversible green coloration of the latter, so they should not be used in pregnant women and children.

Erythromycin estolate is a useful anti-staphylococcal antibiotic but is toxic to the liver in large dosage.

Antibiotics such as streptomycin and kanamycin act on Gram-negative organisms, but are toxic to the ear, causing balance disturbance, especially in patients with impaired renal function, in which there may occur very high blood levels.

Chloramphenicol is highly effective against many organisms, but in view of its toxic effect on the bone marrow should be reserved for typhoid fever and other severe infections.

CYTOTOXIC DRUGS

Cyclophosphamide (Endoxana) is useful in Hodgkin's disease, some forms of leukaemia and secondary malignancy (e.g. ovarian and bronchogenic carcinomatosis). Apart from depression of the white cells, falling of the hair and haemorrhagic cystitis may occur.

Busulphan and chlorambucil, used in myeloid and lymphatic leukaemia respectively, cause dangerous depression of the bone marrow if pushed to excess.

Effect of liver dysfunction

Where liver function or renal excretion is impaired, drugs may have a more prolonged and dangerous effect.

Enzyme induction

Certain drugs such as the barbiturates, stimulate the liver enzymes to destroy other drugs. If the barbiturates are subsequently withdrawn, the remaining drugs will have a more powerful effect. Drug interactions are thus a most important consideration.

The value of drugs

Modern drugs are of the greatest value despite their side effects. They have cured or alleviated many diseases, and their cost should be balanced against this achievement. Their proper use is a major contribution to human welfare.

Index

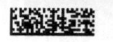